Obstetrics: Clinical Management of Pregnancy

Obstetrics: Clinical Management of Pregnancy

Editor: Tessa Cohen

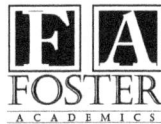

FA FOSTER
ACADEMICS

www.fosteracademics.com

www.fosteracademics.com

FA
FOSTER
ACADEMICS

Cataloging-in-Publication Data

Obstetrics : clinical management of pregnancy / edited by Tessa Cohen.
    p. cm.
Includes bibliographical references and index.
ISBN 978-1-63242-666-6
1. Obstetrics. 2. Pregnancy. 3. Pregnancy--Complications. 4. Obstetrical emergencies.
I. Cohen, Tessa.
RG524 .O27 2019
618.2--dc23

Foster Academics,
118-35 Queens Blvd., Suite 400,
Forest Hills, NY 11375, USA

ISBN 978-1-63242-666-6 (Hardback)

Contents

Preface...IX

Chapter 1   Influence of weight gain, according to Institute of Medicine 2009
            recommendation, on spontaneous preterm delivery in twin pregnancies.....................1
            Paola Algeri, Francesca Pelizzoni, Davide Paolo Bernasconi, Francesca Russo,
            Maddalena Incerti, Sabrina Cozzolino, Salvatore Andrea Mastrolia and
            Patrizia Vergani

Chapter 2   Malignancy during pregnancy in Japan: an exceptional opportunity for early
            diagnosis...8
            Masayuki Sekine, Yoshiyuki Kobayashi, Tsutomu Tabata, Tamotsu Sudo,
            Ryuichiro Nishimura, Koji Matsuo, Brendan H. Grubbs, Takayuki Enomoto and
            Tomoaki Ikeda

Chapter 3   Trajectory of vitamin D status during pregnancy in relation to neonatal birth
            size and fetal survival..13
            Linnea Bärebring, Maria Bullarbo, Anna Glantz, Lena Hulthén, Joy Ellis,
            Åse Jagner, Inez Schoenmakers, Anna Winkvist and Hanna Augustin

Chapter 4   Laparotomy in women with severe acute maternal morbidity: secondary
            analysis of a nationwide cohort study 20
            Tom Witteveen, Athanasios Kallianidis, Joost J. Zwart, Kitty W. Bloemenkamp,
            Jos van Roosmalen and Thomas van den Akker

Chapter 5   Management and obstetric outcomes of 17 heterotopic interstitial pregnancies...........27
            Yuan Jiang, Jie Chen, Huaijun Zhou, Mingming Zheng, Ke Han, Jingxian Ling,
            Xianghong Zhu, Xiaoqiu Tang, Rong Li and Ying Hong

Chapter 6   Maternal bleeding complications following early versus delayed umbilical cord
            clamping in multiple pregnancies..33
            Chayatat Ruangkit, Matthew Leon, Kasim Hassen, Katherine Baker, Debra Poeltler
            and Anup Katheria

Chapter 7   Misoprostol vaginal insert versus misoprostol vaginal tablets for the induction
            of labour..39
            Daniele Bolla, Saskia Vanessa Weissleder, Anda-Petronela Radan,
            Maria Luisa Gasparri, Luigi Raio, Martin Müller and Daniel Surbek

Chapter 8   Pregnancy outcomes in women with gestational diabetes mellitus diagnosed
            according to the WHO-2013 and WHO- 1999 diagnostic criteria......................................45
            Eva A. R. Goedegebure, Sarah H. Koning, Klaas Hoogenberg,
            Fleurisca J. Korteweg, Helen L. Lutgers, Mattheus J. M. Diekman,
            Eva Stekkinger, Paul P. van den Berg and Joost J. Zwart

Chapter 9   **Delayed interval delivery of the second twin in a woman with altered markers of inflammation**..54
George Daskalakis, Panagiotis Fotinopoulos, Vasilios Pergialiotis,
Mariana Theodora, Panagiotis Antsaklis, Michail Sindos, Nikolaos Papantoniou
and Dimitrios Loutradis

Chapter 10   **Signs and symptoms of disordered eating in pregnancy: a Delphi consensus study**..59
Amy Jean Bannatyne, Roger Hughes, Peta Stapleton, Bruce Watt and
Kristen MacKenzie-Shalders

Chapter 11   **Macular choroidal thickness in highly myopic women during pregnancy and postpartum: a longitudinal study**..75
Wei Chen, Li Li, Hongyuan Zhang, Yan Li, Xu Chen and Yue Zhang

Chapter 12   **"If we're here, it's only because we have no money..." discrimination and violence**..81
Rosario Valdez Santiago, Luz Arenas Monreal, Anabel Rojas Carmona and
Mario Sánchez Domínguez

Chapter 13   **Improving shared decision-making in a clinical obstetric ward by using the three questions intervention**..91
S. W. E. Baijens, A. G. Huppelschoten, J. Van Dillen and J. W. M. Aarts

Chapter 14   **The effect of advanced maternal age on perinatal outcomes in nulliparous singleton pregnancies**..99
Bekir Kahveci, Rauf Melekoglu, Ismail Cuneyt Evruke and Cihan Cetin

Chapter 15   **The effect of uterine artery ligation in patients with central placenta pevia**..106
Ahmad Sameer Sanad, Ahmad E. Mahran, Mahmoud Elmorsi Aboulfotouh,
Hany Hassan Kamel, Hashem Fares Mohammed, Haitham A. Bahaa,
Reham R. Elkateeb, Alaa Gamal Abdelazim, Mohamed Ahmed Zeen El-Din and
Hossam El-Din Shawki

Chapter 16   **'If I do 10–15 normal deliveries in a month I hardly ever sleep at home.'
A qualitative study of health providers' reasons for high rates of caesarean deliveries in private sector maternity care**..112
Alison Peel, Abhishek Bhartia, Neil Spicer and Meenakshi Gautham

Chapter 17   **Risk factors for hypertensive disorders of pregnancy among mothers in Tigray region**..123
Hailemariam Berhe Kahsay, Fikre Enquselassie Gashe and
Wubegzier Mekonnen Ayele

Chapter 18   **Towards more accurate measurement of edge to os distance in low-lying placenta using three dimensional transvaginal ultrasound: an innovative technique**..133
Somayya M. Sadek, Reda A. Ahmad, Hytham Atia and Adel G. Abdullah

Chapter 19   **Determinants of client satisfaction to skilled antenatal care services**.. 142
Serawit Lakew, Alaso Ankala and Fozia Jemal

Chapter 20   **Successful preterm pregnancy in a rare variation of Herlyn-Werner-Wunderlich syndrome**... 155
Stefania Cappello, Eleonora Piccolo, Francesco Cucinelli, Luisa Casadei,
Emilio Piccione and Maria Giovanna Salerno

Chapter 21   **Male involvement in the maternal health care system: implication towards decreasing the high burden of maternal mortality** 160
Amanual Getnet Mersha

Chapter 22   **Risk factors associated with the development of postpartum diabetes in Japanese women with gestational diabetes**.. 168
Yukari Kugishima, Ichiro Yasuhi, Hiroshi Yamashita, So Sugimi, Yasushi Umezaki,
Sachie Suga, Masashi Fukuda and Nobuko Kusuda

Chapter 23   **First and second trimester urinary metabolic profiles and fetal growth restriction: an exploratory nested case-control study within the infant development and environment study**.. 176
Gauri Luthra, Ivan Vuckovic, A. Bangdiwala, H. Gray, J. B. Redmon, E. S. Barrett,
S. Sathyanarayana, R. H. N. Nguyen, S. H. Swan, S. Zhang, P. Dzeja, S. I. Macura
and K. S. Nair

Chapter 24   **Development of a tailored strategy to improve postpartum hemorrhage guideline adherence**... 184
Suzan M. de Visser, Mallory D. Woiski, Richard P. Grol,
Frank P. H. A. Vandenbussche, Marlies E. J. L. Hulscher,
Hubertina C. J. Scheepers and Rosella P. M. G. Hermens

Chapter 25   **Avoiding late preterm deliveries to reduce neonatal complications**.. 192
Noémie Bouchet, Angèle Gayet-Ageron, Marina Lumbreras Areta,
Riccardo Erennio Pfister and Begoña Martinez de Tejada

Permissions

List of Contributors

Index

Preface

The field of study involved with pregnancy, childbirth and the postpartum period is known as obstetrics. The chief areas within obstetrics are prenatal and postnatal care. Prenatal care helps to screen for various complications of pregnancy through routine lab tests and physical examinations. CBC tests, general antibody screen test, ultrasound, amniocentesis, MSAFP/quadruple screen test, hematocrit, glucose loading test, etc. are done during the first, second and third trimesters of pregnancy. Some of the pregnancy-related emergencies include ectopic pregnancy, placental abruption, pre-eclampsia, fetal distress, shoulder dystocia, uterine rupture, etc. Postnatal care is provided to mothers following parturition. The mother is examined for bowel and bladder function, and bleeding. This book provides comprehensive insights into the field of obstetrics. It traces the progress of this field and highlights some of its key principles and practices. The extensive content of this book provides the readers with a thorough understanding of the subject.

This book is the end result of constructive efforts and intensive research done by experts in this field. The aim of this book is to enlighten the readers with recent information in this area of research. The information provided in this profound book would serve as a valuable reference to students and researchers in this field.

At the end, I would like to thank all the authors for devoting their precious time and providing their valuable contribution to this book. I would also like to express my gratitude to my fellow colleagues who encouraged me throughout the process.

Editor

Influence of weight gain, according to Institute of Medicine 2009 recommendation, on spontaneous preterm delivery in twin pregnancies

Paola Algeri[1*], Francesca Pelizzoni[1], Davide Paolo Bernasconi[2], Francesca Russo[1], Maddalena Incerti[1], Sabrina Cozzolino[1], Salvatore Andrea Mastrolia[1] and Patrizia Vergani[1]

Abstract

Backgrounds: Maternal total weight gain during pregnancy influences adverse obstetric outcomes in singleton pregnancies. However, its impact in twin gestation is less understood. Our objective was to estimate the influence of total maternal weight gain on preterm delivery in twin pregnancies.

Methods: We conducted a retrospective cohort study including diamniotic twin pregnancies with spontaneous labor delivered at 28 + 0 weeks or later. We analyzed the influence of total weight gain according to Institute of Medicine (IOM) cut-offs on the development of preterm delivery (both less than 34 and 37 weeks). Outcome were compared between under and normal weight gain and between over and normal weight gain separately using Fisher's exact test with Holm-Bonferroni correction.

Results: One hundred seventy five women were included in the study and divided into three groups: under (52.0%), normal (41.7%) and overweight gain (6.3%). Normal weight gain was associated with a reduction in the rate of preterm delivery compared to under and over weight gain [less than 34 weeks: under vs. normal OR 4.97 (1.76–14.02), over vs. normal OR 4.53 (0.89–23.08); less than 37 weeks: OR 3.16 (1.66–6.04) and 6.51 (1.30–32.49), respectively].

Conclusions: Normal weight gain reduces spontaneous preterm delivery compared to over and underweight gain.

Keywords: Twin pregnancy, Preterm delivery, Preterm labor, Weight gain, Institute of medicine recommendation

Background

Pre-gestational body mass index (pBMI), gestational body mass index (gBMI) and total weight gain influence the incidence of preterm delivery and other adverse obstetric outcomes in singletons [1, 2] but their effect on twins is poorly understood, although multiple pregnancies appear to have similar associations between these outcomes, pBMI or weight gain compared to singletons [1, 2]. Indeed, studies evaluating the role of both total and weekly weight gain in twin pregnancies identified a strong correlation between low total weight gain during pregnancy and preterm

delivery (PD) [3, 4]. In 1990, the Institute of Medicine (IOM) proposed ranges of recommended total weight gain correlated to pBMI for singleton pregnancy and an optimal total weight gain between 15.9 and 20.5 kg not related to pBMI for twin pregnancy [5, 6].

In 2009, the IOM revised these guidelines and defined pBMI specific weight gain cut-off, also for twin pregnancies. Optimal ranges proposed for weight gain at term (≥ 37 weeks) are: 17–25 kg for normal weighted women (pBMI 18.5–24.9), 14–23 kg for over weighted women (pBMI 25–29.9) and 11–19 kg for obese women (pBMI 30 or more). No recommendations were given for underweighted women (pBMI less than 18.5) [7].

This is of higher importance due to the rise in the incidence of twin pregnancies in the last three decades because of the older age at childbearing and of the diffusion

* Correspondence: p.algeri@campus.unimib.it
[1]Department of Obstetrics and Gynecology, University of Milano-Bicocca, S. Gerardo Hospital, MBBM Foundation, Via Pergolesi 33, Monza, 20900 Monza, Monza e Brianza, Italy
Full list of author information is available at the end of the article

of assisted reproductive technology [8]. Today, approximately 1 of 80 pregnancies is a multiple gestation, corresponding to 2.6% of all newborns (1–3% in Italy) and they are more frequently diamniotic. Multiple pregnancies present a higher incidence of maternal and fetal adverse outcomes compared to singleton ones [3, 9–13]. Twin pregnancies account for 12.2% of preterm births and 15.4% of neonatal deaths [14–16].

In literature, both pBMI and total weight gain were reported as important influencing factors in pregnancies outcomes. However, the studies took into consideration only one of these parameters at a time. New cut-offs proposed by IOM allowed an easier evaluation of maternal weight influence on obstetrics outcomes, not only in singleton pregnancies but also in twins.

Few studies evaluated the role of the new IOM guidelines in influencing preterm delivery in twins, also considering that IOM gave cut-offs only for gestational age at delivery ≥ 37 weeks [17–19].

In 2010, Fox et al. conducted a study on a cohort of twins divided into subgroups considering pBMI. They show that patients whose weight gain during pregnancy met or exceeded the revised 2009 IOM guidelines had significantly improved pregnancy outcomes such as longer gestation, less overall PD, less spontaneous PD and larger neonates compared to lower weight gain [18]. In 2012, also Quintero et al. found that a weight gain below recommended guidelines was associated with higher rates of spontaneous PD at less than 35 weeks in twin pregnancies [19].

A recent review tried to define the role of absolute total weight gain in the development of adverse pregnancy outcomes. The authors suggested that a higher incidence of PD was correlated with underweight gain and underlined a positive correlation between total weight gain and gestation length [20].

Gestational gain weight and pBMI have been proven to influence not only the risk of PD but also other obstetric outcomes, such as birth weight, hypertensive disorders, gestational diabetes and neonatal adverse outcomes [17].

Contrasting results were instead reported about hypertensive disorders: while some authors described higher incidence of gestational hypertension and preeclampsia in women with excessive weight gain, others showed no differences among different weight gain groups in a series of twin pregnancies delivering at term [5, 17, 20].

In light of the above and due to the scarcity of data available in the literature about this topic, we designed a study with the aim to estimate the influence of total weight gain according to the 2009 IOM recommendations on preterm delivery before 37 and 34 weeks in twin pregnancies with spontaneous onset of labor. Secondary outcomes were the possible correlation with small for gestational age (SGA) and large for gestational age (LGA), pregnancy hypertensive disorders, gestational diabetes, and neonatal adverse outcomes.

Methods

We performed a retrospective cohort study on diamniotic twin pregnancies delivered at more or equal 28 + 0 weeks after spontaneous onset of labor at our Institution (Fondazione MBBM, San Gerardo Hospital, University of Milano Bicocca, Monza, Italy), between January 2010 and December 2013.

Exclusion criteria of our study were induction of labor (15% of all twin pregnancies at our Institution), elective cesarean section (4% of all twin pregnancies at our Institution), monoamniotic twins, intrauterine demise, fetal malformations, twin-to-twin transfusion syndrome, and gestational age at delivery < 28 weeks. We decided to set a gestational age < 28 weeks at delivery as an exclusion criteria in order to have a better definition of the weight gain trend for each patient. A shorter pregnancy duration could be a confounding factor in defining the maternal weight gain.

Patients with pBMI < 18.5 were also excluded since there are no IOM recommendations for underweight patients in case of multiple pregnancies.

All twin gestations were followed according to national guidelines for management of twin pregnancy [21]. The protocol included maternal clinical assessment and ultrasound monitoring every 2 weeks, from 16 weeks, for monochorionic diamniotic pregnancies and every 4 weeks, starting from 20 weeks, for dichorionic diamniotic gestations.

At our Maternal-Fetal Unit, women undergo their first access at obstetric booking that is usually performed during the first trimester after a positive pregnancy test (<8 weeks of gestation). At the first visit we collect patient's medical and obstetric history, define gestational age (calculated based on the last menstrual period and confirmed by ultrasound assessment), as well as chorionicity. Baseline characteristics and pregnancy outcomes were entered into our database by an assigned physician at every patient's access and periodically reviewed by a senior consultant. pBMI was recorded at the first visit, and maternal weight was measured at each obstetric control until delivery.

Since self-report of pBMI can be affected by recall bias, we attempted to reduce the risk of bias with an early assessment of pregnant women as described above.

Total weight gain was calculated as the difference between maternal weight at delivery and pre-gestational weight. This parameter was used to classify women who delivered at 37 weeks or more according to IOM guidelines [7]. In case of preterm delivery (between 28 and 36 + 6 weeks), we calculated a weekly weight gain cut-off as total weight gain during pregnancy in kg/gestational weeks at delivery. We compared this weekly weight gain to a hypothesized weekly IOM cut-off, calculated as IOM cut-off at term/37 weeks, as previously reported, represented for normal-weight women, this was 1.0 lb. per week (37 lbs. over 37 weeks); for overweight women, this was 0.84 lb. per week (31 lbs. over 37 weeks); for obese women, this was 0.68 lb. per week (25 lbs. over 37 weeks) [18].

The data used for the analysis were already available for every patient as part of the clinical report of the Obstetric Department.

SGA and LGA were defined, respectively, as neonatal weight at birth < 10° centile and > 90° centile compared to Italian Neonatal Study (INeS) charts [22]. We considered as separate outcomes the occurrence of at least one twin SGA/LGA and both twins SGA/LGA.

We defined "gestational hypertensive disorders" as the presence of at least one among gestational hypertension, preeclampsia or eclampsia, diagnosed according to American Congress of Obstetricians and Gynecologists (ACOG) criteria [23].

Gestational diabetes was defined as any degree of glucose intolerance with onset or first recognition during pregnancy [24].

We defined composite adverse neonatal outcome as the presence of at least one among: need for neonatal resuscitation, respiratory distress syndrome, disseminated intravascular coagulation, intra-ventricular hemorrhage, leucomalacia, sepsis, necrotizing enteritis, retinopathy of prematurity and neonatal death.

The present work was exempt from IRB approval as per Institutional policy on retrospective studies. At our medical center, women provide a written consent to the use of their clinical anonymized and de-identified data upon admission.

Statistical analysis

Population characteristics were compared among IOM weight gain groups using Chi Square test (categorical variables) or One Way ANOVA (continuous variables). Primary and secondary outcomes rates were compared between under and normal gain and between over and normal gain separately using Fisher's exact test with Holm-Bonferroni correction. Logistic regression analysis was carried out in order to evaluate the independent effect of weight gain adjusted for pBMI on the outcomes. A separate model was built for each primary and secondary outcome. All the analyses were performed using the R software, version 3.0.2. A p value of less than 0.05 was considered significant.

Results

The incidence of twin pregnancies at our Institution was 2.5–3% during the study period.

A cohort of 175 diamniotic twin pregnancies was included in our study, considering exclusion criteria: 91 (52.0%) presented underweight gain, 73 (41.7%) normal weight gain and 11 (6.3%) over weight gain, according to IOM recommendations.

Table 1 shows general population characteristics in the three study groups, considering the IOM classification for total weight gain. The normal weight gain group had a higher mean gestational age at delivery compared with the under and over gain weight ones (respectively 36.5 ± 2.0, 35.3 ± 3.0, 35.3 ± 2.0 weeks). Normal and overweight gain patients presented higher neonatal weight at birth for both twins compared to the under gain ones (respectively 2494.11, 2974.55, 2196.54 g). The over weight gain group presented a higher incidence of pre–gestational over weighted patients (45.5%). The study groups did not differ for other characteristics.

The incidence of primary and secondary adverse outcomes was compared among the three groups, and the results are presented in Tables 2 and 3.

We found that the normal weight gain group presented a significant lower incidence of spontaneous PD compared to both under and over weight gain groups [respectively 39.7% vs 67.0% (p: 0.002); 39.7% vs 81.8% (p: 0.04)]. Underweight gain women presented significantly higher rates of early preterm spontaneous delivery compared to normal weight gain ones; a trend was also reported when overweight gain was compared to normal weight gain group [respectively 25.3% vs. 6.8% (p: 0.005); 27.3% vs. 6.8% (p: 0.13)].

No differences in the occurrence of SGA in one or both twins were observed among the three study groups. In addition, no cases of LGA were recorded. Gestational hypertensive disorders occurred in our population included 1 case of gestational hypertension and seven cases of preeclampsia in the underweight group, five and eight respectively in the normal weight, and one and six in the overweight one. No cases of eclampsia were reported. In the normal weight gain group, women presented a trend toward a higher incidence of hypertensive gestational diseases compared to underweight gain patients, even if not significant (17.8% vs. 7.7%, $p = 0.06$). This complication was significantly less frequent in the normal weight gain group compared with the over weight gain one (17.8% vs. 63.6%, $p = 0.006$). No difference in the incidence of gestational diabetes mellitus and neonatal adverse composite outcomes were reported in the three study groups, and we had no neonatal deaths.

The results of the bivariate analysis on both primary and secondary outcomes were confirmed in the multivariate logistic regression analysis, adjusting for the effect of pBMI (Tables 4 and 5, respectively). Both under and over weight gain increased the risk of PD compared to normal weight gain: ORs were 4.97 (1.76–14.02) and 4.53 (0.89–23.08) for early preterm and 3.16 (1.66–6.04) and 6.51 (1.30–32.49) for PD at less than 37 weeks

Table 1 Population general characteristics, according to weight gain groups

	Under (91)	Normal (73)	Over (11)	P value
Maternal age	34 ± 5.55	34 ± 5.86	34 ± 5.03	0.99
Nulliparity	52 (57.1%)	44 (60.3%)	8 (72.7%)	0.32
Smoker	3 (3.9%)	5 (6.8%)	1 (9.1%)	0.38
Chronic Hypertension	1 (1.1%)	1 (1.4%)	0	0.93
pBMI[a]	22.75 ± 4.44	23.00 ± 3.29	23.97 ± 2.50	0.70
18.5 ≤ pBMI[a] ≤ 24.9	74 (81.3%)	54 (74.0%)	6 (54.5%)	0.11
25 ≤ pBMI[a] ≤ 29.9	10 (11.0%)	15 (20.5%)	5 (45.5%)	*0.01*
pBMI[a] ≥ 30	7 (7.7%)	4 (5.5%)	0	0.57
Medically assisted procreation	16 (17.6%)	18 (24.7%)	4 (36.4%)	0.26
Mono- Chorionicity	13 (14.3%)	11 (15.1%)	2 (18.2%)	0.94
Clinical chorionamnionitis	1 (1.1%)	0	0	0.63
Preterm rupture of membranes[b]	30 (33.0%)	13 (17.8%)	3 (27.3%)	0.09
Gestational age at delivery (weeks)	35.3 ± 3.0	36.5 ± 2.0	35.3 ± 2.0	*0.002*
Vaginal delivery	34 (37.4%)	23 (31.5%)	4 (36.4%)	0.73
1st twin birth weight (gr)	2196.54 ± 592.16	2494.11 ± 426.87	2374.55 ± 471.63	*0.002*
2nd twin birth weight (gr)	2154.89 ± 499.41	2392.95 ± 413.94	2443.50 ± 334.47	*0.002*

Results are reported as means and standard deviations (continuous factors) or numbers and percentages (categorical factors). The p-value of an overall test comparing the three groups is also provided (One-way ANOVA for continuous factors and Chi-square test for categorical factors)
Italic data are statistically significant
[a]pBMI = pre-gestational Body Mass Index; [b]Preterm rupture of membrane = rupture before 37 weeks

(Table 4). Women in the underweight gain group had a lower risk of developing hypertensive gestational disorders compared to the women of the normal weight gain group, even if it was not significant, but only a trend (OR = 0.39, 0.15–1.05). The over weight gain group, instead, presented a significantly higher risk of hypertensive gestational disorders compared to the normal weight gain group (OR = 7.69, 1.94–30.47).

Discussion
Principal findings of the study
In this study, we evaluated the influence of total maternal weight gain, according to the revised IOM recommendations, on the development of spontaneous PD in diamniotic twin gestations [7]. Our results show that 1) normal weight gain is associated with a significant reduction in preterm parturition; and 2) when taking into consideration gestational age at delivery, both under and overweight gain groups presented an increased risk of early

preterm parturition compared to normal weight gain women; and 3) a significantly increased risk for preterm parturition before 37 weeks (three and six times respectively) was present in underweight and overweight women respectively, compared with normal weight gain women.

IOM recommendations for weight gain in twin pregnancies
The important novelty of 2009 IOM recommendations was to give pBMI correlated cut-offs in twin pregnancies. On the other side, a limitation on the clinical use of these guidelines was to refer only to term twin pregnancies, excluding a twin group that delivered before 37 weeks [7, 17]. Therefore, just because IOM guidelines may be used limitedly to term twin pregnancies, we wanted to value how to apply them also in preterm gestations. Thus, we used a weekly gain weight cut-off (IOM cut-off at term/37 weeks), as already done by Fox et al. in a previous study [18].

Table 2 Incidence of the primary outcomes in the weight gain groups

	Under (n. 91)	Normal (n. 73)	p-value§	Over (n. 11)	Normal (n. 73)	p-value§
Preterm delivery < 37 weeks	61 (67.0%)	29 (39.7%)	P = .002	9 (81.8%)	29 (39.7%)	P = .04
Early preterm delivery < 34 weeks	23 (25.3%)	5 (6.8%)	P = .005	3 (27.3%)	5 (6.8%)	P = .13

Results are reported as numbers and percentages. The p-value of an overall test (Chi-square test) correlating the three groups for the two by two comparison
Italic data are statistically significant
§Fisher' exact test with Holm-Bonferroni correction

Table 3 Incidence of the secondary outcomes in the weight gain groups

	Under (n. 91)	Normal (n. 73)	Over (n. 11)	P value[c]
At least one twin SGA[a]	16 (17.6%)	13 (17.8%)	0 (0%)	0.31
Both twins SGA[a]	4 (4.4%)	1 (1.4%)	0 (0%)	0.43
Hypertensive disorders	7 (7.7%)	13 (17.8%)	7 (63.6%)	< 0.001
Gestational diabetes	15 (16.5%)	7 (9.6%)	0	0.18
1st twin adverse outcomes[b]	20 (22.0%)	6 (8.2%)	2 (18.2%)	0.06
2nd twin adverse outcomes[b]	20 (22.0%)	8 (11.0%)	2 (18.2%)	0.18

Results are reported as numbers and percentages
Italic data are statistically significant
[a]SGA = small for gestational age; [b]Adverse outcomes = neonatal resuscitation, respiratory distress syndrome, disseminated intravascular coagulation, intra-ventricular hemorrhage, leucomalacia, sepsis, necrotic enteritis, retinopathy of prematurity; [c]Fisher's exact test with Holm-Bonferroni correction, for all comparison; ns, not significant

Available literature assessing the influence of weight gain on pregnancy outcomes, in twin gestations

Several studies [17–19] analyzed the influence of IOM recommendations on pregnancy outcomes in twin pregnancies. The available literature on the topic is presented herein: 1) Fox et al. [18] collected 297 twin women divided into four groups based on their pBMI (underweight, normal weight, overweight, and obese). They compared pregnancy outcomes for women whose weight gain per week equaled or exceeded the IOM recommendations to women whose weight gain per week was lower than IOM cut-off, in three pBMI-based subgroups (underweight patients were excluded). They found that weight gain was associated with the gestational age at delivery and birth weight of the larger and smaller twin. Specifically, their study showed that, in women with a normal pBMI, patients whose weight gain met or exceeded the IOM recommendations had significantly improved outcomes, such as increment in birthweight of the larger twin and a lower rate of PD before 32 weeks (3.4% vs. 11.5%). In women with an overweight pBMI, if the weight gain met or exceeded the IOM recommendations, they reported higher gestational age at delivery, larger birth weight, and less preterm birth. In pre-gestational obese women, no statistically significant differences were noted; 2) The same authors [17] retrospectively studied a cohort of 170 women restricted to

Table 4 Effect of weight gain on the primary outcomes estimated by logistic regression

	Early preterm delivery OR (95%CI)	Preterm delivery < 37 weeks OR (95%CI)
Under vs normal	4.97 (1.76; 14.02)	3.16 (1.66; 6.04)
Over vs normal	4.53 (0.89; 23.08)	6.51 (1.30; 32.49)

The models were adjusted for pre-pregnancy BMI

twin pregnancies at 37 weeks or more. Their analysis valued pregnancy outcomes in three groups based on IOM recommendations defined as poor, normal, and excessive weight gain. The rate of newborns weighing more than 2500 g was 40%, 60.5% and 79.5% in the three groups, respectively. No differences in gestational hypertension, pre-eclampsia, gestational diabetes or neonatal intensive care unit admission across groups were observed; 3) Gonzalez-Quintero et al. [19], aimed to determine the validity of IOM recommendations for weight gain in twin pregnancies in terms of impact on perinatal outcomes comparing women with mean weight gain per week meeting or exceeding recommendations versus patients who did not meet the suggested weight gain. There was a significantly higher number of both infants weighing > 2500 g or > 1500 g for women gaining weight at or above guidelines. Of interest, women whose gain was below recommended guidelines were 50% more likely to deliver spontaneously at < 35 weeks.

What do our study adds compared to the available literature

Our study follows, in line with the available literature, the idea of assessing whether changes in weight gain during pregnancy in twin gestations, may have an impact on maternal and perinatal outcomes. Moreover, our study design shows several peculiarities, which differentiate it from the previous reports.

Specifically, 1) considering that IOM recommendations were already pBMI correlated, we simplified our analysis and divided our population considering if patients met, exceeded, or presented lower gain weight according to pBMI IOM cut-offs, without performing further stratification of the study groups. The rationale for it was to make the influence of weight gain on PD clearer and useful in clinical practice. Indeed, our analysis showed that a normal weight gain, was correlated with better perinatal and maternal outcomes; 2) Compared with the analysis by Fox et al. [17], our study population also included twins delivered preterm at 28 weeks or more. This was done in order not to lose the effect of prematurity on the analyzed outcomes, since prematurity is common in twin gestations and different outcomes such as preeclampsia and SGA are more frequent in women delivering preterm; 3) In line with Quintero et al., we found that a weight gain below the recommended guidelines was associated with higher rates of spontaneous PD. Moreover, we compared normal weight gain both with under and over gain weight and did not associate patients who met or exceeded IOM recommendations. Of interest, we hypothesized that, both lower and excessive weight gain were associated with worse outcomes; our results confirmed the idea that pregnant women whose weight gain was over recommendation, are at higher risk of hypertensive disorder and PD.

Table 5 Effect of weight gain on the secondary outcomes estimated by logistic regression

	At least one twin SGA[a] OR(95%CI)	Hypertensive gestational disorders OR(95%CI)	Gestational diabetes mellitus OR(95%CI)	Neonatal adverse outcomes[b] OR(95%CI)
Under vs. normal	1.01 (0.45; 2.28)	0.39 (0.15; 1.05)	1.98 (0.75; 5.22)	0.94 (0.29; 3.05)
Over vs. normal	–	7.69 (1.94; 30.47)	–	0.44 (0.05; 3.82)

The model for "neonatal adverse outcomes" was adjusted for pre-pregnancy BMI and gestational age. All the other models were adjusted only for pre-pregnancy BMI

[a]SGA = small for gestational age; [b]Adverse outcomes = neonatal resuscitation, respiratory distress syndrome, disseminated intravascular coagulation, intra-ventricular hemorrhage, leucomalacia, sepsis, necrotic enteritis, retinopathy of prematurity

Strengths and limitations of the study

The novelty of our work was to evaluate if there is an effect of IOM guidelines on the development of spontaneous PD in a cohort of twins at both term and preterm.

Moreover, our study has some limitations, mainly related to its retrospective design and to the small sample size as well as on the fact that it is built on a database registry.

Another possible weakness is the potential for missing data. To minimize this, at our hospital, data is reported by the obstetrician directly after delivery and skilled personnel routinely reviews the information before entering it into the database thereby minimizing recall bias. Coding was done after assessing the medical and prenatal care records together with the routine hospital documents. In addition, since there were no data regarding weekly weight gain cut-offs for twin pregnancies in IOM recommendations, we decided to apply linearity to weekly gain cut-offs as performed within IOM recommendations for single pregnancies [25].

Conclusions

Our findings suggest that normal weight gain, according to revised IOM recommendations, is associated with a reduction of spontaneous PD and, in a selected population, with better pregnancy course and better obstetrics outcomes. This information could be useful for early counseling in twin pregnancy.

Abbreviations

IOM: Institute of medicine; LGA: Large for gestational age; pBMI: Pre-gestational body mass index; PD: Preterm delivery; SGA: Small for gestational age

Acknowledgments
None.

Funding
None.

Authors' contributions

PA Protocol/project development; manuscript writing/editing; data collection or management; data analysis. FP Protocol/project development; manuscript writing/editing; data collection or management. DPB data analysis; manuscript writing/editing. FR manuscript writing/editing. MI Protocol/project development; manuscript writing/editing. SC manuscript writing/editing. SAM/manuscript editing. PV Protocol/project development; manuscript writing/editing. All authors have read and approved the final version of the manuscript.

Competing interests

The authors declare that they have no competing interests.

Author details

Department of Obstetrics and Gynecology, University of Milano-Bicocca, S. Gerardo Hospital, MBBM Foundation, Via Pergolesi 33, Monza, 20900 Monza, Monza e Brianza, Italy. [2]Department of Health Sciences, Center of Biostatistic for Clinical Epidemiology, University of Milan-Bicocca, Via Pergolesi 33, Monza, 20900 Monza, Monza e Brianza, Italy.

References

1. Abenhaim HA, Kinch RA, Morin L, Benjamin A, Usher R. Effect of prepregnancy body mass index categories on obstetrical and neonatal outcomes. Arch. Gynecol. Obstet. 2007;**275**(1):39–43.
2. Menacker F, Hamilton BE. Recent trends in cesarean delivery in the United States. NCHS Data Brief. 2010;35:1–8.
3. Brown JE, Carlson M. Nutrition and multifetal pregnancy. J Am Diet Assoc. 2000;100(3):343–8.
4. Kanadys WM, Oleszczuk J. Maternal weight gain during twin pregnancy. Its relationship to the incidence of preterm delivery. Ginekol Pol. 2000;71(11): 1355–9.
5. Yeh J, Shelton JA. Association of pre-pregnancy maternal body mass and maternal weight gain to newborn outcomes in twin pregnancies. Acta Obstet Gynecol Scand. 2007;86(9):1051–7.
6. Institute of Medicine. Subcommittee on nutritional status and weight gain during pregnancy. Washington, DC: National Academy Press; 1990.
7. Institute of Medicine. Weight gain during pregnancy: reexamining the guidelines. Washington, DC: National Academies Press; 2009.
8. Vayssiere C, Benoist G, Blondel B, Deruelle P, Favre R, Gallot D, Jabert P, Lemery D, Picone O, Pons JC, et al. Twin pregnancies: guidelines for clinical practice from the French College of Gynaecologists and Obstetricians (CNGOF). Eur J Obstet Gynecol Reprod Biol. 2011;156(1):12–7.
9. Luke B, Gillespie B, Min SJ, Avni M, Witter FR, O'Sullivan MJ. Critical periods of maternal weight gain: effect on twin birth weight. Am J Obstet Gynecol. 1997;177(5):1055–62.
10. Lantz ME, Chez RA, Rodriguez A, Porter KB. Maternal weight gain patterns and birth weight outcome in twin gestation. Obstet Gynecol. 1996;87(4):551–6.
11. Luke B, Minogue J, Witter FR, Keith LG, Johnson TR. The ideal twin pregnancy: patterns of weight gain, discordancy, and length of gestation. Am J Obstet Gynecol. 1993;169(3):588–97.
12. Luke B. The evidence linking maternal nutrition and prematurity. J Perinat Med. 2005;33(6):500–5.
13. Russo FM, Pozzi E, Pelizzoni F, Todyrenchuk L, Bernasconi DP, Cozzolino S, Vergani P. Stillbirths in singletons, dichorionic and monochorionic twins: a comparison of risks and causes. Eur J Obstet Gynecol Reprod Biol. 2013; 170(1):131–6.

14.　Ghai V, Vidyasagar D. Morbidity and mortality factors in twins. An epidemiologic approach. Clin Perinatol. 1988;15(1):123–40.

15.　Gardner MO, Goldenberg RL, Cliver SP, Tucker JM, Nelson KG, Copper RL. The origin and outcome of preterm twin pregnancies. Obstet Gynecol. 1995;85(4):553–7.

16.　Lee CM, Yang SH, Lee SP, Hwang BC, Kim SY. Clinical factors affecting the timing of delivery in twin pregnancies. Obstet Gynecol Sci. 2014;57(6):436–41.

17.　Fox NS, Saltzman DH, Kurtz H, Rebarber A. Excessive weight gain in term twin pregnancies: examining the 2009 Institute of Medicine definitions. Obstet Gynecol. 2011;118(5):1000–4.

18.　Fox NS, Rebarber A, Roman AS, Klauser CK, Peress D, Saltzman DH. Weight gain in twin pregnancies and adverse outcomes: examining the 2009 Institute of Medicine guidelines. Obstet Gynecol. 2010;116(1):100–6.

19.　Gonzalez-Quintero VH, Kathiresan AS, Tudela FJ, Rhea D, Desch C, Istwan N. The association of gestational weight gain per institute of medicine guidelines and prepregnancy body mass index on outcomes of twin pregnancies. Am J Perinatol. 2012;29(6):435–40.

20.　Bodnar LM, Pugh SJ, Abrams B, Himes KP, Hutcheon JA. Gestational weight gain in twin pregnancies and maternal and child health: a systematic review. J Perinatol. 2014;34(4):252–63.

21.　Nicola C, Mariarosaria DT, Giovanni BLS, Anna MM, Antonio R, Nicola R, Tamara S, Alessandro S, Bianiamino T, Patrizia V. In collaborations with: Pietro A, Maria EB, Giuseppe C, Giancarlo C, Marzia M, Stefano P, Giuliana S. Revised by: Paolo S, Vito T, Nicola C, Fabio S. Gestione della gravidanza multipla - Linee guida italiane, Fondazione Confalonieri Ragonese su mandato SIGO, AOGOI, AGUI. 2016. Online at http://www.sigo.it/wp-content/uploads/2016/03/Gestione-della-Gravidanza-Multipla.pdf.

22.　Bertino E, Spada E, Occhi L, Coscia A, Giuliani F, Gagliardi L, Gilli G, Bona G, Fabris C, De Curtis M, et al. Neonatal anthropometric charts: the Italian neonatal study compared with other European studies. J Pediatr Gastroenterol Nutr. 2010;51(3):353–61.

23.　ACOG Committee on Obstetric Practice. ACOG practice bulletin. Diagnosis and management of preeclampsia and eclampsia. Number 33, January 2002. American College of Obstetricians and Gynecologists. Int J Gynaecol Obstet. 2002;77(1):67-75.

24.　American Diabetes Association (2004). Gestational diabetes mellitus. Diabetes Care. Jan;27 Suppl 1:S88–90.

25.　Weight Gain During Pregnancy: Reexamining the guidelines. Editors Institute of Medicine (US) and National Research Council (US) committee to reexamine IOM pregnancy weight guidelines; Rasmussen KM, Yaktine AL, editors. Source Washington (DC): National Academies Press (US); 2009. The National Academies Collection: Reports funded by National Institutes of Health.

Malignancy during pregnancy in Japan: an exceptional opportunity for early diagnosis

Masayuki Sekine[1], Yoshiyuki Kobayashi[2], Tsutomu Tabata[2], Tamotsu Sudo[3], Ryuichiro Nishimura[3], Koji Matsuo[4], Brendan H. Grubbs[4], Takayuki Enomoto[1*] and Tomoaki Ikeda[2]

Abstract

Background: Malignancy during pregnancy has become a significant cause of maternal death in developed countries, likely due to both an older pregnant population, and increases of cervical cancer in younger women. Our aim is to investigate the clinical aspects of malignancy during pregnancy in Japan and to use this information to identify opportunities for earlier detection and treatment.

Methods: We provided a questionnaire to 1508 secondary or tertiary care hospitals in Japan. We reviewed the clinical characteristics of cases with malignancy during pregnancy for the period of January to December, 2008. From the 760 institutions which responded, we obtained clinical information for 227 unique cases. The questionnaire provided clinical information, including disease site, pregnancy outcome and how the disease was detected.

Results: The most common type of malignancy was cervical cancer ($n = 162$, 71.4%) followed by ovarian ($n = 16$, 7.0%) and breast cancer ($n = 15$, 6.6%). Leukemia ($n = 7$, 3.1%), colon cancer ($n = 5$, 2.2%), gastric cancer ($n = 5$, 2.2%), malignant lymphoma ($n = 4$, 1.8%), thyroid cancer ($n = 3$, 1.3%), brain cancer ($n = 3$, 1.3%), endometrial cancer ($n = 2$, 0.9%), and head and neck cancer ($n = 2$, 0.9%) accounted for the remaining cases. Overall, gynecological malignancies accounted for 79. 3% (95% confidence interval 74.0–84.6) of pregnancy associated malignancies diagnosed in the present study. The majority of cervical cancers, 149 (92.0%) of 162, were diagnosed by a Pap (Papanicolaou) smear during early gestation. Ten (62.5%) of the ovarian cancer cases were diagnosed by ultrasonography during a prenatal checkup or at the time of initial pregnancy diagnosis. Out of 14 breast cancers, only one (7.1%) was diagnosed by screening breast exam.

Conclusions: From this study, we reaffirm the clear and significant benefits of prenatal checkups starting at an early gestational age for the detection of gynecological cancers during pregnancy. Conversely, breast cancer detection during pregnancy was poor, suggesting new strategies for early identification of this disease are required.

Keywords: Malignancy, Pregnancy, Cervical cancer, Early diagnosis

Background

Malignancy during pregnancy has recently become a major cause of maternal death in developed countries. The incidence of malignancies coinciding with pregnancy increased from 1:2000 in 1964 to 1:1000 deliveries in 2000 [1–4]. The increase is attributed to not only higher rates of cancer in general but also to delays in childbearing to the third and fourth decades of life for women [5]. This is also associated with increase in the incidence rate of cervical cancer in 20 to 49-year-olds has been seen in Japan

[6–8]. This is assumed to be a result of a decline in the age of initial incidence of HPV (Human papillomavirus) infection due to a decline in the age of first sexual intercourse, in addition to low screening rate.

It is noteworthy that a nationwide investigation of pregnancy-linked malignancy has yet to be performed in Japan, so the underlying causes of this increase are uncertain. Several reports on malignancies during pregnancy have been published [3, 9–13] (e.g. Cancer Statistics of American Cancer Society's Epidemiology Research Program, a population-based cohort study from the Cancer Registry and the Medical Birth Registry of Norway, and an international collaborative setting of institutional registry in Belgium, the Netherlands and Czech Republic).

* Correspondence: enomoto@med.niigata-u.ac.jp
[1]Department of Obstetrics and Gynecology, Niigata University Graduate School of Medical and Dental Science, 1-757 Asahimachi-dori, Niigata 951-8510, Japan
Full list of author information is available at the end of the article

In these reports, gynecological tumors are among the malignancies most frequently diagnosed during pregnancy [9–12], particularly those of cervical and ovarian origin [13]. When managing such tumors, the physician must consider both potential fetal effects, as well as the potential loss of the patient's future reproductive capacity as a result of any chosen cancer therapy.

In this study, we have investigated the clinical characteristics of malignancy during pregnancy in Japan, with the goal that our findings will contribute to the earlier detection and better management of malignant diseases during pregnancy.

Methods

This study was performed under ethics committee approval of National Cerebral and Cardiovascular Center in Japan. We developed a questionnaire to investigate the clinical characteristics of all cases of pregnancy associated malignancy and distributed copies of this questionnaire to all training hospitals within the Japanese Society of Obstetrics and Gynecology (1475 institutions) and the Japanese Association of Clinical Cancer Centers (32 institutions). Most of the cases has been collected in hospital-based tumor registries. Subsequently, the attending obstetrician or gynecologist has examined the clinical information of the cases from medical records. Over the period of January to December 2008, 760 responding institutions provided information for 227 relevant cases, which we analyzed for clinical characteristics including the site of disease, method of disease detection, and pregnancy outcome.

Results

The clinical backgrounds and obstetrical characteristics of the 227 malignant cases reported during pregnancy for this study are shown in Table 1. The median age of the cases was 31.0 years (range: 14–41); 94 patients (41.4%) were nulliparous, 130 (57.3%) were primiparous or multiparous, and 3 were unknown. Pregnancy outcomes were available for all 227 of the cases, and 133 (58.6%) of them delivered at term. As shown in Table 1, the remaining pregnancies resulted in either: iatrogenic preterm delivery (18.9%), elective termination (10.6%), spontaneous abortion (5.3%), or spontaneous preterm delivery (4.4%).

The distribution of gestational age at iatrogenic preterm delivery (after 22 weeks of gestation) is shown in Fig. 1. None occured between 22 and 27 weeks gestation. The gestational age at delivery was distributed almost uniformly from 27 weeks until 36 weeks.

The majority of cases identified were cervical cancer (71.4%) followed by ovarian cancer (7.0%) and breast cancer (6.6%). Small numbers of malignancies at various sites account for the remaining cases as seen in Fig. 2.

Table 1 Obstetrical characteristics of malignancy during pregnancy (n = 227)

age (range)	31.0	(14–41)
parity		
nulliparaous	94	(41.4%)
multiparaous	130	(57.3%)
unknown	3	(1.3%)
pregnancy outcome		
abortion		
artificial	24	(10.6%)
spontanious	12	(5.3%)
preterm delivery		
iatrogenic	43	(18.9%)
spontanious	10	(4.4%)
term delivery	133	(58.6%)
unknown	5	(2.2%)

Overall, gynecological malignancies accounted for 79.3% (95% confidence interval 74.0–84.6) of pregnancy associated cancer diagnosed in the present study. The stage at diagnosis of 162 cases with cervical cancer in this study was as follows: 102 cases (63%) in CIN3 (cervical intraepithelial neoplasia: CIN), 16 cases (10%) in stage Ia, 33 cases (20%) in stage Ib, 5 cases (3%) in stage II, 2 cases (1%) in stage IV and 4 cases (3%) with unknown clinical stage. The histologic type of 16 cases with ovarian cancer in this study was as follows: 5 cases with adenocarcinoma (2 endometrioid, 1 serous, 1 clearcell, and 1 mucinous type), 2 with serous borderline tumor, 4 with germcell tumor (3 immature teratoma and 1 dysgerminoma), 1 with malignant transformation of mature teratoma, 1 with sertoli-leidich tumor, and 3 with unknown histology.

Table 2 demonstrates how the most common types of malignancy identified during pregnancy were diagnosed. Routine Pap (Papanicolaou) smear screening detected 92.0% of the cervical cancer cases, with the remainder identified due to vaginal bleeding, abnormal discharge, or abdomino-pelvic pain. Over half of the ovarian cancer cases (62.5%) were incidentally diagnosed by ultrasonography performed as part of a routine fetal assessment. Three cases (18.8%) were diagnosed at the time of a Caesarean section, with the remaining 3 cases identified either due to abdominal distention or palpation of swollen lymph nodes. Only one of the breast cancer cases (7.1%) was identified by a healthcare provider at the time of routine screening. The remainder were identified by patients performing self-examinations.

Discussion

In our study, we found that gynecological malignancies accounted for approximately 80% of all malignant diseases

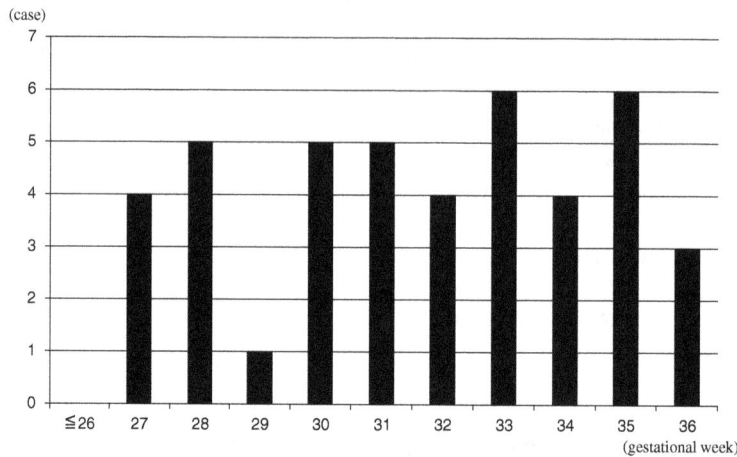

Fig. 1 Distribution of gestational age at induced termination after 22 weeks gestation ($n = 43$). There was no case of an induced termination before 27 weeks gestation. The gestational age of termination was almost equally divided from 27 weeks until 36 weeks gestation

with pregnancy during 2008. The most common pregnancy associated malignancies worldwide are cervical cancer, breast cancer, lymphoma, ovarian cancer, and melanoma [12, 14, 15]. Of these, cervical and breast cancers account for 50% of all cancers occurring during pregnancy [15], which is a lower rate than is seen in the present study (78%). The obstetrician will often have the best opportunity to make the diagnosis of malignancy during pregnancy, so awareness of the associated symptoms is required during regular pre-natal checkups.

We found that conducting a Pap smear during the early pregnancy period was very effective in early detection of cervical cancer, the most common pregnancy associated cancer in Japan. The prevalence of cervical

cancer for women in their twenties and thirties has risen dramatically over the past decade in several studies in Japan [6–8]. Based on the findings of this study, it is essential that the obstetrician ask each pregnant patient about her past Pap smear and examination history and strongly recommend this test for any patient who is not up to date on her screening.

In order to detect ovarian cancer during pregnancy, assessment of the adnexae is important at the time of all prenatal ultrasounds. In review of the literature, up to one third of ovarian cancers diagnosed during pregnancy were identified incidentally by ultrasonography, making it the most common method of tumor diction [16–18]. As gestational age increases, use of

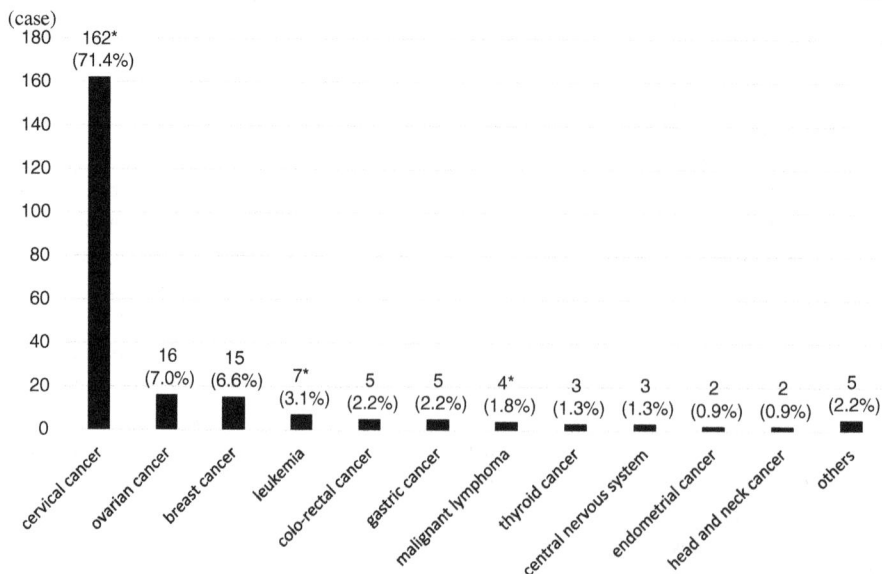

Fig. 2 Site of malignant disease during pregnancy ($n = 227$). Most cases were cervical cancer (162 out of 227, 71.4%), ovarian cancer (16 cases, 7.0%), and breast cancer (15 cases, 6.6%). *Two cases with cervical cancer were affected with other malignancy; leukemia or malignant lymphoma, respectively

Table 2 Opportunity to detect malignancy during pregnancy

Malignancy during pregnancy	number of cases (%)
Cervical cancer (n = 162)	
screening Pap cytology	149 (92.0%)
abnormal vaginal bleeding	11 (6.8%)
abnormal vaginal discharge	1 (0.6%)
abdomino-pelvic pain	1 (0.6%)
Ovarian cancer (n = 16)	
ultrasonography (routine prenatal care)	10 (62.5%)
incidental (during cesarian section)	3 (18.8%)
abdominal distension	2 (12.5%)
abnormal lymphadenopathy	1 (6.3%)
Breast cancer (n = 14)	
self-detection of a palpable mass	13 (92.9%)
health care screening	1 (7.1%)

transabdominal ultrasound observation to detect an ovarian tumor becomes more difficult, so this is particularly important at the time of the first trimester examination. In cases where the ovaries are not adequately visualized, or characterized by transabdominal ultrasound, a vaginal probe can often provide a better assessment.

In some cases MRI (Magnetic Resonance Imaging) subsequent to an unclear or suspicious ultrasound finding may be necessary to help differentiate whether an ovarian mass is malignant or benign [19]. As the progression of ovarian cancer can be very rapid, at our institution we use a combination of early pregnancy vaginal ultrasonography with a follow-up MRI scan in all cases where there is any suspicion of malignancy.

We found that the majority of breast cancer cases were found following self-detection of a palpable mass and not by a health care provider. Increased breast cancer awareness during pregnancy may contribute to this finding. Additionally, pregnant women are generally not yet at an age where routine mammography is recommended, skewing the results towards initial breast tumor discovery by self-examination. Regular prenatal checkups did not appear to be useful for detecting breast masses, however this may be an area where improvement may come from stressing the importance of a thorough examination, with appropriate close follow up of any suspicious findings. It is a general practice in Japan for midwives, rather than obstetricians to perform breast examinations during prenatal care. Thus, several strategies may be needed to improve the early detection of breast cancer during pregnancy. These might include development of a universal training guideline for breast examination by obstetricians with possible assistance by the midwife service.

Conclusions

From this study, we reaffirm the significant benefits of pre-natal checkups at an early gestational age for early detection of gynecologic cancer during pregnancy. On the other hand, the detection of non-gynecologic cancers tends to be delayed, and it is clear that we need new strategies as to how to improve screening, particularly for breast cancer in pregnant women.

Abbreviations
CIN: Cervical intraepithelial neoplasia; HPV: human papillomavirus; MRI: Magnetic resonance imaging; Pap: Papanicolaou

Funding
The present study was financially supported by Grant-in-Aid for Scientific Research from the Ministry of Health, Labour and Welfare, Japan.

Authors' contributions
TI, TS, RN, TE contributed to the design of this study. MS, YK, TT collected the data and were involved in data analysis. MS drafted the manuscript, performed the data analysis and wrote the primary version of the manuscript. YK, TE, TT, KM, BHG, TI interpreted the data and gave relevant scientific input during the conduction of the study and worked to set up the final version of the manuscript. All authors reviewed the manuscript and approved the final version.

Competing interests
The authors declare that they have no competing interests.

Author details
[1]Department of Obstetrics and Gynecology, Niigata University Graduate School of Medical and Dental Science, 1-757 Asahimachi-dori, Niigata 951-8510, Japan. [2]Departments of Obstetrics and Gynecology, Mie University Graduate School of Medicine, Mie, Japan. [3]Department of Gynecology, Hyogo Cancer Center, Hyogo, Japan. [4]Department of Obstetrics and Gynecology, University of Southern California, Los Angeles, CA, USA.

References
1. Salani R, Billingsley CC, Crafton SM. Cancer and pregnancy: an overview for obstetricians and gynecologists. Am J Obstet Gynecol. 2014;211:7–14.
2. Williams TJ, Turnbull KE. Carcinoma in situ and pregnancy. Obstet Gynecol. 1964;24:857–64.
3. Pavlidis NA. Coexistence of pregnancy and malignancy. Oncologist. 2002;7:279–87.
4. Smith LH, Danielsen B, Allen ME, Cress R. Cancer associated with obstetric delivery: results of linkage with the California cancer registry. Am J Obstet Gynecol. 2003;189:1128–35.
5. Voulgaris E, Pentheroudakis G, Pavlidis N. Cancer and pregnancy: a comprehensive review. Surg Oncol. 2011;20:e175–85.
6. Matsuda A, Matsuda T, Shibata A, Katanoda K, Sobue T, Nishimoto H, Japan Cancer Surveillance Research Group. Japan cancer surveillance research group : cancer incidence and incidence rates in Japan in 2007: a study of 21 population-based cancer registries for the monitoring of cancer incidence in Japan (MCIJ) project. Jpn J Clin Oncol. 2013;43:328–36.

7. Vaccarella S, Lortet-Tieulent J, Plummer M, Franceschi S, Bray F. Worldwide trends in cervical cancer incidence: impact of screening against changes in disease risk factors. Eur J Cancer. 2013;49:3262–73.

8. Banzai C, Yahata T, Tanaka K. Trends in the incidence of uterine cancer in Niigata, Japan: a population-based study from 1982 to 2007. Eur J Gynaecol Oncol. 2011;32:521–4.

9. Stensheim H, Moller B, van Dijk T, Fossa SD. Cause-specific survival for women diagnosed with cancer during pregnancy or lactation: a registry-based cohort study. J Clin Oncol. 2009;27:45–51.

10. Van Calsteren K, Heyns L, De Smet F, et al. Cancer during pregnancy: an analysis of 215 patients emphasizing the obstetrical and the neonatal outcomes. J Clin Oncol. 2010;28:683–9.

11. Zanotti KM, Belinson JL, Kennedy AW. Treatment of gynecologic cancers in pregnancy. Semin Oncol. 2000;27:686–98.

12. Morice P, Uzan C, Gouy S, Verschraegen C, Haie-Meder C. Gynaecological cancers in pregnancy. Lancet. 2012;379:558–69.

13. Latimer J. Gynaecological malignancies in pregnancy. Curr Opin Obstet Gynecol. 2007;19:140–4.

14. Amant F, Loibl S, Neven P, Van Calsteren K. Breast cancer in pregnancy. Lancet. 2012;379:570–9.

15. Ji YI, Kim KT. Gynecologic malignancy in pregnancy. Obstet Gynecol Sci. 2013;56:289–300.

16. Blake EA, Kodama M, Yunokawa M, Ross MS, Ueda Y, Grubbs BH, Matsuo K. Feto-maternal outcomes of pregnancy complicated by epithelial ovarian cancer: a systematic review of literature. Eur J Obstet Gynecol Reprod Biol. 2015;186:97–105.

17. Kodama M, Grubbs BH, Blake EA, Cahoon SS, Murakami R, Kimura T, Matsuo K. Feto-maternal outcomes of pregnancy complicated by ovarian malignant germ cell tumor: a systematic review of literature. Eur J Obstet Gynecol Reprod Biol. 2014;181:145–56.

18. Blake EA, Carter CM, Kashani BN, Kodama M, Mabuchi S, Yoshino K, Matsuo K. Feto-maternal outcomes of pregnancy complicated by ovarian sex-cord stromal tumor: a systematic review of literature. Eur J Obstet Gynecol Reprod Biol. 2014;175:1–7.

19. Patenaude Y, Pugash D, Lim K, Morin L, Lim K, Bly S, Butt K, Cargill Y, Davies G, Denis N, Hazlitt G, Morin L, Naud K, Ouellet A, Salem S. The Use of Magnetic Resonance Imaging in the Obstetric Patient. J Obstetr Gynaecol Can. 2014;36(4):349–55.

Trajectory of vitamin D status during pregnancy in relation to neonatal birth size and fetal survival

Linnea Bärebring[1*] , Maria Bullarbo[2,3], Anna Glantz[4], Lena Hulthén[1], Joy Ellis[5], Åse Jagner[4], Inez Schoenmakers[6,7], Anna Winkvist[1] and Hanna Augustin[1]

Abstract

Background: We investigated the associations between vitamin D status in early and late pregnancy with neonatal small for gestational age (SGA), low birth weight (LBW) and preterm delivery. Furthermore, associations between vitamin D status and pregnancy loss were studied.

Methods: Serum 25-hydroxyvitamin D (25OHD) was sampled in gestational week ≤ 16 (trimester 1 (T1), $N = 2046$) and > 31 (trimester 3 (T3), $N = 1816$) and analysed using liquid chromatography tandem mass spectrometry. Pregnant women were recruited at antenatal clinics in south-west Sweden at latitude 57–58°N. Gestational and neonatal data were retrieved from medical records. Multiple gestations and terminated pregnancies were excluded from the analyses. SGA was defined as weight and/or length at birth < 2 SD of the population mean and LBW as < 2500 g. Preterm delivery was defined as delivery < 37 + 0 gestational weeks and pregnancy loss as spontaneous abortion or intrauterine fetal death. Associations between neonatal outcomes and 25OHD at T1, T3 and change in 25OHD (T3-T1) were studied using logistic regression.

Results: T1 25OHD was negatively associated with pregnancy loss and 1 nmol/L increase in 25OHD was associated with 1% lower odds of pregnancy loss (OR 0.99, $p = 0.046$). T3 25OHD ≥ 100 nmol/L (equal to 40 ng/ml) was associated with lower odds of SGA (OR 0.3, $p = 0.031$) and LBW (OR 0.2, $p = 0.046$), compared to vitamin D deficiency (25OHD < 30 nmol/L, or 12 ng/ml). Women with a ≥ 30 nmol/L increment in 25OHD from T1 to T3 had the lowest odds of SGA, LBW and preterm delivery.

Conclusions: Vitamin D deficiency in late pregnancy was associated with higher odds of SGA and LBW. Lower 25OHD in early pregnancy was only associated with pregnancy loss. Vitamin D status trajectory from early to late pregnancy was inversely associated with SGA, LBW and preterm delivery with the lowest odds among women with the highest increment in 25OHD. Thus, both higher vitamin D status in late pregnancy and gestational vitamin D status trajectory can be suspected to play a role in healthy pregnancy.

Keywords: Vitamin D, 25-hydroxyvitamin D, Small for gestational age, Low birth weight, Preterm delivery, Miscarriage, Intrauterine fetal death

* Correspondence: linnea.barebring@gu.se
[1]The Department of Internal Medicine and Clinical Nutrition, Sahlgrenska Academy, University of Gothenburg, Box 459, 405 30 Gothenburg, Sweden
Full list of author information is available at the end of the article

Background

Placental pathology is often found in pregnancies complicated by intrauterine growth restriction, preeclampsia or intrauterine fetal death. It is associated with inadequate invasion of extravillous trophoblasts and inadequate angiogenesis, with insufficient conversion of arterial spiral arteries in the decidua [1]. These processes are complex and normal development is dependent on several factors. Vitamin D status (measured as 25-hydroxyvitamin D (25OHD)) of pregnant women has been inversely associated with adverse gestational outcomes and associated with uteroplacental dysfunction [2].

We have previously shown that higher vitamin D status in late pregnancy and larger increase in vitamin D status during pregnancy is associated with lower risk of preeclampsia [3]. Associations have also been shown between vitamin D insufficiency (< 50 nmol/L) and increased risk of infant small for gestational age (SGA) and low birth weight (LBW) [4]. Circulating concentrations of 25OHD below 25 or 30 nmol/L have been associated with 50–300% increased odds of SGA, compared to higher concentrations [5–7]. Also, maternal 25OHD < 28 nmol/L in late, but not early, pregnancy have been associated with lower infant birth size and shorter gestational length in a smaller longitudinal study [8]. However, there is also limited evidence for a U-shaped association where high 25OHD concentrations (> 80 nmol/L) may be related to higher risk of SGA [9]. Thus, the association between vitamin D status and neonatal birth size is not clear and warrants further investigation. A recent meta-analysis of 10 studies concluded that 25OHD concentrations < 50 nmol/L were associated with an approximately 30% increased risk of preterm delivery [10]. Bodnar et al. found that early pregnancy 25OHD concentrations < 75 nmol/L were associated with higher risk of both medically indicated and spontaneous preterm delivery [11]. Lower vitamin D status has also been associated with a medical history of recurrent miscarriage [12] but only two prospective studies have investigated this, without finding that lower 25OHD concentrations increases the risk of pregnancy loss [5, 13]. Both these prospective studies had relatively few cases of pregnancy loss and may therefore have been insufficiently powered to study this association. Thus, the association between vitamin D status and risk of miscarriage needs further investigation.

To our knowledge, no previous study has related 25OHD concentration in both early and late pregnancy to neonatal outcomes related to placental dysfunction. Therefore, it has not been possible to ascertain whether the associations at implantation in early pregnancy differ from those during the fetal growth spurt in late pregnancy.

Our objectives were to study the associations between vitamin D status in both early and late pregnancy, as well as change in vitamin D status during pregnancy with neonatal SGA, LBW and preterm delivery. Associations between vitamin D status in early pregnancy and pregnancy loss were also studied.

Methods

The GraviD study is a prospective cohort study, conducted in parts of the Västra Götaland region in the southwest of Sweden, at latitude 57–58°N [3]. Pregnant women were recruited from gestational week 4 during fall 2013 and spring 2014, when registering at one of the participating antenatal care units. The only exclusion criterion was pregnancy exceeding 16 gestational weeks at inclusion. Gestational age at delivery and data collection was determined by routine ultrasound in the second trimester, but gestational age at inclusion was based on the date of the last menstrual period. Women who terminated the pregnancy ($N = 31$), were lost to follow-up ($N = 13$) or carried more than one foetus ($N = 26$) were excluded from the present analyses. Pregnancy termination was mostly due to fetal malformations. Women who were lost to follow-up had moved and their medical records could not be retrieved. This study was conducted according to the Declaration of Helsinki and all procedures were approved by the Regional Ethics Committee in Gothenburg, Sweden. Written informed consent was obtained from all participants.

Outcomes

SGA was defined as either weight or length at birth below 2 SD of the gender-specific population mean [14]. LBW was defined as weight at birth < 2500 g. Preterm delivery was defined as delivery before gestational week +days 37 + 0, including both induced and spontaneous preterm delivery. Pregnancy loss was defined as both spontaneous abortions from gestational week 4 and intrauterine fetal death (IUFD). Late pregnancy loss was defined as spontaneous abortion at gestational week ≥ 14 + 0, including IUFD. IUFD was defined as pregnancy loss at gestational week ≥ 22 + 0. Pregnancy loss before gestational week 22 was based on self-report data and medical records to verify miscarriage were not available. Information on IUFD was collected from medical records from the obstetrics care.

Exposure

Maternal blood samples were collected from each participant at two time points; before gestational week 16 (predominantly week 8–12, first trimester, T1) and after gestational week 31 (predominantly week 32–35, third trimester, T3). Non-fasting venous blood samples were drawn in gel serum separating tubes and centrifuged for 10 min within 2 h of sampling. Serum was stored at – 70 °C until analysis of 25OHD. Analyses were performed by liquid chromatography tandem mass spectrometry (LC-MS/MS,

Mass spectrometer API 4000) by the clinical chemistry laboratory in Region Skåne, Sweden, certified by the Vitamin D External Quality Assessment Scheme [15]. The LC-MS/MS method has a measuring range of 6–450 nmol/L for $25OHD_3$ and of 6–225 nmol/L for $25OHD_2$. The interassay coefficient of variation is 6% at 40 nmol/L for both $25OHD_3$ and $25OHD_2$. Sampling and laboratory analyses have been described previously [3]. Maternal serum T1 and T3 samples were analysed in sequence. At T1 and T3, participants answered questionnaires regarding lifestyle factors and background data. Neonatal and gestational data were obtained from antenatal and obstetrics medical records. Information on BMI at T1 and season of conception (December–May or June–November) was obtained from the medical records. Season was coded as a binary variable, since this explained 30% of vitamin D status in a previous study in pregnant women at the same latitude [16]. Data on education level (≤primary level, secondary level or university level) and origin (continent of birth: Northern Europe, Continental Europe, America, Asia, Africa) were collected from study questionnaires.

Statistical analysis

Concentrations of 25OHD at T1 and T3 were used as categorical variables, grouped into 25OHD < 30 (used as reference category), 30–49.9, 50–74.9, 75–99.9 and ≥ 100 nmol/L. These groups were chosen to study whether vitamin D insufficiency (30–50 nmol/L), sufficiency (≥ 50 nmol/L) or high status (≥ 75 or ≥ 100 nmol/L) was associated with the outcomes studied, compared to vitamin D deficiency (< 30 nmol/L). Quartiles were not used because the distribution of 25OHD was different at T1 and T3. T1 25OHD was also investigated as a continuous variable as there were few cases in some categories. Change in 25OHD was calculated as the difference between T3 and T1 (T3-T1) and was coded into 3 groups: decrease in 25OHD (≤ 0 nmol/L), small increase (0.1–29.99 nmol/L) or large increase (≥30 nmol/L).

Multivariable logistic regression analyses of the outcome variables SGA, LBW and preterm delivery were performed with 25OHD at T1, T3 and change in 25OHD during pregnancy as the independent variables. For SGA, appropriate for gestational age and large for gestational age were combined as reference. Potential confounders for the associations studied were identified using directed acyclic graphs (www.dagitty.net) [17]. Variables BMI, season of conception, education level and origin were identified and included in the final models. Tobacco use and vitamin D supplement use were also investigated as potential confounders but did not show any confounding effect and were thus not included in the final models. In the multivariable analysis with change in 25OHD as the independent variable, T1 25OHD was also included as a confounder. Correlation between continuous T1 25OHD

and continuous change in 25OHD was low ($r = -0.22$, $p < 0.001$) and it was therefore considered acceptable to include both variables in the same model. Multivariable logistic regression analysis of the outcome pregnancy loss was also performed with 25OHD at T1 (continuous and categorical) as independent variable. These models were adjusted for BMI, season of conception, education level, origin and gestational age at registration to antenatal care (based on last menstrual period). Unadjusted logistic regression analysis was used to assess the association between T1 25OHD (< 30 nmol/L; no/yes) and IUFD. Here, no confounders were included due to the small number of cases ($N = 9$). Significance was accepted at $p < 0.05$. Computer software IBM SPSS Statistics version 22.0 was used for all statistical analyses.

Results

In total, 2052 women were included in this study, 2046 with a blood sample at T1 and 1816 at T3 (Fig. 1). In total, 1810 women had samples collected both in T1 and T3. Characteristics of the women and the live born infants are shown in Table 1. Mean infant birth weight was 3542 (538) grams and mean gestational age at delivery was 280 (12.4) days. Mean (SD) maternal 25OHD at T1 was 64 (24.4) nmol/L and 75 (34.4) nmol/L at T3. At T1, 10% had 25OHD concentrations < 30 nmol/L and 9% at T3 (Table 2).

Birth size and preterm delivery

In total, 93 (4.5%) infants were born SGA. Of the SGA deliveries, 37 were SGA by weight and 56 by length. Also, 58 (2.8%) infants had LBW, while 78 (3.8%) infants were delivered preterm (Table 1). Of those who delivered preterm, 10 delivered before gestational week 31 and thus before the T3 blood sample could be drawn.

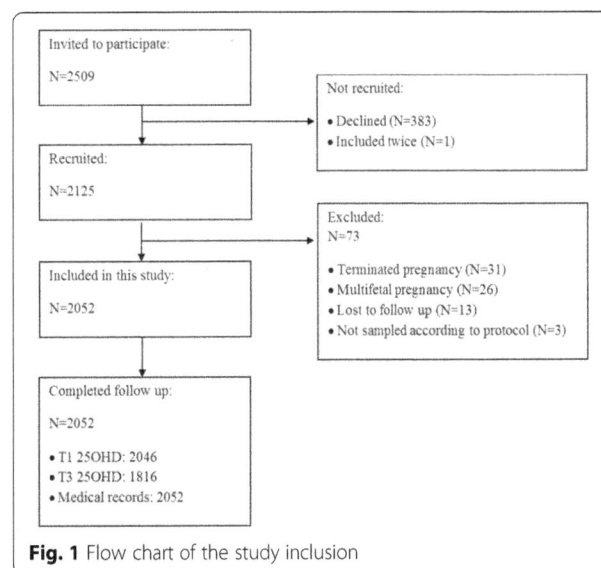

Fig. 1 Flow chart of the study inclusion

Table 1 Characteristics of the pregnant women and their infants at birth

	Mean	SD
Birth weight (grams)[a]	3542	537.7
Birth length (cm)[a]	50	2.3
Gestational age at delivery (days)	280	12.4
Gestational age T1 (days)	76	13.8
Gestational age T3 (days)	234	12.9
Maternal s-25OHD T1 (nmol/L)	64	24.4
Maternal s-25OHD T3 (nmol/L)	75	34.4
	N (%)	
Male gender of infant[a]	976 (49.8)	
Small for gestational age (weight or length)	93 (4.5)	
Low birth weight (< 2500 g)	58 (2.8)	
Preterm delivery (< 37 weeks)	78 (3.8)	
Spontaneous preterm delivery (< 37 weeks)	55 (2.7)	
Pregnancy loss	97 (4.7)	
Intrauterine fetal death (≥ 22 weeks)	9 (0.5)	

T1 first trimester, *T3* third trimester, *25OHD* 25-hydroxyvitamin D
[a]Live born infants only

Among these women, one (10%) had 25OHD concentration < 30 nmol/L in T1.

There were no associations between the predictor T1 25OHD and the outcomes SGA, LBW and preterm delivery (Table 3). Women with T3 25OHD ≥ 100 nmol/L had a lower OR for SGA (OR = 0.32, $p = 0.031$) compared to those with vitamin D deficiency (< 30 nmol/L). Women with T3 25OHD concentrations ≥ 100 nmol/L and 30–50 nmol/L had lower OR for LBW (OR = 0.22, $p = 0.046$ and OR = 0.07, $p = 0.017$, respectively), compared to vitamin D deficiency. However, T3 25OHD was not significantly associated with preterm delivery. The results were not meaningfully affected by additional adjustment for tobacco use or vitamin D supplementation or by excluding cases of preeclampsia (data not shown).

Vitamin D status trajectory between T1 and T3 was inversely related to SGA, preterm and LBW (Table 3). Compared to women with a large increase in 25OHD (≥30 nmol/L), women with a decrease in 25OHD had significantly higher OR of having a child born SGA (OR = 3.7, $p = 0.002$), with LBW (OR = 4.7, $p = 0.014$) as well as a trend toward higher odds of preterm delivery (OR = 2.9, $p = 0.061$). Women with a small increase in 25OHD (0–30 nmol/L) had significantly higher OR of SGA (OR = 2.6, $p = 0.019$) and preterm delivery (OR = 2.9, $p = 0.047$) as well as a trend toward significance for LBW

Table 2 The pregnant women's vitamin D status in the first (T1) and third (T3) trimester of pregnancy, and their characteristics (mean or percent) grouped by 25OHD concentration in (T1)

T1 25OHD (nmol/L)	< 30	30–49.9	50–74.9	75–99.9	≥ 100
N	198	291	788	565	125
%	10.1	14.8	40.1	28.7	6.4
BMI T1 (kg/m^2)	25.1	24.9	24.4	23.9	24.4
Age T1 (years)	29.4	30.9	31.6	32.0	32.4
Born in Sweden (%)	14.1	54.6	83.3	87.8	93.5
Tobacco use T1 (%)	6.8	4.6	4.0	4.6	1.6
Nulliparous T1 (%)	34.8	42.0	42.6	43.1	42.7
Vitamin D supplement use T1 (%)	10.6	28.2	45.2	56.6	62.9
University level education (%)	32.3	54.9	61.3	67.3	66.1
Small for gestational age (%)	5.7	4.2	5.3	4.1	4.0
Preterm delivery (%)	4.1	5.2	3.8	3.9	1.6
Low birth weight (%)	3.0	4.5	3.1	2.1	1.6
Pregnancy loss (%)	6.3	5.6	4.5	5.1	0
T3 25OHD (nmol/L)	< 30	30–49.9	50–74.9	75–99.9	≥ 100
N	163	330	473	409	443
%	9.0	18.2	26.0	22.5	24.4
Small for gestational age (%)	7.5	5.5	4.7	4.6	2.3
Preterm delivery (%)	4.3	1.2	3.6	2.2	1.6
Low birth weight (%)	4.3	0.3	2.7	1.2	1.4

T1 first trimester, *T3* third trimester, *25OHD* 25-hydroxyvitamin D

Table 3 Association between vitamin D status in pregnancy with birth size and pregnancy loss (adjusted logistic regression analysis)

	Small for gestational age[a]		Preterm delivery (< 37 weeks)[b]		Low birth weight (< 2500 g)[c]		Pregnancy loss[d]	
	OR	CI 95%	OR	CI 95%	OR	CI 95%	OR	CI 95%
T1 25OHD[e]								
Continuous nmol/L	1.003	0.99–1.01	0.996	0.99–1.01	0.999	0.99–1.01	0.989*	0.98–1.00
< 30 (ref)	1.0		1.0		1.0		1.0	
30–49.9	1.078	0.44–2.66	1.647	0.63–4.33	2.549	0.88–7.38	1.030	0.44–2.41
50–74.9	1.632	0.69–3.85	1.260	0.47–3.36	2.287	0.77–6.83	0.688	0.29–1.62
75–99-9	1.292	0.51–3.27	1.332	0.48–3.73	1.665	0.51–5.49	0.809	0.33–1.96
≥ 100	1.294	0.38–4.42	0.502	0.09–2.72	1.255	0.22–7.27	0.000[f]	
T3 25OHD[e]								
< 30 (ref)	1.0		1.0		1.0			
30–49.9	0.771	0.34–1.75	0.302	0.08–1.14	0.071*	0.01–0.63		
50–74.9	0.623	0.27–1.45	0.933	0.31–2.79	0.584	0.17–1.98		
75–99-9	0.657	0.27–1.61	0.614	0.18–2.14	0.237	0.06–1.01		
≥ 100	0.318*	0.11–0.90	0.446	0.11–1.76	0.215*	0.05–0.97		
Δ25OHD[g]								
Large increase (≥ 30 nmol/L) (ref)	1.0		1.0		1.0			
Small increase (0–30 nmol/L)	2.564*	1.16–5.67	2.905*	1.01–8.34	3.122	0.97–10.09		
Decrease (< 0 nmol/L)	3.679**	1.60–8.44	2.894	0.95–8.85	4.722*	1.37–16.28		

T1 first trimester, *T3* third trimester, *25OHD* 25-hydroxyvitamin D
*$p < 0.05$ **$p < 0.01$
[a]Models include 92 (T1) and 80 (T3 and Δ25OHD) cases of small for gestational age
[b]Models include 77 (T1) and 43 (T3 and Δ25OHD) cases of preterm delivery
[c]Models include 57 (T1) and 31 (T3 and Δ25OHD) cases of low birth weight
[d]Models include 96 cases of pregnancy loss
[e]Adjusted for education, origin, season of conception and BMI at T1. Pregnancy loss models are also adjusted for gestational age at registration for antenatal care
[f]No case of pregnancy loss in category
[g]Adjusted for education, origin, season of conception, BMI at T1 and 25OHD at T1

(OR = 3.1, $p = 0.056$), compared to women with a large increase. Neither of these results changed after adjustment for tobacco use and vitamin D supplementation at T3 or after excluding cases of preeclampsia.

Pregnancy loss
The total rate of pregnancy loss was 4.7% and the rate of late pregnancy loss (gestational week ≥ 14 + 0) was 1.5% (Table 1). There were nine cases of IUFD at gestational week ≥ 22 + 0. Overall, lower T1 25OHD (as a continuous but not categorical variable) was associated with pregnancy loss (Table 3). In unadjusted analysis, T1 25OHD was associated with IUFD and women with 25OHD < 30 nmol/L at T1 had more than fourfold higher odds of IUFD (OR = 4.52, $p = 0.034$).

Discussion
We found that higher vitamin D status among women in late, but not early, pregnancy was associated with lower probability of SGA and LBW. Vitamin D status trajectory during pregnancy was inversely associated with SGA, LBW and preterm delivery. Women with an increase in 25OHD ≥30 nmol/L from T1 to T3 had the lowest odds of SGA, LBW and preterm delivery. We also found that lower vitamin D status in early pregnancy was related to pregnancy loss.

Previous findings from the GraviD study show lower odds of preeclampsia among women with a large increase (≥ 30 nmol/L) in 25OHD [3]. As SGA, LBW and preterm delivery are related to preeclampsia; these results are consistent with the current findings. However, excluding preeclampsia cases from the analysis did not change the results. Thus, preeclampsia does not seem to mediate the associations between vitamin D status trajectory and neonatal birth size or preterm birth. We have previously shown that the determinants of season-corrected change in 25OHD during pregnancy include origin, sun-exposure and dietary as well as supplementary vitamin D intake [18]. Supplements containing vitamin D were used by 43% in T1 and 39% in T3- mainly multivitamins [19]. As the results between change in 25OHD and neonatal birth size and preterm delivery remained after adjustment for season of conception, origin and vitamin D supplementation, vitamin D status trajectory can be suspected to play a role in healthy pregnancy. Vitamin D has been shown to facilitate the transport of nutrients across the placenta [20, 21], which could contribute to fetal growth [22]. Vitamin D status could also facilitate fetal development by regulating placental inflammation [23]. It is also possible that the associations between fetal growth and maternal vitamin D status are due to residual confounding or reverse causation. Whether vitamin D metabolism is altered in placental dysfunction in unclear and warrants further investigation.

Our results indicates that 25OHD at T3 but not at T1 is associated with SGA and LBW, despite better statistical power at T1 due to more 25OHD samples and subsequently more cases of SGA, LBW and preterm birth. This finding is partly consistent with previous studies where 25OHD concentrations of 25–30 nmol/L were associated with higher probability of SGA [5–7]. The study by Burris et al. [6] sampled women in gestational week 26–28, and found a higher OR for SGA than the two studies that sampled women in T1. This could be interpreted as support of our finding that late rather than early pregnancy vitamin D status is the stronger predictor of fetal growth restriction. Our results also concur with findings by Morley et al. that late but not early pregnancy 25OHD was related to gestational length and neonatal birth size [8]. Our results could also indicate that it takes time for changes in vitamin D metabolism to manifest as changes in circulating 25OHD. We did not see a U-shaped association between early pregnancy vitamin D status and SGA, as previously indicated [9]. We found the lowest odds of SGA among women with the highest T3 25OHD concentration, ≥100 nmol/L. A total of 25% of the women had 25OHD concentrations ≥100 nmol/L at T3. Sampling was evenly distributed across the seasons and time of year cannot explain the high proportion with high 25OHD concentrations. Also, vitamin D supplements were used by almost half of the women but most (88%) used multivitamins containing 5–10 μg of vitamin D3. Supplementation can therefore only partly explain the large proportion with high vitamin D status, and other likely contributors are pregnancy associated endocrine changes and possibly lifestyle factors.

To our knowledge, ours is one of the first studies to find associations between vitamin D status and pregnancy loss. The 25OHD concentration has been shown to have immunological effects in women with a history of recurrent pregnancy loss [12]. Two previous studies have investigated but not found any association between 25OHD and miscarriage [5, 13]. In those studies, 25OHD was used as a categorical variable. One earlier study, from Denmark, found that lower vitamin D status in early pregnancy was associated with pregnancy loss in the first trimester [24]. We found that pregnancy loss was associated with lower 25OHD when expressed on a continuous but not categorical scale. As most women with high vitamin D status were born in Sweden and thus more likely to be familiar with the Swedish health-

care system, it is possible that they registered earlier for antenatal care and were more likely to report pregnancy loss. However, the models were adjusted for gestational age at registration for antenatal care. Despite few cases of IUFD in the GraviD cohort, our results suggest that vitamin D deficiency in early pregnancy may be linked to IUFD. These results need confirmation, preferably by adjusted statistical analysis as confounding can be expected, which was not possible in our present study due to few cases.

Strengths of this study are that the GraviD cohort is representative of the general pregnant population in terms of origin, education, parity, BMI and tobacco use [25], which increases the external validity of the findings. Also, gestational age at delivery was estimated by routine ultrasound, which is considered more accurate than dating by last menstrual period [26]. A limitation of this study is that information on pregnancy loss, except IUFD, was self-reported. The information on pregnancy loss is likely correct, albeit without conclusive information on the time of fetal demise. Survival analysis could therefore not be performed, as time to event data were missing. In addition, vitamin D status among women who terminated the pregnancy was not assessed. Data on SGA, LBW and preterm delivery were collected from obstetrics charts based on standardized measures. Since there were few cases of SGA based on birth weight alone, the definition of SGA used in this study was based on birth weight and/or length. Among the SGA cases defined by length only, most were close to also meeting the SGA definition for birth weight. Therefore, the definition used in this study is likely to be relevant. Another limitation is that data on physical activity during pregnancy was only available for a subset of the women and was therefore not used.

While the GraviD study indicates an association between T3 25OHD and consequences of placental insufficiency, change in 25OHD during pregnancy might be a stronger predictor of placental dysfunction, as it is associated with SGA, LBW and preterm delivery. The lowest odds of SGA and LBW are found among women with the largest increments in 25OHD (≥ 30 nmol/L). Interestingly, vitamin D status at T1- around the time the maternal blood flow of the placenta is fully developed- is only related to pregnancy loss.

Conclusion

In conclusion, lower early pregnancy 25OHD was associated with pregnancy loss. High vitamin D status in late, but not early, pregnancy was associated with lower odds of SGA and LBW. Change in 25OHD during pregnancy was associated with SGA, LBW and preterm delivery, with the lowest odds for women with an increment in 25OHD ≥ 30 nmol/L. Both higher late pregnancy vitamin D status and gestational vitamin D status trajectory can be suspected to play a role in healthy pregnancy.

Abbreviations

25OHD: 25-hydroxyvitamin D; IUFD: Intrauterine fetal death; LBW: Low birth weight; SGA: Small for gestational age; T1: First trimester of pregnancy; T3: Third trimester of pregnancy

Acknowledgements

The authors would like to thank the women who participated in the study, as well as the midwives and nurses whose contributions were pivotal in the realization of the study.

Funding

This research was funded by the Swedish Research Council for Health, Working Life and Welfare (HA, Forte, Dnr 2012–0793) and Regional Research and Development grants (MB, FoU, Dnr VGFOUREG-388201 and VGFOUREG-229331). Inez Schoenmakers was funded by the Medical Research Council, programme U105960371. The funders had no role in study design, data collection and analysis, decision to publish, or preparation of the manuscript.

Authors' contributions

HA MB AG JE LH conceived and designed the study. LB ÅJ HA collected the data. LB analyzed the data. LB MB AG AW ÅJ JE LH IS HA wrote the paper and all authors have contributed substantially in drafting and revising the manuscript. All authors read and approved the final manuscript.

Competing interests

The authors declare that they have no competing interests.

Author details

[1]The Department of Internal Medicine and Clinical Nutrition, Sahlgrenska Academy, University of Gothenburg, Box 459, 405 30 Gothenburg, Sweden. [2]Södra Älvsborg Hospital, Borås, Sweden. [3]The Department of Obstetrics and Gynecology, Sahlgrenska Academy, University of Gothenburg, Gothenburg, Sweden. [4]Department of Antenatal Care, Närhälsan, Primary Care, Gothenburg, Sweden. [5]Department of Antenatal Care, Närhälsan, Primary Care, Södra, Bohuslän, Sweden. [6]MRC Human Nutrition Research, Nutrition and Bone Health Group, Cambridge, UK. [7]The Department of Medicine, Faculty of Medicine and Health Sciences, University of East Anglia, Norwich, UK.

References

1. Hacker NF, Gambone JC, Hobel CJ. Hacker and Moore's essentials of obstetrics and gynecology. 5th ed. Philadelphia: Saunders Elsevier; 2010.
2. Kiely ME, Zhang JY, Kinsella M, Khashan AS, Kenny LC. Vitamin D status is associated with uteroplacental dysfunction indicated by pre-eclampsia and small-for-gestational-age birth in a large prospective pregnancy cohort in Ireland with low vitamin D status. Am J Clin Nutr. 2016;104(2):354–61.
3. Bärebring L, Bullarbo M, Glantz A, Leu Agelii M, Jagner A, Ellis J, et al. Preeclampsia and blood pressure trajectory during pregnancy in relation to vitamin D status. PLoS One. 2016;11(3):e0152198.
4. Chen YH, Fu L, Hao JH, Yu Z, Zhu P, Wang H, et al. Maternal vitamin D deficiency during pregnancy elevates the risks of small for gestational age and low birth weight infants in Chinese population. J Clin Endocrinol Metab. 2015;100(5):1912–9.
5. Schneuer FJ, Roberts CL, Guilbert C, Simpson JM, Algert CS, Khambalia AZ, et al. Effects of maternal serum 25-hydroxyvitamin D concentrations in the first trimester on subsequent pregnancy outcomes in an Australian population1-3. Am J Clin Nutr. 2014;99(2):287–95.
6. Burris HH, Rifas-Shiman SL, Camargo CA, Litonjua AA, Huh SY, Rich-Edwards JW, et al. Plasma 25-hydroxyvitamin D during pregnancy and small-for-gestational age in black and white infants. Ann Epidemiol. 2012;22(8):581–6.
7. Leffelaar ER, Vrijkotte TGM, Van Eijsden M. Maternal early pregnancy vitamin D status in relation to fetal and neonatal growth: results of the multi-ethnic Amsterdam born children and their development cohort. Br J Nutr. 2010;104(1):108–17.
8. Morley R, Carlin JB, Pasco JA, Wark JD. Maternal 25-hydroxyvitamin D and parathyroid hormone concentrations and offspring birth size. J Clin Endocrinol Metab. 2006;91(3):906–12.
9. Bodnar LM, Catov JM, Zmuda JM, Cooper ME, Parrott MS, Roberts JM, et al. Maternal serum 25-hydroxyvitamin D concentrations are associated with small-for-gestational age births in white women. J Nutr. 2010;140(5):999–1006.
10. Qin LL, Lu FG, Yang SH, Xu HL, Luo BA. Does maternal vitamin D deficiency increase the risk of preterm birth: a meta-analysis of observational studies. Nutrients. 2016;8:5.
11. Bodnar LM, Platt RW, Simhan HN. Early-pregnancy vitamin D deficiency and risk of preterm birth subtypes. Obstet Gynecol. 2015;125(2):439–47.
12. Ota K, Dambaeva S, Han AR, Beaman K, Gilman-Sachs A, Kwak-Kim J. Vitamin D deficiency may be a risk factor for recurrent pregnancy losses by increasing cellular immunity and autoimmunity. Hum Reprod. 2014;29(2):208–19.
13. Zhou J, Su L, Liu M, Liu Y, Cao X, Wang Z, et al. Associations between 25-hydroxyvitamin D levels and pregnancy outcomes: a prospective observational study in southern China. Eur J Clin Nutr. 2014;68(8):925–30.
14. Clayton PE, Cianfarani S, Czernichow P, Johannsson G, Rapaport R, Rogol AD. Consensus statement: management of the child born small for gestational age through to adulthood: a consensus statement of the international societies of pediatric endocrinology and the growth hormone research society. J Clin Endocrinol Metab. 2007;92(3):804–10.
15. Metodbeskrivning S-25-OH Vitamin D3, S-25-OH Vitamin D2, Malmö [Internet]. 2014 [cited 2015-08-19]. Available from: http://analysportalen-labmedicin.skane.se/pics/Labmedicin/Verksamhetsomr%E5den/Klinisk%20kemi/Analyser/Skane/S-25-OH%20Vitamin%20D3,%20S-25-OH%20Vitamin%20D2.pdf.
16. Brembeck P, Winkvist A, Olausson H. Determinants of vitamin D status in pregnant fair-skinned women in Sweden. Br J Nutr. 2013;110(5):856–64.
17. Textor J, Hardt J, Knuppel S. DAGitty: a graphical tool for analyzing causal diagrams. Epidemiology. 2011;22(5):745.
18. Bärebring L, Schoenmakers I, Glantz A, Hulthén L, Jagner Å, Ellis J, et al. Vitamin D status during pregnancy in a multi-ethnic population-representative Swedish cohort. Nutrients. 2016 22;8(10):655.
19. Bärebring L, Mullally D, Glantz A, Elllis J, Hulthen L, Jagner A, et al. Sociodemographic factors associated with dietary supplement use in early pregnancy in a Swedish cohort. Br J Nutr 2017:1–6.
20. Chen YY, Powell TL, Jansson T. 1,25-Dihydroxy vitamin D3 stimulates system a amino acid transport in primary human trophoblast cells. Mol Cell Endocrinol. 2017;442:90–7.
21. Cleal JK, Day PE, Simner CL, Barton SJ, Mahon PA, Inskip HM, et al. Placental amino acid transport may be regulated by maternal vitamin D and vitamin D-binding protein: results from the Southampton Women's survey. Br J Nutr. 2015;113(12):1903–10.
22. Cetin I. Placental transport of amino acids in normal and growth-restricted pregnancies. Eur J Obstet Gynecol Reprod Biol. 2003;110(Suppl 1):S50–4.
23. Liu NQ, Kaplan AT, Lagishetty V, Ouyang YB, Ouyang Y, Simmons CF, et al. Vitamin D and the regulation of placental inflammation. J Immunol. 2011;186(10):5968–74.
24. Andersen LB, Jorgensen JS, Jensen TK, Dalgard C, Barington T, Nielsen J, et al. Vitamin D insufficiency is associated with increased risk of first-trimester miscarriage in the Odense child cohort. Am J Clin Nutr. 2015;102(3):633–8.
25. OFFICIAL STATISTICS OF SWEDEN. Pregnancies, deliveries and newborn infants the Swedish medical birth register 1973–2014; 2015. p. 1400–3511.
26. Dietz PM, England LJ, Callaghan WM, Pearl M, Wier ML, Kharrazi MA. Comparison of LMP-based and ultrasound-based estimates of gestational age using linked California livebirth and prenatal screening records. Paediatr Perinat Epidemiol. 2007;21(Suppl 2):62–71.

Laparotomy in women with severe acute maternal morbidity: secondary analysis of a nationwide cohort study

Tom Witteveen[1], Athanasios Kallianidis[1,2], Joost J. Zwart[3], Kitty W. Bloemenkamp[4], Jos van Roosmalen[1,5] and Thomas van den Akker[1*] (iD)

Abstract

Background: Although pregnancy-related laparotomy is a major intervention, literature is limited to small case-control or single center studies. We aimed to identify national incidence rates for postpartum laparotomy related to severe acute maternal morbidity (SAMM) in a high-income country and test the hypothesis that risk of postpartum laparotomy differs by mode of birth.

Methods: In a population-based cohort study in all 98 hospitals with a maternity unit in the Netherlands, pregnant women with SAMM according to specified disease and management criteria were included from 01/08/2004 to 01/08/2006. We calculated the incidence of postpartum laparotomy after vaginal and cesarean births. Laparotomies were analyzed in relation to mode of birth using all births in the country as reference. Relative risks (RR) were calculated for laparotomy following emergency and planned cesarean section compared to vaginal birth, excluding laparotomies following births before 24 weeks' gestation and hysterectomies performed during cesarean section.

Results: The incidence of postpartum laparotomy in women with SAMM in the Netherlands was 6.0 per 10,000 births. Incidence was 30.1 and 1.8 per 10,000 following cesarean and vaginal birth respectively. Compared to vaginal birth, RR of laparotomy after cesarean birth was 16.7 (95% confidence interval [95% CI] 12.2-22.6). RR was 21.8 (95% CI 15.8-30.2) for emergency and 10.5 (95% CI 7.1-15.6) for planned cesarean section.

Conclusions: Risk of laparotomy, although small, was considerably elevated in women who gave birth by cesarean section. This should be considered in counseling and clinical decision making.

Keywords: Childbirth, Obstetric surgical procedures, Cesarean section, Laparotomy, Severe acute maternal morbidity, Maternal mortality, High-risk pregnancy, Obstetrics, Cohort studies

Background

According to the World Health Organization (WHO), laparotomy is a critical intervention required in the management of life-threatening and potentially life-threatening conditions [1]. In this study, laparotomy is defined as a surgical procedure involving an incision through the abdominal wall to gain access into the abdominal cavity other than cesarean section. Its use is indicative of severe maternal outcome and may be applied as a quality marker for obstetric care [1]. Although it is clear that laparotomy during pregnancy and after childbirth is a major intervention, literature is sparse and limited to case-control or single center studies with limited numbers of cases.

Previous studies only address 're-laparotomy' after cesarean section. Reported incidence rates of 're-laparotomy' are low, varying between 0.2 and 0.9% [2–11]. Although data on laparotomy after vaginal birth are not reported, it has been suggested that the incidence of laparotomy may be higher after cesarean section, since operative birth is associated with a higher risk of maternal morbidity and mortality [12, 13].

* Correspondence: t.h.van_den_akker@lumc.nl; thomas_vd_akker@hotmail.com
[1]Department of Obstetrics, Leiden University Medical Center, building 1, room K-6-P-35, P.O. Box 9600, 2300 RC Leiden, The Netherlands
Full list of author information is available at the end of the article

In this paper, we report national incidence rates of postpartum laparotomy, using a nationwide cohort of women with severe acute maternal morbidity (SAMM), and test the hypothesis that the risk of pregnancy-related laparotomy in the postpartum period differs by mode of birth.

Methods

This study is part of a well-known two-year nationwide cohort study to assess SAMM during pregnancy, labour and puerperium in the Netherlands, called the 'LEMMoN-study' (Landelijke studie naar Ethnische determinanten van Maternale Morbiditeit in Nederland). Pregnant women sustaining SAMM were included from all 98 hospitals with a maternity unit, in the period 1st August 2004 until 1st August 2006. These were eight tertiary care hospitals, 35 non-academic teaching hospitals and 55 general hospitals. Detailed information regarding data collection was described previously [14].

Inclusion criteria for SAMM were categorized in five groups: admission into an intensive care unit, uterine rupture, eclampsia, major obstetric hemorrhage (defined as four or more units of pack red blood cells or hysterectomy or arterial embolization) and a miscellaneous group with SAMM in the opinion of the treating clinician, which could not be classified in any of the other four groups. Women could be included into more than one group, therefore: one woman could have more than one indication for laparotomy, and more than one co-morbidity. For all calculations of risk and incidence, we used the number of women as the denominator. Laparotomy was not a specific inclusion criterion in the LEMMoN-study.

All women in the nationwide SAMM cohort who had a laparotomy after vaginal or cesarean birth were included in this specific study. Incidence of postpartum laparotomy and relative risks with regard to mode of birth were calculated. Only women with a birth after 24 weeks' gestational age were included, and only those who had a laparotomy within six weeks after birth. Women who had hysterectomy or other surgery during cesarean birth were excluded.

The main outcome measure was relative risk (RR) related to cesarean birth (with vaginal birth as reference) and associated risk factors. The Dutch Perinatal Register was used as the source for background denominator data. Clinical characteristics and birth data were analyzed in search of predisposing factors. Maternal characteristics included age, body mass index, parity, gestational age, and previous cesarean section. Data concerning birth included: mode of birth, blood loss, number of units of blood transfused, indication for laparotomy, timing of laparotomy after birth (< 24 h, 2-7 days or >7 days), number of laparotomies and

duration of hospital admission. Indications for laparotomy were clustered into six groups: severe postpartum hemorrhage, intra-abdominal bleeding, (suspected) uterine rupture, sepsis, hematoma and miscellaneous (i.e. removal of purposely-left sterile gauze, bladder damage, rectovaginal fistula). Therapeutic interventions were clustered into: bleeding control, which was then subdivided by location (abdominal wall, intra-abdominal and uterine scar-related), compression sutures such as the B-lynch procedure, ligation of large vessels, hysterectomy, hematoma/abscess drainage, negative laparotomy (exploration without therapeutic intervention) and miscellaneous. More than one indication or intervention could be assigned.

RRs with 95% confidence intervals (CI) were calculated where appropriate. Differences in characteristics between modes of birth were tested with a chi-square test or Fisher's exact test for categorical data and independent t-test or Mann-Whitney U test for numerical data where appropriate. Statistical analysis was performed using SPSS statistics, version 20.0 (SPSS, Chicago, IL).

Results

During the two years, 355,841 births were registered in the Netherlands Perinatal Register: 302,689 (85.1%) vaginal births and 53,152 (14.9%) cesarean sections, of which 24,580 (46.2%) planned and 28,572 (53.8%) emergency sections. Among 2552 women with SAMM in the cohort, 325 laparotomies were reported in 276 women. This gives a total incidence of laparotomy in women with SAMM in the Netherlands of 7.8 per 10,000 births. Sixty-one women were excluded from analysis of risk as they did not fit the inclusion criteria: 37 had the (initial) laparotomy before birth, 15 had a cesarean section with additional procedures including 11 hysterectomies, 6 had delivered before 24 weeks' gestational age and 3 were more than 42 days postpartum at the time of laparotomy.

The 215 remaining women were included for risk analysis, of whom 160 (74.4%) had laparotomies following cesarean section (10 out of these 160 were failed vacuum extractions) and 55 (25.6%) following vaginal birth (14 out of these 55 were instrumental births -all vacuum extractions, forceps are rarely used in the Netherlands).

One hundred and forty-five women (67.4%) were admitted into an intensive care unit. Comorbidity included major obstetric hemorrhage in 192 (89.3%), uterine rupture in 22 (10.2%), eclampsia in 8 (3.7%) and miscellaneous morbidity in six (2.8%) out of the 215 women. These 'miscellaneous comorbidities' were (A) postoperative adhesion ileus (twice), (B) large abdominal wall hematoma after cesarean section, (C) incarcerated hernia one day postpartum requiring ilio-caecal resection, (D) rectovaginal fistula nine days after anal sphincter rupture requiring colostomy, (E) a large wound defect with multiple abscesses.

One hundred thirty-eight women had more than one comorbidity (118 had two, 19 had three and one woman had four co-morbidities). The incidence of laparotomy after childbirth in women with SAMM in the Netherlands, who fitted our inclusion criteria for risk analysis in relation to mode of birth, was 6.0 per 10,000. Incidence was 30.1 per 10,000 cesarean births and 1.8 per 10,000 vaginal births (Table 1). This gives a RR of 16.7 (95% CI 12.2-22.6). The absolute risk of laparotomy was 39.5 per 10,000 births for emergency cesarean section and 19.1 per 10,000 for planned section. Compared to vaginal birth, RRs for emergency and planned cesarean section were 21.8 (95% CI 15.8-30.2) and 10.5 (95% CI 7.1-15.6) respectively (Table 1).

Women who had laparotomy after cesarean section, were more often nulliparous, had pregnancies of lower gestational age and longer hospital admissions compared to those who gave birth vaginally (Table 2). Large proportions in both groups were found to have scarred uteri: 32.7% of women who delivered by cesarean section and 34.0% of women who delivered vaginally. Among women who had laparotomy after cesarean section the proportion of women with a scarred uterus secondary to previous cesarean section was larger in the planned cesarean section group (emergency 20.4%, planned 61.7%; $p < 0.01$). There were 103 women (48%) who needed to be transfused nine or more units of red blood cell concentrates: 30 following vaginal and 73 following cesarean birth.

SAMM occurred before childbirth in 14 (6.5%) and after childbirth in 198 (92.1%) women; in three women this information was unknown (Table 2). In 99 women (46.0%), the indication for laparotomy after birth was intra-abdominal bleeding, followed by severe postpartum hemorrhage (83 women, 38.6%) (Table 3). For cesarean section, the main indication was intra-abdominal bleeding (93 women, 58.1%). For vaginal birth, main indications were severe postpartum hemorrhage (34 women, 61.8%) or suspected uterine rupture (12 women, 21.8%).

A total of 147 (68.4%) laparotomies were performed within 24 h after birth (cesarean section 63.1% vs. vaginal birth 83.6%; $p < 0.05$). Late laparotomies (within 2-7 days) were more likely to happen following cesarean section (26.9% vs. vaginal birth 9.1%; $p < 0.05$).

During the first laparotomy, hysterectomy was the most frequently performed intervention (63 women, 29.3%), followed by control of intra-abdominal (53 women, 24.7%) and caesarean scar-related bleeding (34 women, 15.8%). In 21 (9.8%) women, no therapeutic intervention was done during laparotomy.

Forty out of the 215 women included in the risk analysis (18.6%) had more than one laparotomy: 32 out of these 40 (80.0%) had two, seven (17.5%) had three and one (2.5%) had four laparotomies. In 21 (52.5%) of these 40 women, the operation was due to intra-abdominal bleeding and in 5 (12.5%) re-laparotomy resulted in hysterectomy.

Three out of the 215 women died shortly after or during laparotomy (case fatality rate 1.4%): one woman died in the intensive care unit after hysterectomy for severe hemorrhage following vaginal birth. Another woman, who had a history of cardiac disease, died due to massive intra-peritoneal hemorrhage from iatrogenic perforation of the iliac artery during uterine embolization following vaginal birth. Laparotomy was performed as a last resort, but she died shortly afterwards in the intensive care unit. The third maternal death was due to puerperal sepsis with group-A streptococcus. The woman had delivered a stillbirth vaginally and suffered persistent postpartum hemorrhage despite embolization. She died during hysterectomy.

Discussion

This study, using a nationwide cohort of women who suffered SAMM, is the first to report national incidence rates of laparotomy after vaginal and cesarean birth. The risk of postpartum laparotomy was more than 16 times higher in women who gave birth by cesarean section compared to those who gave birth vaginally. The risk for laparotomy is lower when cesarean section is planned, but nevertheless still 10 times higher compared to vaginal birth.

Our results also indicate that laparotomy after childbirth may be an appropriate indicator of severe maternal outcome and quality marker for obstetric care. For example, 183 of 215 women (85.1%), fulfill the WHO Maternal Near Miss criterion of having had five or more units of blood transfused [1]. Based on a previously performed hypothetical experiment based study, 113 out of the 215 women (52.6%) would have died if massive

Table 1 Incidence of laparotomy after childbirth, related to mode of birth

		Births (n)	Laparotomy (n)	Incidence*	RR (95% CI)
Total		355,841	215	6.0	
CS		53,152	160	30.1	16.7 (12.2-22.6)
	Planned	24,580	47	19.1	10.5 (7.1-15.6)
	Emergency	28,572	113	39.5	21.8 (15.8-30.2)
VD		302,689	55	1.8	Reference

RR relative risk, *CI* confidence interval, *CS* cesarean section, *VD* vaginal birth
*per 10,000 births

Table 2 Maternal characteristics and birth information

	VD $N = 55$	CS $N = 160$	P	Emergency CS $N = 113$	Elective CS $N = 47$	P
Age (y)	34.1 (3.4)	33.0 (5.3)	0.08	32.8 (5.5)	33.6 (4.8)	0.35
BMI (kg/m^2)	24.6 (6.7)	24.7 (5.5)	0.55	24.1 (4.7)	25.8 (6.8)	0.37
Nulliparity	13 (24.1%)	72 (45.3%)	**< 0.001**	61 (54.0%)	11 (23.4%)	**< 0.001**
Gestational age (w)	39.4 (2.6)	38.2 (3.4)	**< 0.05**	38.5 (3.7)	37.5 (2.5)	**< 0.001**
Previous CS	18 (34.0%)	52 (32.7%)	0.87	23 (20.4%)	29 (61.7%)	**< 0.001**
Hospital admission (d)	11.7 (13.1)	14.4 (10.9)	**< 0.05**	14.6 (10.5)	13.8 (11.9)	0.18
Blood loss (mL)	5556 (4532)	4262 (3432)	0.053	4166 (3342)	4303 (3486)	0.81
Units of RBC (n)	12.4 (9.4)	10.8 (9.0)	0.19	11.6 (9.6)	9.1 (7.1)	0.18
SAMM before birth (n)	3 (5.5%)	11 (6.9%)	0.52	10 (8.9%)	1 (2.1%)	0.275

CS cesarean section, VD vaginal birth, RBC red blood cells. Data is presented as mean (SD) or number (%)

Table 3 Detailed information of laparotomies after childbirth

Total		VD $N = 55$	CS $N = 160$	P	Emergency $N = 113$	Elective $N = 47$	P
Indication[*]	Intra-abd. Bleeding	6 (10.9)	93 (58.1)	**< 0.001**	65 (57.5)	28 (59.6)	0.777
	sPPH	34 (61.8)	49 (30.6)		36 (31.9)	13 (27.7)	
	Suspected rupture	12 (21.8)	1 (0.6)		1 (0.9)	0 (0.0)	
	Sepsis	4 (7.2)	7 (4.4)		6 (5.3)	1 (2.1)	
	Hematoma	0 (0.0)	4 (2.5)		3 (2.7)	1 (2.1)	
	Miscellaneous	9 (16.4)	11 (7.5)		6 (5.3)	5 (10.6)	
	Unknown	0 (0.0)	1 (0.6)		1 (0.9)	0 (0.0)	
Time[*]	< 24 h	46 (83.6)	101 (63.1)	**< 0.05**	71 (62.8)	30 (63.8)	**< 0.05**
	2-7d	5 (9.1)	43 (26.9)		30 (26.5)	13 (27.7)	
	>7d	4 (7.3)	12 (7.5)		11 (9.7)	1 (2.1)	
	Unknown	0 (0.0)	4 (2.9)		1 (0.9)	3 (6.4)	
Intervention[*]	Arrest of bleeding:						
	-Abdominal wall	0 (0.0)	13 (8.1)	**< 0.001**	10 (8.9)	3 (6.4)	0.591
	-Intra-abdominal	13 (23.6)	40 (25.0)		28 (24.8)	12 (25.5)	
	-CS scar	2 (3.6)	32 (20.0)		22 (19.5)	10 (21.3)	
	B-lynch procedure	1 (1.8)	8 (5.0)		7 (6.2)	1 (2.1)	
	Ligation	6 (10.9)	11 (6.9)		8 (7.1)	3 (6.4)	
	Hysterectomy	31 (56.4)	32 (20.0)		21 (18.6)	11 (23.4)	
	Drainage	3 (5.5)	9 (5.6)		7 (6.2)	2 (4.3)	
	Negative	2 (3.6)	19 (11.9)		16 (14.2)	3 (6.4)	
	Miscellaneous	10 (18.2)	24 (15.0)		18 (15.9)	6 (12.8)	
	Unknown	0 (0.0)	6 (3.8)		3 (2.7)	3 (6.4)	
Number	1	43 (78.2)	129 (80.6)	0.26	88 (77.9)	41 (87.2)	0.44
	≥2	10 (18.2)	30 (18.8)		24 (21.2)	6 (12.8)	
	Unknown	2 (3.6)	1 (0.6)		1 (0.9)	0 (0.0)	

CS cesarean section, VD vaginal birth, sPPH severe postpartum hemorrhage. Data is presented as number (%)
[*]for 1st laparotomy

blood transfusion had not been available, as is the case in many low-income countries [15].

The rate of laparotomy after cesarean section in women with SAMM in the Netherlands (0.3%) appears relatively low compared to the literature (0.2-0.9%) [2–11]. Since laparotomy after vaginal birth has not been studied before, the incidence we found for laparotomy following vaginal birth cannot be compared to other studies. The largest study of laparotomy following cesarean section was conducted in a single university medical center in Israel and included 80 women over a period of 20 years. Our study is unique because of its large sample size ($n = 215$), included in a relatively short time frame, and its prospective nationwide design.

Postpartum hemorrhage, placental abruption, uterine rupture and previous cesarean section were previously found to be associated with increased risk of re-laparotomy [2, 4, 5, 10]. We confirmed that the main proportion (68.4%) of all laparotomies was performed within 24 h after birth due to either intra-abdominal bleeding (46.0%) or postpartum hemorrhage (38.6%). One third of women (32.6%) had a previous cesarean section. Although placental abruption was not an endpoint, the majority of these cases are likely represented in the group of major obstetric hemorrhage since women would generally receive at least four units of blood. Thirteen women underwent laparotomy due to (suspected) uterine rupture. Infection or sepsis were not reported as outcomes of interest in previous studies. In our study, sepsis was the indication for laparotomy in 11 cases.

Our results need to be interpreted with caution since our study has several important limitations. First, the data from the LEMMoN-study are rather old and changes in incidence and risk may have occurred since data collection took place. However, we are not aware of any currently ongoing studies of postpartum laparotomy and think that our data are therefore still of considerable importance, since more up-to-date information is unlikely to become available for some time. A second limitation is that laparotomy was not a separate inclusion criterion as having severe acute maternal morbidity. This may introduce selection bias, since women who were transfused less than five units of blood, those who did not have hysterectomy, embolization, or uterine rupture and those who were not admitted into intensive care may have been missed. These women would only have been included if the treating obstetrician still decided to include her as severe acute maternal morbidity. Nevertheless, the fact that laparotomies in women with SAMM will have been included validates our conclusions for this group. The fact that the overwhelming majority (149, 93.1%) of SAMM in our cohort occurred after birth provides an additional argument for the hypothesis that SAMM may often be related to the mode of birth. Some of these SAMM conditions may be more common after (difficult) cesarean versus vaginal birth and this is precisely what should be included in any clinical counseling about risks of cesarean section. We analyzed all vaginal births as one group and did not subdivide between instrumental and spontaneous births, postulating that the risk of laparotomy following a successful instrumental birth would not be elevated.

With regard to mode of birth (vaginal birth, emergency and planned cesarean section) there are some noteworthy results. In contrast with what is commonly assumed, the proportion of re-laparotomy due to intra-abdominal bleeding was comparable for planned and emergency cesarean section. The timing to perform laparotomy is more often between two and seven days after cesarean section than after vaginal birth, where laparotomy is performed earlier. In total, 140 out of 160 (88%) laparotomies after cesarean birth were performed within four days. This means that clinicians should be particularly cautious of the occurrence of complications that may lead to laparotomy in the first four days after cesarean section. It should also be underlined that almost 20% of women had more than one laparotomy after birth and that in 10% of all laparotomies exploration was performed without any therapeutic intervention.

Cesarean birth rates have been increasing for the past decades up to 47.6% in China and 50% in Brazil [16, 17]. In the Netherlands, although rates are relatively low, the proportion of cesarean section has risen from 11% to 16% between 1999 and 2012 [18]. A recent study in China showed that 40% of cesarean sections were performed without medical indication [19]. Considering the elevated risk of laparotomy after cesarean section, such developments will inevitably lead to a rise in unfavorable outcomes. This adds to the results of previous studies in which cesarean birth was also found to be associated with a clearly elevated risk of maternal morbidity and mortality compared to vaginal birth, regardless of the indication [12, 13, 20]. Our study addresses both short- and long-term adverse effects of cesarean section: the complications as a result of initial surgery requiring laparotomy, and the complications in subsequent pregnancies, such as abnormally invasive placentation and the risks of birth in presence of a uterine scar [21–23]. Women with vaginal birth after previous cesarean section are over-represented (18/55 women, 34.0%) compared to the general Dutch pregnant population (6.0%) [14].

WHO has recently stated again that national cesarean birth rates above 10% are not associated with a further decrease in maternal or neonatal mortality [24]. It is alarming that cesarean rates are still on the rise in most countries [16]. These rates may be difficult to curb, but it is important to realize that every cut may have its cost.

Adverse maternal outcome, including laparotomy, should be kept in mind when cesarean section is considered and women are counselled for mode of birth, particularly when maternal request is the only indication.

Conclusion

Main finding of this nationwide cohort study is that the risk of postpartum laparotomy in women with severe acute maternal morbidity in the Netherlands was much higher after cesarean section compared to vaginal birth. This information must be taken into account by clinicians when considering mode of birth and can be interpreted as yet another reason to reduce unnecessary cesarean sections.

Abbreviations
CI: Confidence interval; RR: Relative risk; SAMM: Severe acute maternal morbidity; WHO: World Health Organization

Acknowledgements
We greatly thank all local LEMMoN-coordinators who kindly participated.

Funding
The LEMMoN-study was supported by the Dutch Organization for Health Research (ZonMw; grant 3610.0024) and the Matty Brand Foundation. No specific funding was obtained for this study.

Authors' contributions
JZ and JvR designed and performed the LEMMoN-study. TW and JvR conceived and designed this specific analysis. Data analysis and interpretation was done by TW, AK, KB, JZ, JvR and TvdA. TW drafted a first version of a manuscript with help from TvdA. All authors (TW, AK, KB, JZ, JvR and TvdA) then edited subsequent drafts and approved of the final version. This study was previously presented as part of a dissertation by TW for a PhD degree, at Leiden University, the Netherlands.

Competing interests
Two of the authors are members of the editorial board of the journal: JvR is a section editor and TvdA an associate editor.

Author details
[1]Department of Obstetrics, Leiden University Medical Center, building 1, room K-6-P-35, P.O. Box 9600, 2300 RC Leiden, The Netherlands. [2]Department of Obstetrics and Gynecology, Haga Teaching Hospital, Els Borst-Eilersplein 275, 2545 AA Den Haag, The Netherlands. [3]Department of Obstetrics and Gynecology, Deventer Ziekenhuis, Nico Bolkesteinlaan 75, 7416 SE Deventer, The Netherlands. [4]Department of Obstetrics, Wilhelmina Children's Hospital Birth Centre, University Medical Centre Utrecht, Lundlaan 6, 3584 EA Utrecht, The Netherlands. [5]Athena Institute, Faculty of Science, VU University Amsterdam, De Boelelaan 1085, 1081 HV Amsterdam, The Netherlands.

References
1. World Health Organization, Department of Reproductive Health and Research. Evaluating the quality of care for severe pregnancy complications. In: The WHO near-miss approach for maternal health. Geneva: World Health Organization; 2011.
2. Ashwal E, Yogev Y, Melamed N, Khadega R, Ben-Haroush A, Wiznitzer A, Peled Y. Characterizing the need for re-laparotomy during puerperium after cesarean section. Arch Gynecol Obstet. 2014;290(1):35–9.
3. Gedikbasi A, Akyol A, Asar E, Bingol B, Uncu R, Sargin A, Ceylan Y. Re-laparotomy after cesarean section: operative complications in surgical birth. Arch Gynecol Obstet. 2008;278(5):419–25.
4. Kessous R, Danor D, Weintraub YA, Wiznitzer A, Sergienko R, Ohel I, Sheiner E. Risk factors for relaparotomy after cesarean section. J Matern Fetal Neonatal Med. 2012;25(11):2167–70.
5. Levin I, Rapaport AS, Salzer L, Maslovitz S, Lessing JB, Almog B. Risk factors for relaparotomy after cesarean birth. Int J Gynaecol Obstet. 2012;119(2):163–5.
6. Lurie S, Sadan O, Golan A. Re-laparotomy after cesarean section. Eur J Obstet Gynecol Reprod Biol. 2007;134(2):184–7.
7. Ragab A, Mousbah Y, Barakat R, Zayed A, Badawy A. Re-laparotomy after cesarean births: risk factors and how to avoid? J Obstet Gynaecol. 2014;24:1–3.
8. Seal SL, Kamilya G, Bhattacharyya SK, Mukherji J, Bhattacharyya AR. Relaparotomy after cesarean birth: experience from an Indian teaching hospital. J Obstet Gynaecol Res. 2007;33(6):804–9.
9. Seffah JD. Re-laparotomy after cesarean section. Int J Gynaecol Obstet. 2005; 88(3):253–7.
10. Shinar S, Hareuveni M, Ben-Tal O, Many A. Relaparotomies after cesarean sections: risk factors, indications, and management. J Perinat Med. 2013; 41(5):567–72.
11. Levitt L, Sapir H, Kabiri D, Ein-Mor E, Hochner-Celnikier D, Amsalem H. Re-laparotomy following cesarean birth - risk factors and outcomes. J Maternal Fetal Neonatal Med. 2015;24:1–3.
12. Hall MH, Bewley S. Maternal mortality and mode of birth. Lancet. 1999; 354(9180):776.
13. van Dillen J, Zwart JJ, Schutte J, Bloemenkamp KW, van Roosmalen J. Severe acute maternal morbidity and mode of birth in the Netherlands. Acta Obstet Gynecol Scand. 2010;89(11):1460–5.
14. Zwart JJ, Richters JM, Ory F, de Vries JI, Bloemenkamp KW, van Roosmalen J. Severe maternal morbidity during pregnancy, birth and puerperium in the Netherlands: a nationwide population-based study of 371,000 pregnancies. BJOG. 2008;115(7):842–50.
15. Hendriks J, Zwart JJ, Briët E, Brand A, van Roosmalen J. The clinical benefit of blood transfusion: a hypothetical experiment based on a nationwide survey of severe maternal morbidity. Vox Sang. 2013;104(3):234–9.
16. Vogel JP, Betrán AP, Vindevoghel N, Souza JP, Torloni MR, Zhang J, Tunçalp Ö, Mori R, Morisaki N, Ortiz-Panozo E, Hernandez B, Pérez-Cuevas R, Qureshi Z, Gülmezoglu AM. Temmerman M; WHO multi-country survey on maternal and newborn Health Research network. Use of the Robson classification to assess caesarean section trends in 21 countries: a secondary analysis of two WHO multicountry surveys. Lancet Glob Health. 2015;3(5):e260–70. https:// doi.org/10.1016/S2214-109X(15)70094-X. Epub 2015 Apr 9
17. Ramires de Jesus G, Ramires de Jesus N, Peixoto-Filho F, Lobato G. Cesarean rates in Brazil: what is involved? BJOG. 2015;122(5):606–9.
18. Stichting Perinatale Registratie Nederland. Perinatale Registratie Nederland Grote Lijnen 1999 - 2012 [The Netherlands Perinatal Registry Trends 1999-2012]. Utrecht: Stichting Perinatale Registratie Nederland; 2011:26-27.
19. Deng W, Klemetti R, Long Q, Wu Z, Duan C, Zhang WH, Ronsmans C, Zhang Y, Hemminki E. Cesarean section in shanghai: women's or healthcare provider's preferences? BMC Pregnancy Childbirth. 2014;14:285.
20. Schuitemaker N, van Roosmalen J, Dekker G, van Dongen P, van Geijn H, Gravenhorst JB. Maternal mortality after cesarean section in The Netherlands. Acta Obstet Gynecol Scand. 1997;76:332–4.
21. Nederlandse Vereniging voor Obstetrie & Gynecologie. Zwangerschap en bevalling na een voorgaande sectio cesarea [Pregnancy and birth after previous cesarean section]. [http://www.nvog-documenten.nl/]. Accesed 30 Jul 2016.

22.   van Ham MA, van Dongen PW, Mulder J. Maternal consequences of
      cesarean section. A retrospective study of intra-operative and postoperative
      maternal complications of cesarean section during a 10-year period. Eur J
      Obstet Gynecol Reprod Biol. 1997;74:1–6.
23.   Zelop C, Heffner LJ. The downside of cesarean birth: short- and long-term
      complications. Clin Obstet Gynecol. 2004;47:386–93.
24.   Ye J, Zhang J, Mikolajczyk R, Torloni MR, Gulmezoglu AM, Betran AP.
      Association between rates of cesarean section and maternal and neonatal
      mortality in the 21st century: a worldwide population-based ecological
      study with longitudinal data. BJOG. 2015;123:745–53.

Management and obstetric outcomes of 17 heterotopic interstitial pregnancies

Yuan Jiang[1,2†], Jie Chen[1,2†], Huaijun Zhou[1,2†], Mingming Zheng[2], Ke Han[2], Jingxian Ling[2], Xianghong Zhu[2], Xiaoqiu Tang[2], Rong Li[2] and Ying Hong[1,2*] (iD)

Abstract

Background: Heterotopic interstitial pregnancy is a rare variant of heterotopic pregnancies, and it poses challenges in treating the heterotopic pregnancy and preserving the intrauterine pregnancy. However, there is no clear consensus regarding the optimal management. The aim of this study was to investigate the pregnancy outcomes of women diagnosed with heterotopic interstitial pregnancy.

Methods: A total of 17 women diagnosed with heterotopic interstitial pregnancy between July 2010 and December 2015 were included. General characteristics of each patient, including age, gravidity and parity, history of pelvic inflammatory disease or surgery, and especially the corresponding therapeutic interventions, were retrospectively analyzed. Moreover, pregnancy outcomes were further followed by face-to-face interview.

Results: Of the 17 patients, 10 (58.5%) underwent surgical treatment (7 laparoscopic cornual resection, and 3 laparotomy); and 3 cases simultaneously terminated the intrauterine pregnancy by suction evacuation. Compared with laparotomy, laparoscopic cornual section showed shorter operative time (median 40 vs. 70 min), less blood loss (150 vs. 400 ml) and shorter hospital stay (2 vs. 4 days). In addition, 4 (23.5%) patients underwent selective embryo reduction under transvaginal ultrasound guidance. Expectant management was chosen in the remaining 3 patients. In the follow-up study, other than a case of missed miscarriage, the other 13 women who remained committed to their pregnancies all delivered healthy babies either by caesarean section or vaginal birth. No congenital anomalies were reported, and all the infants were in good growth and development.

Conclusions: Laparoscopic cornual resection is a feasible approach with favorable surgical and long-term pregnancy outcomes. Additionally, medical or expectant management may be a viable treatment option for selected symptom-free patient. Although the survival of the intrauterine pregnancy could not always be assured, the prognosis for a woman with heterotopic interstitial pregnancy is generally good.

Keywords: Heterotopic interstitial pregnancy, Laparoscopic cornual resection, Selective embryo reduction, Expectant management

Background

Heterotopic interstitial pregnancy, a rare form of pregnancy that involves the coexistence of an ectopic interstitial pregnancy and intrauterine pregnancy, is one of the most life-threatening types of all the ectopic gestations [1]. The calculated incidence is documented to be as high as 1/3600 in pregnancies after assisted reproductive technology (ART) [2].

However, most of these women were asymptomatic or only showed non-specific symptoms such as abdominal pain and vaginal bleeding [3]. The clinicians might not consider the possibility of extrauterine pregnancy in the case of a confirmed intrauterine gestation by ultrasonography. Therefore, the diagnosis of heterotopic interstitial pregnancy is often delayed, even after its rupture [2] and meticulous care is required, especially in the patients with relevant risk factors associated with heterotopic

* Correspondence: hongyingglyy@tom.com
†Equal contributors
[1]Department of Obstetrics and Gynecology, Nanjing Drum Tower Hospital, Nanjing Medical University, Nanjing 210008, China
[2]Department of Obstetrics and Gynecology, Nanjing Drum Tower Hospital, Affiliated Hospital of Nanjing University Medical School, Nanjing 210008, China

pregnancy such as previous history of ectopic pregnancy, pelvic surgery, or pelvic inflammatory diseases [2, 4].

The treatment of heterotopic interstitial pregnancy aims to preserve the intrauterine pregnancy while removing or interrupting the evolution of the ectopic interstitial pregnancy using a minimally invasive method. The therapeutic modalities include surgical, medical or expectant treatment [2]. However, there is no consensus for the treatment of heterotopic interstitial pregnancy. Therefore, in the present study, we aimed to investigate the therapeutic interventions and corresponding obstetric outcomes of women diagnosed with heterotopic interstitial pregnancy.

Methods
Study population
We retrospectively analyzed all the inpatients in the department of obstetrics and gynecology from Nanjing Drum Tower Hospital between July 2010 and December 2015. A total of 17 patients with diagnosed heterotopic interstitial pregnancy were included in the present study, suggesting an overall incidence of 0.04% for all the deliveries (n = 40,761) at our institution over the same study period. The Reproductive medicine center of our hospital is the first batch approved by the Ministry of health to carry out ART, and therefore it serves for infertility patients throughout the country. Nearly 18,000 patients conceived by ART during the study period. The heterotopic interstitial pregnancy was diagnosed by experienced radiologist using 2-D ultrasound.

The criteria included an intrauterine pregnancy along with feature of a co-exisiting interstitial pregnancy, i.e. a gestational sac visualized high in the fundus, and not surrounded by 5 mm of myometrium in all planes; and a gestational sac seen separately and < 1 cm from the most lateral edge of the uterine cavity [5]. Exclusion criteria referred to an ectopic gestational sac observed in another location such as fallopian tube, ovary, cervix, or abdominal cavity. This study was performed according to the Declaration of Helsinki and approved by the institutional review boards of Nanjing Drum Tower Hospital (NJDTH20160810).

Data collection
Each patient's age, gravidity and parity, history of pelvic inflammatory disease or surgery, gestational weeks at diagnosis, and clinical symptoms of abdominal pain and vaginal bleeding was retrospectively collected by reviewing the medical records. We also recorded whether the current pregnancy had been conceived naturally or by ART. The gestational age was calculated by adding 14 days to the date of embryo transfer. Routine transvaginal ultrasound examination was performed at approximately 6 weeks of gestation (i.e. 4 weeks after embryo transfer) in all the pregnant women, and a repeat ultrasound scan was performed after a two weeks interval, or promptly if the patient presented with clinical symptoms of abdominal pain or vaginal bleeding at any time.

The therapeutic intervention, including surgery (either laparoscopy (KARL STORZ ENDOSKOPE) or laparotomy with cornual resection, or hysterectomy), medical treatment, or expectant management, was collected from each patient. The operative time, volume of intra-operative haemorrhage, length of hospital stay and incidence of intra-operative and postoperative complications were recorded. A transvaginal ultrasound scan was performed on the third day postoperative or before discharge to confirm the fetal viability of intrauterine gestation in each patient who continued with their intrauterine pregnancy.

Medical treatment comprised aspiration of ectopic fetal heart along with products of conception and local injection of 10% potassium chloride (KCl) into cornual gestational sac under transvaginal ultrasound guidance (SIEMENS G50). In the patients under medical or expectant management, due to the possibility of miscarriage of intrauterine pregnancy and rupture of extrauterine pregnancy, repeated clinical and ultrasound examinations were performed weekly until a complete resolution of interstitial pregnancy was confirmed.

Furthermore, to investigate the pregnancy outcome, we invited each patient to a face-to-face interview conducted during August 2016 to January 2017. Of the 17 patients, 16 women gave their oral and written informed consent on behalf of themselves and their children during the face-to-face interview. Nevertheless, one case refused our face-to-face invitation over the telephone because she underwent a missed miscarriage at 8 gestational weeks following expectant management; but she provided the verbal informed consent for participation in the study and publication, and also agreed to sign the written informed consent if requested. The median child's age was 3.5 years (range, 1–6 years) at our follow-up study. Data recorded for all the live births comprised of gestational age, mode of delivery, the infant's birth weight, height and gender, which were collected from the child health record. This parent held record contained details of the child's vaccinations, growth, and development, which was assessed by professional child health care doctor. During the face-to-face interview, based on the child health and development record, we evaluated the infant's overall health condition including congenital malformations, intelligence, hearing, and language. Each infant's height and weight was measured.

Statistical analysis
Statistical analysis was performed with the SPSS software (SPSS Standard version 17.0, SPSS Inc., Chicago, IL). Quantitative data non-normally distributed were presented as median (range) and compared by Wilcoxon rank sum test between two groups; categorical variables were reported as number (percentage). A two-sided P value< 0.05 is considered statistically significant.

Results

From July 2010 through December 2015, a total of 17 inpatients were diagnosed with heterotopic interstitial pregnancy in our institution. As shown in Table 1, all 17 women achieved the current pregnancies by in-vitro fertilization and embryo transfer. The median mother's age and gestational age at diagnosis was 29 years (range, 24–35 years) and 7 weeks (range, 6–14 weeks), respectively. None of the pregnant women were multiparous. Of the 17 patients, 13 (76.5%) had previously undergone at least one pelvic surgical intervention such as salpingectomy, hystero-laparoscopy, and pelvic adhesiolysis; and 6 (35.3%) patients had previously undergone either unilateral or bilateral salpingectomy for ectopic pregnancy (Table 1). The clinical manifestations of abdominal pain or vaginal bleeding were observed in 8 (47.1%) of the 17 cases, but neither hypovolaemic shock nor maternal death was reported due to timely diagnosis and treatment. However, the remaining 9 asymptomatic patients were diagnosed incidentally on routine ultrasound examination after ART procedure.

Of the total 17 patients, 10 (58.5%) underwent surgical treatment (7 laparoscopic cornual resection, and 3 laparotomy). Laparotomy in those three patients was mainly attributed to poor family economic situation or restriction of laparoscopic operation on weekends or holidays in our institution. However, three cases simultaneously terminated the intrauterine pregnancy by suction evacuation, as they were aware of the risk of uterine rupture later in pregnancy. The median operative time was 45 min (range, 28–135 min) and estimated blood loss in the operation was 175 ml (range, 20–750 ml). Only one case had blood transfusion (2 units of red blood cells) after the operation. The median length of postoperative hospital stay was 2.5 days (range 2–7 days) without any intraoperative and postoperative complications such as miscarriage or uterine rupture. Furthermore, compared with laparotomy, the laparoscopic treatment showed shorter operative time (median 40 vs. 70 min), less blood loss in the operation (150 vs. 400 ml) and shorter hospital stay (2 vs. 4 days), although the difference was not statistically significant ($P = 0.11$, 0.11 and 0.09 respectively). It was likely due to the small sample size of the study.

After fully informed consent, 4 (23.5%) patients (including 3 with no clinical symptoms and 1 with mild abdominal pain) underwent selective embryo reduction, i.e. aspiration of the ectopic fetal heart and local injection of 10% KCl into the interstitial pregnancy sac under direct transvaginal ultrasound guidance. Expectant management was chosen in the remaining 3 (17.6%) patients with no symptoms or only a small amount of vaginal bleeding (Table 1). Importantly, only a crown rump length or yolk sac was shown in either case, but no fetal cardiac activity in ectopic interstitial gestation was seen by ultrasound scan. All of these 7 patients were followed up closely by weekly clinical and ultrasound assessment. Unfortunately, missed miscarriage of intrauterine gestation at 8 gestational weeks was confirmed in one case with expectant management. However, no surgical treatment was indicated due to persistent existence of ectopic cardiac activity or rupture of interstitial gestation in the other six patients.

In the follow-up study, the three pregnant women, who had simultaneously terminated intrauterine pregnancy, all recovered well after the surgery. In addition, as shown in Table 1, only one of the 14 cases who had an ongoing intrauterine pregnancy was diagnosed with a missed miscarriage at 8 gestational weeks; but the other 13 patients all delivered healthy live babies vaginally or by cesarean section. However, only one case attempted vaginal delivery because the dilatation of cervix was 3 cm when seeing the doctor. The other 12 women all delivered their babies by elective cesarean section due to fears of uterine rupture or cultural factors. It was worthy that no congenital anomalies were reported, and all the infants were in normal growth and development.

Discussion

The incidence of heterotopic interstitial pregnancy has considerably increased, with the widespread use of assisted reproductive technology and the rising frequency of tubal and pelvic inflammatory diseases. However, the optimal management of heterotopic interstitial pregnancy still remains controversial. There are currently limited clinical data or only several case reports in the literature, especially in developing countries. In the present study, we conducted a retrospective review of the therapeutic interventions and further investigated the corresponding obstetric outcomes of all the 17 patients diagnosed with heterotopic interstitial pregnancy over the past five years in our centre.

Previous history of pelvic inflammatory disease, pelvic surgery, and ART are associated with the incidence of heterotopic interstitial pregnancy [2]. Consistent with these studies, we found that all of the 17 pregnant women had been conceived through ART, and 76.5% (13/17) had a history of ectopic pregnancy, pelvic inflammatory disease or surgery. In the present study, neither hypovolemic shock nor maternal death was reported. It seemed that this was not a typical population presenting with ectopic pregnancy. We speculated that it may be related to the fact that all these patients after embryo transfer were provided with detailed health education on red flag symptoms of ectopic pregnancy; and therefore they sought medical advice and received timely professional assessment and treatment.

The feasibility of surgical cornual resection has been demonstrated in treating heterotopic interstitial pregnancy. However, most of these studies were only case reports and mainly conducted in the developed countries or regions [3, 6–10]. Some authors indicated that the

Table 1 Characteristics and pregnancy outcomes of the patients diagnosed with heterotopic interstitial pregnancy ($n = 17$)

No.	Age (years)	Gravidity/parity	Risk factors	Gestational age (week + days)	Symptoms	Interstitial gestation	Treatment	Pregnancy Outcome
1	30	5/0	IVF-ET	6	Asymptomatic	Fetal cardiac activity	Explo-left cornual resection + suction evacuation	NA
2	25	1/0	IVF-ET, LSC-RS, LTL	6	Vaginal bleeding	Fetal cardiac activity	Same as above	NA
3	34	4/0	IVF-ET, LSC-RS, LTL (Ectopic pregnacy)	6 + 2	Abdominal pain	Yolk sac (20*23*19 mm)	LSC-right cornual resection + suction evacuation	NA[a]
4	28	2/0	IVF-ET, LSC-RS (Ectopic pregnancy)	6	Asymptomatic	Fetal cardiac activity	LSC-right cornual resection	CS at 35 + 4 weeks due to preterm labor, female, 2305 g
5	28	1/0	IVF-ET, LSC-BS	7 + 6	Asymptomatic	Fetal cardiac activity	Explo-right cornual resection	CS at 38 weeks, male, 3540 g
6	27	2/0	IVF-ET, LSC-BS	6	Abdominal pain	Yolk sac (16*19*16 mm)	LSC-left cornual resection	CS at 38 + 1 weeks, male, 3020 g
7	35	3/0	IVF-ET, LSC-LS (Ectopic pregnancy)	8	Asymptomatic	Yolk sac (21*22*23 mm)	LSC-left cornual resection	CS at 38 + 2 weeks, male, 2980 g
8	30	3/0	IVF-ET, LSC-RS (Ectopic pregnancy)	7 + 5	Vaginal bleeding	Yolk sac (17*16*16 mm)	LSC-left cornual resection	CS at 38 + 4 weeks, male, 3480 g
9	32	1/0	IVF-ET	12	Vaginal bleeding	Yolk sac (41*38*43 mm)	LSC-right cornual resection	CS at 39 weeks, female,3100 g
10	29	3/0	IVF-ET	6 + 5	Asymptomatic	Fetal cardiac activity	LSC-right cornual resection	CS at 39 + 1 weeks, female,3460 g
11	24	1/0	IVF-ET, LSC-RS, Pelvic adhesiolysis	6 + 5	Asymptomatic	Fetal cardiac activity	cornual embryo reduction	CS at 38 weeks, male, 2670 g
12	28	3/0	IVF-ET, LSC-BS (Ectopic pregnancy)	6 + 1	Abdominal pain	Fetal cardiac activity	cornual embryo reduction	CS at 38 + 5 weeks, female, 2800 g
13	26	1/0	IVF-ET	6 + 3	Asymptomatic	Fetal cardiac activity	cornual embryo reduction	CS at 39 weeks, female, 2730 g
14	33	2/0	IVF-ET, LSC	7	Asymptomatic	Fetal cardiac activity	cornual embryo reduction	CS at 39 + 2 weeks, male, 3020 g
15	33	3/0	IVF-ET, LSC-RS (Ectopic pregnancy)	6	Vaginal bleeding	Yolk sac (8*9*9 mm)	Conservative	Missed miscarriage at 8 weeks
16	34	3/0	IVF-ET, LSC-BS	14	Asymptomatic	Yolk sac (25*23*23 mm)	Conservative	CS at 38 + 2 weeks, female, 2940 g
17	27	1/0	IVF-ET, H-LSC	6 + 4	Abdominal pain	Yolk sac (20*19*19 mm)	Conservative	VD at 35 + 6 weeks due to PROM, male, 2230g[b]

LSC laparoscopy, LTL left tubal ligation, LSC-RS laparoscopic right salpingectomy, LSC-BS laparoscopic bilateral salpingectomy, H-LSC hystero-laparoscopy, LSC-LS laparoscopic left salpingectomy, Explo- exploratory, NA not available, PROM premature rupture of membrane

[a]The woman conceived again by ART procedure; and it was confirmed to be normal intrauterine gestation of 15 weeks in the telephone follow-up study

[b]She refused emergency cesarean section but attempted vaginal delivery because the cervix was 3 cm wide when seeing the doctor

long operative time and altered intraperitoneal carbon dioxide environment throughout the laparoscopic operation may involve surgical and anesthetic risk, causing an adverse effect on maternal morbidity and the surviving intrauterine pregnancy [10]. In the present study, we found that all the infants born to the seven pregnant women, who had undergone laparoscopic cornual resection or laparotomy, were in good health and no congenital conformations were reported. In addition, compared with laparotomy, laparoscopic treatment showed the shorter hospital stay, fewer surgical wounds, and reduced use of antibiotics and analgesics. Therefore, laparoscopic cornual resection appears to be a safe and viable treatment option and should be considered, especially in the patients without signs of cornual rupture [11]. The other three women had selected laparotomy only because of poor family economic situation or restriction of laparoscopic operation at night time, weekends or holidays in our institution. We hope that improved access to laparoscopic treatment can be offered in the future.

Surgical cornual resection may increase the risk of delayed haemorrhage and uterine rupture. Compared with surgical treatment, the medical approach is less expensive, less invasive with minimal blood loss and quicker recovery. Therefore, medical embryo reduction of interstitial gestation has been recommended in the patient with hemodynamically stable status [12, 13]. It consists of injecting methotrexate, prostaglandin, or KCL directly into ectopic gestational sac under the guidance of transvaginal ultrasonography. Kim et al. suggested that KCl has reportedly been associated with intrauterine damage, periventricular leukomalacia, and limb anomalies [3]. However, more studies confirmed that no teratogenicity secondary to local injection of KCl was reported [14]. Therefore, selective embryo reduction using local injection of 10% KCl has been performed in four patients after fully informed consent at our centre. To ascertain whether KCl may have adverse effects on the pregnancy outcomes, we further evaluated the infant's overall health condition during face-to-face interview. No congenital malformation was found, and all the infants were in normal growth and development. Therefore, it indicated that selective embryo reductionby local injection of KCl during the first trimester might be a viable treatment approach.

Expectant management seems to offer a third possible and safe therapeutic alternative [2]. Nevertheless, the current reported clinical studies were limited [15, 16]. In the present study, expectant management had been chosen in three patients (Table 1). Other than a single case of missed miscarriage, an uneventful ongoing pregnancy was documented in the other two cases. Therefore, expectant management might be a viable alternative for the interstitial pregnancy with absence of fetal cardiac activity and limited gestational sac size. Nevertheless, because of the potential risk of continued growth of interstitial gestation and subsequent rupture, cornual gestation and subsequent rupture, serial ultrasound scans and close clinical assessment are necessary [2].

Conclusion

In summary, laparoscopic cornual resection is a feasible approach with favorable surgical and long-term pregnant outcomes. Medical or expectant management may be an efficient treatment alternative for selected symptom-free patient. Although the survival of the intrauterine pregnancy could not always be assured, the prognosis for a woman with heterotopic interstitial pregnancy is generally good.

Acknowledgements
None.

Funding
None.

Authors' contributions
YJ, JC, HZ, and YH designed the study, collected the patients' information, performed statistical analysis, and drafted the manuscript. MZ and KH collected the patients' information and drafted the manuscript. JL, XZ,XT, and RL collected the patients' information and performed statistical analysis. All authors read and approved the final manuscript.

Competing interests
The authors declare that they have no competing interests.

References
1. Parker VL, Srinivas M. Non-tubal ectopic pregnancy. Arch Gynecol Obstet. 2016;294(1):19–27.
2. Habana A, Dokras A, Giraldo JL, Jones EE. Cornual heterotopic pregnancy: contemporary management options. Am J Obstet Gynecol. 2000;182(5):1264–70.
3. Kim MJ, Jung YW, Cha JH, Seok HH, Han JE, Seong SJ, Kim YS. Successful management of heterotopic cornual pregnancy with laparoscopic cornual resection. Eur J Obstet Gynecol Reprod Biol. 2016;203:199–203.
4. Strandell A, Thorburn J, Hamberger L. Risk factors for ectopic pregnancy in assisted reproduction. Fertil Steril. 1999;71(2):282–6.
5. Lin EP, Bhatt S, Dogra VS. Diagnostic clues to ectopic pregnancy. Radiographics. 2008;28(6):1661–71.
6. Sills ES, Perloe M, Kaplan CR, Sweitzer CL, Morton PC, Tucker MJ. Uncomplicated pregnancy and normal singleton delivery after surgical excision of heterotopic (cornual) pregnancy following in vitro fertilization/embryo transfer. Arch Gynecol Obstet. 2002;266(3):181–4.

7.   Loret DMJ, Austin CM, Judge NE, Assel BG, Peskin B, Goldfarb JM. Cornual heterotopic pregnancy and cornual resection after in vitro fertilization/embryo transfer. A report of two cases. J Reprod Med. 1995;40(8):606–10.

8.   Divry V, Hadj S, Bordes A, Genod A, Salle B. Case of progressive intrauterine twin pregnancy after surgical treatment of cornual pregnancy. Fertil Steril. 2007;87(1):190–1.

9.   Blazar AS, Frishman GN, Winkler N. Heterotopic pregnancy after bilateral salpingectomy resulting in near-term delivery of a healthy infant. Fertil Steril. 2007;88(6):1671–6.

10. Peker N, Aydeniz EG, Gündo An S, Enda F. Laparoscopic Management of Heterotopic Istmocornual Pregnancy: a different technique. J Miniminvas Gyn. 2017;24(1):8–9.

11. Eom JM, Choi JS, Ko JH, Lee JH, Park SH, Hong JH, Hur CY. Surgical and obstetric outcomes of laparoscopic management for women with heterotopic pregnancy. J Obstet Gynaecol Res. 2013;39(12):1580–6.

12. Park HR, Moon MJ, Ahn EH, Baek MJ, Choi DH. Heterotopic quadruplet pregnancy: conservative management with ultrasonographically-guided KCl injection of cornual pregnancy and laparoscopic operation of tubal pregnancy. Fetal Diagn Ther. 2009;26(4):227–30.

13. Verma U, English D, Brookfield K. Conservative management of nontubal ectopic pregnancies. Fertil Steril. 2011;96(6):1391–5.

14. Guan Y, Ma C. Clinical outcomes of patients with heterotopic pregnancy after surgical treatment. J Miniminvas Gyn. 2017;24(7):1111–5.

15. Sentilhes LC, Bouet P, Gromez A, Poilblanc M, Lefebvre-Lacoeuille C, Descamps P. Successful expectant management for a cornual heterotopic pregnancy. Fertil Steril. 2009;91(3):911–34.

16. Fernandez H, Lelaidier C, Doumerc S, Fournet P, Olivennes F, Frydman R. Nonsurgical treatment of heterotopic pregnancy: a report of six cases. Fertil Steril. 1993;60(3):428–32.

Maternal bleeding complications following early versus delayed umbilical cord clamping in multiple pregnancies

Chayatat Ruangkit[1], Matthew Leon[2], Kasim Hassen[2], Katherine Baker[2], Debra Poeltler[2] and Anup Katheria[2*]

Abstract

Background: In 2015, the American Academy of Pediatrics recommended delayed umbilical cord clamping for at least 30–60 s for all infants. However, there is limited data regarding the maternal safety of delayed cord clamping in multiple pregnancies. We aimed to compare the maternal bleeding complications following early cord clamping (ECC) versus of delayed cord clamping (DCC) in multiple pregnancies.

Methods: A retrospective cohort study of pregnant women with multiples who delivered live-born infants at Sharp Healthcare Hospitals in San Diego, CA, USA during January 1st, 2016 – September 30th, 2017. Bleeding complications of 295 women who underwent ECC (less than 30 s) were compared with 154 women who underwent DCC (more than 30 s). ECC or DCC was performed according to individual obstetrician discretion.

Results: Four hundred forty-nine women with multiple pregnancies ($N = 910$ infants) were included in the study. 252 (85.4%) women underwent cesarean section in ECC group vs. 99 (64.3%) in DCC group. 58 (19.7%) women delivered monochorionic twins in ECC group vs. 32 (20.8%) women in DCC group. There was no increase in maternal estimate blood loss when DCC was performed comparing to ECC. There were no differences in operative time, post-delivery decrease in hematocrits, rates of postpartum hemorrhage, bleeding complications, maternal blood transfusions and therapeutic hysterectomy between the two groups.

Conclusions: No differences in maternal bleeding complications were found with DCC in multiple pregnancies compared to ECC. Delayed cord clamping can be done safely in multiple pregnancies without any increased maternal risk.

Keywords: Delayed umbilical cord clamping, Multiple pregnancy, Postpartum hemorrhage

Background

Evidence from multiple randomized controlled trials and metanalysis suggest that delayed umbilical cord clamping results in significant health benefits for term and preterm infants [1, 2]. Maintaining placenta-to-infant circulation during delayed clamping and cutting the umbilical cord after the onset of ventilation provides a more physiologic transition from fetal to neonatal life [3]. In term infants, delayed cord clamping (DCC) increases hemoglobin at birth, improves iron storage and decreases iron deficiency anemia during the first year of life when compared to early cord clamping (ECC) [2].

These effects have translated into improved neurodevelopmental outcomes at 4 years of age [4]. In preterm infants, DCC has been shown to reduce mortality [5]. Despite these neonatal benefits, there are limited data on maternal outcomes. While previous systematic reviews have reported no association between DCC and maternal risk of postpartum hemorrhage, blood loss at delivery, or need for blood transfusion [2] they have only included vaginal singleton births [6–12].

Multiple pregnancy is associated with a higher risk of maternal and neonatal complications compared to singleton pregnancy [13]. Multiple pregnancy is known to be risk factors for maternal bleeding complications [14]. Moreover, when combined with the operative delivery that is frequently performed in this patient population, the risk for bleeding complication is expected to be

* Correspondence: anup.katheria@sharp.com
[2]Neonatal Research Institute at Sharp Mary Birch Hospital for Women and Newborns, 8555 Aero Dr., Suite 104, San Diego, CA 92123, USA
Full list of author information is available at the end of the article

even higher. Our institution holds theoretical concerns regarding performing DCC in this patient population that DCC can significantly increase the duration of labor due to the delayed time spent with multiple infants which could result in increased blood loss from operation site as well as may precipitate uterine atony.

The lack of sufficient evidence in the literature in multiple gestations leads to variation in obstetric practice in this patient population. Different cord management techniques were used in previous clinical trials in this patient population including ECC, DCC, or umbilical cord milking (UCM) [15, 16]. In our institution, like most places, the decision to perform any of these procedures is based on obstetrics provider's discretion.

We, therefore, sought to evaluate the effect of DCC in multiple pregnancies at our institution. We hypothesized that DCC in multiple pregnancies increased the risk of maternal blood loss and bleeding complication when comparing to ECC.

Methods

We performed a retrospective cohort study by reviewing electronic medical records of all women with multiple pregnancies who delivered live-born infants at Sharp Healthcare Hospitals in San Diego, California from January 1st, 2016 to September 30th, 2017. All multiple deliveries in Sharp Healthcare Hospitals that provided obstetrics service, including Sharp Mary Birch Hospital for Women & Newborns, Sharp Grossmont Hospital, and Sharp Chula Vista Medical Center, were reviewed. Since no written protocol is available regarding umbilical cord management technique in multiple pregnancies in our institution, the umbilical cord was managed according to individual obstetrician preference in each hospital. The information on umbilical cord management technique for each delivery was extracted from the delivery record that documented the duration of umbilical cord clamping and cutting. The patients were categorized into two groups; ECC, defined as a mother who received umbilical cord clamping before 30 s in all infants and DCC, defined as a mother who received umbilical cord clamping at least after 30 s in one or more infants. 30 s was selected as the cutoff point between ECC and DCC for both term and preterm deliveries in our study to be in accordance with national recommendation [17, 18]. UCM could have been performed in either group but it was not felt to increase maternal morbidity, so it was included. Only patients with incomplete information on umbilical cord management technique during delivery were excluded. This study was approved by Sharp Mary Birch Hospital for Women & Newborns Human Research Protection Office, IRB No. 1712804. Waiver of individual patient informed consent was granted.

Patient records were reviewed for baseline characteristics including age, race, gestational age, antenatal complications, mode of delivery, anesthesia method, body mass index (BMI) at the time of delivery, number of infants, total fetal (infants) weight, and placental pathology. Outcomes of interest including estimated blood loss (EBL), post-delivery decrease in maternal hemoglobin and hematocrit, operative time (as defined by start of skin incision to complete skin closure), post-partum hemorrhage (PPH) defined as EBL > 500 mL for vaginal delivery or EBL > 1000 mL for a cesarean delivery, etiology of bleeding complications (e.g., uterine atony, placental abruption, or uterine rupture), maternal blood transfusion and therapeutic hysterectomy were reviewed. Infants mortality before hospital discharge were recorded.

Statistics

Univariate analyses were performed to identify significant differences between the groups. Student's t-test were used for parametric continuous variables and results were presented as mean ± standard deviation; SD. Mann-Whitney U test were used for non-parametric continuous variables. Results were specified accordingly wherever it is used and presented as median (interquartile ranges). Pearson's Chi-square tests or Fisher Exact tests were used for categorical variables and results were presented as total number (%). A p-value < 0.05 was considered statistically significant. SPSS (version 23, IBM, Chicago, IL) was used for all statistical analysis.

Results

During the study period, 506 women with multiple pregnancies delivered 910 live-born infants in Sharp Healthcare Hospitals (372 women at Sharp Mary Birch Hospital for Women & Newborns, 68 women at Sharp Grossmont Hospital, 66 women at Sharp Chula Vista Medical Center). Fifty-seven women had incomplete information on umbilical cord management during the delivery and were excluded from the study. The medical records of 449 women with complete delivery information were reviewed, and the patients were categorized into two groups as previously described. Figure 1, the lowest gestational age of the women in the study was 22 + 0 weeks, and the highest gestational age was 40 + 1 weeks. Two hundred ninety-five women in ECC group gave birth to 600 infants, and 154 women in DCC group gave birth to 310 infants. One hundred seventy-six women (59.7%) in ECC group and 113 women (73.4%) in DCC group delivered before 37 weeks. DCC more than 30 s was performed successfully in all infants at the delivery in 122 women (79.2%) in DCC group and in the remaining 32 women (20.8%), DCC was successfully performed only with one of the infants. During the study

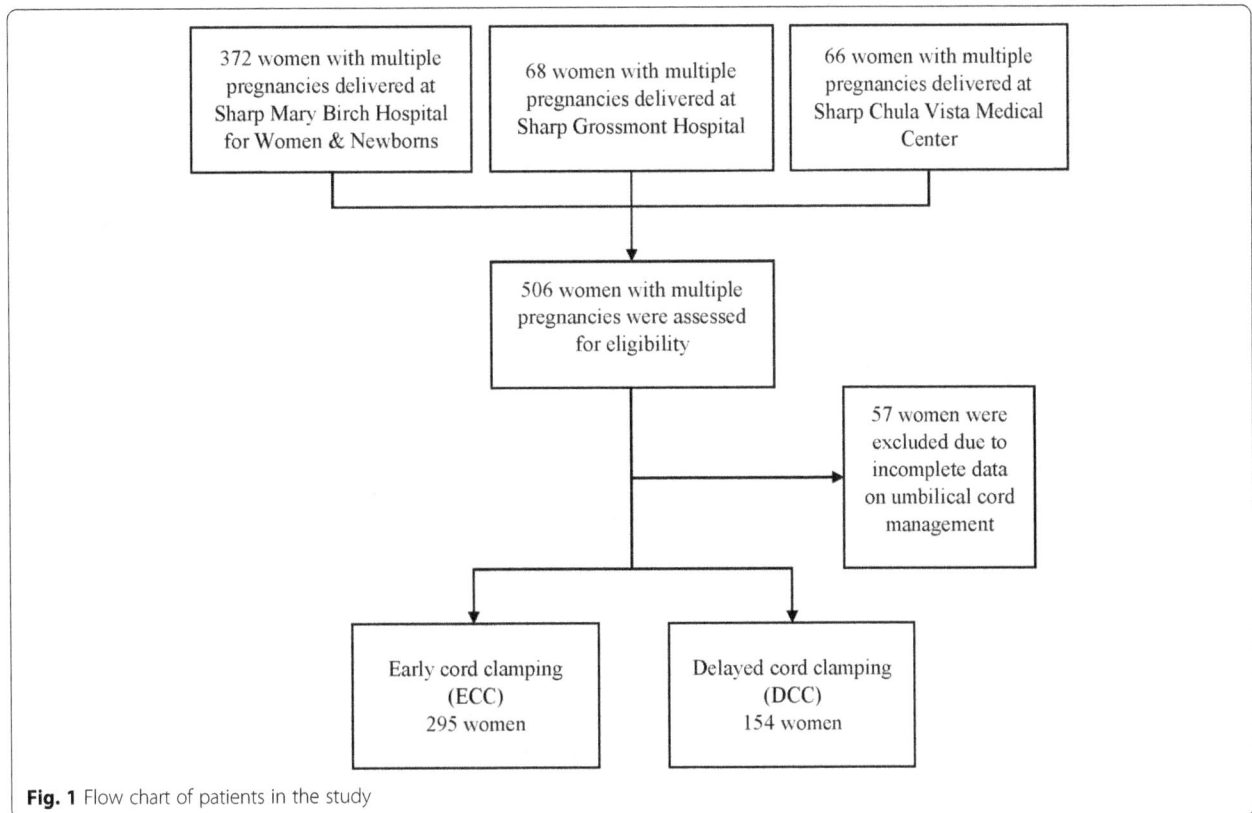

Fig. 1 Flow chart of patients in the study

period, UCM was performed concurrently in 336 infants (36.9%), and 901 infants (99.0%) survived to hospital discharge.

Patients demographic and baseline clinical characteristics were comparable between the two groups. However, the mean gestational age and the mean total fetal weight in the ECC group were statistically higher than the DCC group. Patients in ECC group were more likely to deliver by cesarean section and less likely to be in active labor at the time of delivery. There were 10 triplets (8 in ECC group and 2 in DCC) and 1 quadruplets (ECC group) in the cohort. There were similar rates monochorionic twins in each group (19.7% in ECC group and 20.8% in DCC group (Table 1).

At the time of delivery, 253 (85.8%) women underwent cesarean section in ECC group vs. 99 (64.3%) in DCC group. There was a significant difference in overall maternal estimate blood loss between the two groups (809.5 ± 400.0 mL in ECC vs. 728.8 ± 312.6 mL in DCC, $p = 0.02$). No significant differences in operative time (35.3 ± 18.2 min in ECC vs. 37.4 ± 13.2 min in DCC, $p = 0.23$), post-delivery decrease in hemoglobin (2.0 ± 1.5% in ECC vs. 2.1 ± 1.6% in DCC, $p = 0.72$), post-delivery decrease in hematocrits (6.0 ± 4.6% in ECC vs. 6.2 ± 4.8% in DCC, $p = 0.77$), rates of PPH (11.9% in ECC vs 14.3% in DCC, $p = 0.46$), and maternal blood transfusion (7.8% in ECC vs. 5.8% in DCC, $p = 0.45$). No patients in ECC group underwent

hysterectomy for treatment for post-partum hemorrhage. However, the procedure was performed in 3 patients in DCC group (1.0%). In multivariable linear regression model to predict EBL, operative delivery ($\beta = 0.323$, $p < 0.001$) and maternal age ($\beta = 0.166$, $p < 0.001$) significantly predicated EBL while DCC was not a significant predictor ($\beta = -0.008$, $p = 0.86$).

Even though uterine atony was the most common cause of PPH in our study, not all patients with PPH received the diagnosis of uterine atony, and not all patients with the diagnosis of uterine atony experienced PPH. There was no significant difference in the rates of bleeding complication diagnosis between the two group (13.9% in ECC vs. 18.2% in DCC, $p = 0.23$). Uterine atony was diagnosed in 35 (11.9%) of patients in ECC group and 26 (16.9%) patients in DCC group. Other causes of bleeding complications were diagnosed in 6 (2.0%) patients in ECC group (1 placenta accreta, 1 abruptio placenta, 1 uterine rupture, 2 retain placental tissue, and 1 unspecified hemorrhage) and 2 (1.3%) patients in DCC group (1 abruptio placenta and 1 intrauterine hematoma).

When maternal outcomes were analyzed according to mode of delivery, there was no significant difference in EBL between ECC and DCC both in vaginal delivery and cesarean section. Similarly, post-delivery decrease in hemoglobin and hematocrits, PPH, bleeding

Table 1 Maternal demographic and baseline clinical characteristics

	ECC (N = 295)	DCC (N = 154)	p-values
Maternal age (years)	32.2 ± 5.9	31.1 ± 6.1	0.05
Gestational age (weeks)	35.2 ± 2.9	34.5 ± 3.0	0.02
Race/Ethnicity			
White, non-Hispanic	114 (38.6)	74 (48.1)	
White, Hispanic	111 (37.6)	54 (35.1)	
Others (Black, Asian, or other race)	70 (23.7)	26 (16.8)	0.10
Multigravida	228 (77.3)	106 (68.8)	0.05
Multiparous	193 (65.4)	87 (56.5)	0.06
Monochorionic twins	58 (19.7)	32 (20.8)	0.78
3 or more multiples	9 (3.0)	2 (1.3)	0.25
Antenatal complications			
PIH	49 (16.6)	24 (15.6)	0.78
GDM	44 (14.9)	28 (18.8)	0.37
Initial hemoglobin (g/dL)	11.9 ± 1.4	11.9 ± 1.3	0.58
Initial hematocrit (%)	35.7 ± 3.8	35.7 ± 3.5	0.98
BMI (kg/m2)	32.3 ± 5.6	32.0 ± 6.4	0.64
Anesthesia method			
Local	4 (1.4)	3 (1.9)	
Epidural/Spinal	288 (97.6)	150 (97.4)	
General	3 (1.0)	1 (0.6)	0.38
In labor at the time of delivery	164 (55.6)	113 (73.4)	< 0.01
Operative delivery	253 (85.8)	99 (64.3)	< 0.01
Total fetal weight (g)	4813.3 ± 1129.7	4490.8 ± 1057.2	< 0.01

BMI body mass index, GDM Gestational diabetes mellitus, PIH pregnancy-induced hypertension
The results are reported as the mean ± standard deviation (SD) and frequency (percentage), and p < 0.05 is statistically significant

complications, maternal blood transfusion, and therapeutic hysterectomy were not significantly different between ECC and DCC groups both in vaginal delivery (Table 2) and cesarean section (Table 3).

Discussion

Contrary to our hypothesis, we did not find an increased rate of maternal blood loss and bleeding complications when DCC was performed in multiple pregnancies compared to ECC. Despite the theoretical concerns of increased risk of maternal blood loss secondary to increase time spent performing DCC in multiple infants which may result in delayed hysterotomy closure as well as may precipitate uterine atony, no significant increase in morbidity was found in terms of EBL, post-cesarean decreases in maternal hemoglobin and hematocrit, operative time, rate of PPH, diagnosis of other bleeding complication, maternal blood transfusion or therapeutic hysterectomy between the two groups. While overall

Table 2 Maternal outcomes in vaginal delivery

	ECC (n = 43)	DCC (n = 55)	p-values
EBL (mL)	581.5 ± 469.2	509.3 ± 332.7	0.40
Mean hemoglobin decrease (g/dL)[a]	2.2 ± 2.1	1.9 ± 1.6	0.63
Mean hematocrit decrease (%)[a]	6.6 ± 6.5	5.8 ± 5.1	0.67
Bleeding complications diagnosed	9 (20.9)	14 (25.5)	0.60
Uterine atony	8 (18.6)	14 (25.5)	0.42
Others	1 (2.3)	0 (0)	0.44
Postpartum hemorrhage	11 (25.6)	11 (20.0)	0.51
Blood transfusion	3 (7.0)	3 (5.5)	1.00
Hysterectomy	0 (0)	0 (0)	1.00

[a]Blood work was not routinely performed in vaginal delivery, ECC n = 22, DCC n = 23
The results are reported as the mean ± standard deviation (SD) and frequency (percentage), and p < 0.05 is statistically significant. EBL estimated blood loss

mean EBL was higher in the ECC group, this is most likely unrelated to umbilical cord management technique. The higher EBL in ECC group most likely can be explained by significantly higher cesarean section rate in ECC group comparing to DCC group. In our study, patients who underwent cesarean section, on average, tend to lose more blood than patients who undergo vaginal delivery. Therefore, increase in cesarean section rate resulted in EBL increases in ECC group. This association was confirmed in the multivariable linear regression model. Moreover, when the data was analyzed by mode of delivery, there was no significant difference in EBL between ECC and DCC both in vaginal delivery and cesarean section.

Table 3 Maternal outcomes in cesarean section

	ECC (n = 252)	DCC (n = 98)	p-values
Operation time (min)[a]	35.3 ± 18.2	37.4 ± 13.2	0.23
EBL (mL)	848.4 ± 374.3	848.5 ± 255.1	0.99
Mean hemoglobin decrease (g/dL)	2.0 ± 1.5	2.1 ± 1.6	0.55
Mean hematocrit decrease (%)	6.0 ± 4.1	6.2 ± 4.7	0.61
Bleeding complications diagnosed	32 (12.7)	14 (14.2)	0.69
Uterine atony	27 (10.7)	12 (12.2)	0.68
Others	5 (2.0)	2 (2.0)	1.00
Postpartum hemorrhage	24 (9.5)	11 (11.2)	0.63
Blood transfusion	20 (7.9)	6 (6.1)	0.56
Hysterectomy	3 (1.2)	0 (0)	0.55

[a]Operation time only recorded in cesarean section, defined by time from surgical incision to complete skin closure
The results are reported as the mean ± standard deviation (SD) and frequency (percentage), and p < 0.05 is statistically significant. EBL estimated blood loss

The absence of adverse maternal outcomes when DCC was performed in multiple pregnancies could be due to a relatively short time in performing DCC compared to the entire time spent during the delivery procedure. Many obstetricians in our group are delivering the second or third infant even before the first infant has his or her cord clamped, minimizing the total length of delay. In addition, it is also possible that obstetricians may be more attentive to bleeding as a major complication when performing DCC in multiples and they may have acted to maintain hemostasis during the procedure.

As previously mentioned the rate of cesarean section was higher in ECC group compared to DCC group in our study. This is most likely secondary to the theoretical risk and logistic difficulty of performing the DCC procedure in operative delivery, so the procedure was less likely to be performed during cesarean section. The higher rate of cesarean section in ECC may also be associated with multiple pregnancies with advanced gestational age that elective caesarian section was selected as a delivery method. The higher mean total fetal weight in ECC group also support this association. An alternative explanation for the difference in maternal baseline characteristics given the earlier recommendations for DCC only in premature infants, obstetrician and neonatologists attending deliveries may have increased preference for DCC with the lower gestational ages. This may have resulted in lower average gestational age and total fetal weight in DCC group. The higher rate of the patients who were in active labor at the time of delivery in DCC group and the lower rate of operative delivery are possibly due to more preterm labor in this group as an indication for the delivery.

The overall rate of PPH in multiple pregnancies during the study period in our institution was 12.7% (11.8% in ECC and 14.4% in DCC). Our numbers were comparable to those previously reported in the literature which ranges from 4 to 24% in multiple pregnancies [19–24]. It is unclear whether DCC technique was performed in any patients of those reports, however as the number of PPH in our study falls within ranges without significant difference between both ECC and DCC methods, we are quite reassured that DCC has been performed safely in multiple pregnancies in our institution.

The fact that there were similar rates of monochorionic twins in both groups (19.7% in ECC group and 20.9% in DCC group) is worth noting. There has been a theoretical concern regarding acute placenta-fetal transfusion that may occur during the delivery of monochorionic twins [25]. This is possibly the reasons why most DCC trial excluded monochorionic twins from their study. Despite this concern, our data indicate that DCC was performed routinely in these infants by many obstetric providers in our institution as well as in other

institution without any significant detrimental infant outcomes [26].

To the best of our knowledge, our study is the largest cohort to report maternal outcomes following different umbilical cord management techniques in multiple pregnancies. Previous trials on DCC have primarily excluded women (and infants) with multiple pregnancies. Many trials on DCC, however, included women with multiple pregnancies, but the focus was to evaluate and report only on infant outcomes with insufficient maternal safety outcomes [15, 16, 27]. In 2016, Kuo et al. evaluated maternal outcomes before and after implementation of an institutional DCC protocol which included singleton and twin pregnancies and found no increase in the risk of excessive maternal bleeding or other adverse maternal outcomes, but the number of women with multiples pregnancies in the study was too small to perform any subgroup analyses [28]. Our study has large enough numbers to increase our certainty that there would be minimal maternal risk with DCC in multiple pregnancies. Many DCC trials previously reported EBL or rates of PPH which can be subjective and inaccurate [29]; therefore, we also collected data on hemoglobin and hematocrit values before and after the delivery to provide objective and relatively precise information on the degree of maternal blood loss. However, we acknowledge this is a retrospective dataset which has several limitations and still would need to be validated in a prospective randomized controlled trial.

UCM was performed concurrently during the delivery to increase placental transfusion in more than one-third of the infants. Since UCM would not affect maternal outcomes, we did not include UCM in our analysis. The data on the benefits of UCM has been previously reported, and this was outside of the intent and scope of our study [15, 30].

Due to the recent American Academy of Pediatrics and The American College of Obstetricians and Gynecologists recommending universal implementation of delayed umbilical cord clamping for at least 30–60 s for vigorous infants [17, 18], the number of obstetrician performing DCC has increased. However, it is unclear whether multiples and cesarean section delivery fall into this category. High-risk patients such as those who deliver by operative delivery or multiple pregnancies should be prospectively studied in a well-controlled, adequate- powered, randomized controlled trial. Moreover, not only infant outcomes but also maternal health outcomes should be evaluated before DCC can be generalized to those patient populations. Although this study provides more evidence to support that DCC can be performed in multiple pregnancies without detrimental maternal outcomes when compared to ECC, other technique to facilitate placental transfusion that may be more efficient, practical and timely, such as UCM, should be investigated in future clinical trials.

Conclusions

In our study, no significant difference in maternal bleeding complications was found when DCC more than 30 s were performed in multiple pregnancies compared to ECC.

Abbreviations

BMI: Body mass index; DCC: Delayed cord clamping; EBL: Estimated blood loss; ECC: Early cord clamping; GDM: Gestational diabetes mellitus; PIH: Pregnancy-induced hypertension; PPH: Postpartum hemorrhage; UCM: Umbilical cord milking

Acknowledgements

The authors thank the clinical and research staff at Neonatal Research Institute at Sharp Mary Birch Hospital for Women and Newborns for their hospitality and their support.

Funding

This Research was funded by Career Development Grant, Faculty of Medicine Ramathibodi Hospital Mahidol University, Bangkok Thailand and Neonatal Research Institute at Sharp Mary Birch Hospital for Women and Newborns, San Diego, CA, USA.

Authors' contributions

CR, KB, and AK designed the present study. CR, ML, and KH performed data collection. AK and DP were involved in data analysis. CR drafted the original manuscript. AK was involved in revising the final manuscript and supervising the overall project. All authors read and approved the final manuscript.

Competing interests

The authors declare that they have no competing interests.

Author details

[1]Chakri Naruebodindra Medical Institute, Faculty of Medicine Ramathibodi Hospital, Mahidol University, Samut Prakan, Thailand. [2]Neonatal Research Institute at Sharp Mary Birch Hospital for Women and Newborns, 8555 Aero Dr., Suite 104, San Diego, CA 92123, USA.

References

1. Rabe H, Diaz-rossello JL, Duley L, Dowswell T. Effect of timing of umbilical cord clamping and other strategies to influence placental transfusion at preterm birth on maternal and infant outcomes. Cochrane Database Syst Rev. 2012;8:CD003248.
2. Mcdonald SJ, Middleton P, Dowswell T, Morris PS. Effect of timing of umbilical cord clamping of term infants on maternal and neonatal outcomes. Cochrane Database Syst Rev. 2013;7:CD004074.
3. Bhatt S, Alison BJ, Wallace EM, et al. Delaying cord clamping until ventilation onset improves cardiovascular function at birth in preterm lambs. J Physiol. 2013;591(8):2113–26.
4. Andersson O, Lindquist B, Lindgren M, Stjernqvist K, Domellöf M, Hellström-westas L. Effect of delayed cord clamping on neurodevelopment at 4 years of age: a randomized clinical trial. JAMA Pediatr. 2015;169(7):631–8.
5. Fogarty M, Osborn DA, Askie L, et al. Delayed vs early umbilical cord clamping for preterm infants: a systematic review and meta-analysis. Am J Obstet Gynecol. 2017; [Epub ahead of print]
6. Oxford Midwives Research Group. A study of the relationship between the delivery to cord clamping interval and the time of cord separation. Midwifery. 1991;7(4):167–76.
7. McDonald SJ. Management in the third stage of labour [dissertation]. Perth: University of Western Australia; 1996.
8. Geethanath RM, Ramji S, Thirupuram S, Rao YN. Effect of timing of cord clamping on the iron status of infants at 3 months. Indian Pediatr. 1997;34(2):103–6.
9. Ceriani Cernadas JM, Carroli G, Pellegrini L, et al. The effect of timing of cord clamping on neonatal venous hematocrit values and clinical outcome at term: a randomized, controlled trial. Pediatrics. 2006;117(4):e779–86.
10. Chaparro CM, Neufeld LM, Tena Alavez G, et al. Effect of timing of umbilical cord clamping on iron status in Mexican infants: a randomised controlled trial. Lancet. 2006;367(9527):1997–2004.
11. Van Rheenen P, De Moor L, Eschbach S, De Grooth H, Brabin B. Delayed cord clamping and haemoglobin levels in infancy: a randomised controlled trial in term babies. Tropical Med Int Health. 2007;12(5):603–16.
12. Andersson O, Hellström-westas L, Andersson D, Domellöf M. Effect of delayed versus early umbilical cord clamping on neonatal outcomes and iron status at 4 months: a randomised controlled trial. BMJ. 2011;343:d7157.
13. Su RN, Zhu WW, Wei YM, et al. Maternal and neonatal outcomes in multiple pregnancy: a multicentre study in the Beijing population. Chronic Dis Transl Med. 2015;1(4):197–20.
14. Nyfløt LT, Sandven I, Stray-Pedersen B, et al. Risk factors for severe postpartum hemorrhage: a case-control study. BMC Pregnancy and Childbirth. 2017;17:17.
15. Katheria AC, Truong G, Cousins L, Oshiro B, Finer NN. Umbilical cord milking versus delayed cord clamping in preterm infants. Pediatrics. 2015;136(1):61–9.
16. Tarnow-mordi W, Morris J, Kirby A, et al. Delayed versus immediate cord clamping in preterm infants. N Engl J Med. 2017; [Epub ahead of print]
17. Weiner G, Zaichkin J, Kattwinkel J. Textbook of neonatal resuscitation. 7th ed. Elk Grove Village, IL: American Academy of Pediatrics; 2016.
18. Committee on Obstetric Practice. Committee Opinion No. 684: delayed umbilical cord clamping after birth. Obstet Gynecol. 2017;129(1):e5–e10.
19. Santana DS, Cecatti JG, Surita FG, et al. Twin pregnancy and severe maternal outcomes: the World Health Organization multicountry survey on maternal and newborn health. Obstet Gynecol. 2016;127(4):631–41.
20. Conde-agudelo A, Belizán JM, Lindmark G. Maternal morbidity and mortality associated with multiple gestations. Obstet Gynecol. 2000;95(6 Pt 1):899–904.
21. Qazi G. Obstetric and perinatal outcome of multiple pregnancy. J Coll Physicians Surg Pak. 2011;21(3):142–5.
22. Su RN, Zhu WW, Wei YM, et al. Maternal and neonatal outcomes in multiple pregnancy: a multicentre study in the Beijing population. Chronic Dis Transl Med. 2015;1(4):1.
23. Rather S, Habib R, Sharma P. Studying pregnancy outcome in twin gestation in developing world. IOSR Journal of Dental and Medical Sciences. 2014;13(5):62–5.
24. Suzuki S, Kikuchi F, Ouchi N, et al. Risk factors for postpartum hemorrhage after vaginal delivery of twins. J Nippon Med Sch. 2007;74(6):414–7.
25. Lopriore E, Sueters M, Middeldorp JM, Vandenbussche FP, Walther FJ. Haemoglobin differences at birth in monochorionic twins without chronic twin-to-twin transfusion syndrome. Prenat Diagn. 2005;25(9):844–50.
26. Ruangkit C, Moroney V, Viswanathan S, Bhola M. Safety and efficacy of delayed umbilical cord clamping in multiple and singleton premature infants - a quality improvement study. J Neonatal Perinatal Med. 2015; 8(4):393–40.
27. Kugelman A, Borenstein-levin L, Riskin A, et al. Immediate versus delayed umbilical cord clamping in premature neonates born < 35 weeks: a prospective, randomized, controlled study. Am J Perinatol. 2007;24(5):307–15.
28. Kuo K, Gokhale P, Hackney DN, Ruangkit C, Bhola M, March M. Maternal outcomes following the initiation of an institutional delayed cord clamping protocol: an observational case-control study. J Matern Fetal Neonatal Med. 2018;31(2):197–201.
29. Hancock A, Weeks AD, Lavender DT. Is accurate and reliable blood loss estimation the "crucial step" in early detection of postpartum haemorrhage: an integrative review of the literature. BMC Pregnancy and Childbirth. 2015;15:230.
30. Katheria A, Mercer J, Brown M, et al. Umbilical cord milking at birth for term newborns with acidosis: neonatal outcomes. J Perinatol. 2017; [Epub ahead of print]

Misoprostol vaginal insert versus misoprostol vaginal tablets for the induction of labour: a cohort study

Daniele Bolla[1]*[ID], Saskia Vanessa Weissleder[1], Anda-Petronela Radan[1], Maria Luisa Gasparri[1], Luigi Raio[1], Martin Müller[1,2] and Daniel Surbek[1]

Abstract

Background: Misoprostol vaginal insert for induction of labor has been recently reported to be superior to dinoprostone vaginal insert in a phase III trial, but has never been compared to vaginal misoprostol in another galenic form. The aim of this study was to compare misoprostol vaginal insert (MVI) with misoprostol vaginal tablets (MVT) for induction of labor in term pregnancies.

Methods: In this retrospective cohort study we compared 200 consecutive women induced with 200-μg misoprostol 24-h vaginal insert (Misodel®) with a historical control of 200 women induced with Misoprostol 25-μg vaginal tablets (Cytotec®) every 4-6 h. Main outcomes variables included induction-to-delivery interval, vaginal delivery within 24-h, incidence of tachysystole, mode of delivery, and neonatal outcome. A subanalysis in the MVI group was performed in order to identify predictive factors for tachysistole and vaginal delivery within 24 h.

Results: The time from induction to vaginal delivery was 1048 ± 814 min in the MVI group and 1510 ± 1043 min in the MVT group (p < 0.001). Vaginal delivery within 24-h occurred in 127 (63.5%) patients of the MVI group and in 110 (55%) patients of the MVT group (p < 0.001). Tachysystole was more common in the MVI group (36% vs. 18%; p < 0.001). However, no significant predictors of uterine tachysystole in MVI group have been identified in crude and fully adjusted logistic regression models. Bishop score was the only predictor for vaginal delivery within 24 h (p < 0.001) in MVI group. Caesarean delivery rate (27% vs. 20%) and vaginal-operative deliveries (15.5% vs. 15.5%) did not differ significantly between the two groups. Neonatal outcomes were similar in both groups.

Conclusions: MVI achieves a more vaginal delivery rate within 24 h and Tachysystole events compared to MVT. However, no differences in caesarean section, operative vaginal delivery, and neonatal outcomes are reported. No predictors of tachysistole after MVI administration have been identified. Bishop score and parity are the only predictors of vaginal delivery within 24 h after MVI administration.

Keywords: Misoprostol vaginal insert, Misoprostol vaginal tablets, Induction of labour, Tachysytole, Misoprostol, Caesarean section, Neonatal outcomes

* Correspondence: d.bolla@sro.ch
[1]Department of Obstetrics and Gynaecology, Inselspital, Bern University Hospital, University of Bern, Effingerstrasse 102, CH-3010 Bern, Switzerland
Full list of author information is available at the end of the article

Background

Labour induction is a commonly performed procedure in obstetrics with an increasing incidence of approximately 25% [1–3]. In the latest decades, several pharmacological and mechanical methods of labour induction have been developed. Success of labour induction is linked to the Bishop score. An unfavourable cervix characterized by low cervical Bishop score decreases the success of labour induction and therefore is associated with a higher incidence of caesarean sections (CS) [4–7]. In this context, the use of prostaglandins has proven to be more effective for cervical ripening in women with low Bishop score as compared to other commonly used methods (oxytocin, Foley catheter, amniotomy), but is associated with an increased rate of uterine tachysystole, hyperstimulation syndrome, and uterine rupture [8, 9].

Misoprostol is a prostaglandin E_1 analogue currently marketed as oral tablets for the prophylaxis and treatment of peptic ulcer disease. Although the obstetrical use of Misoprostol is off-label in most countries, an extensive literature have proven its safety, efficacy, and dose-response effect in labour induction at term pregnancies [8]. Its pharmacological characteristics compared to prostaglandins E2, along with its easiness of storage led to the widespread use in obstetrics [10, 11]. Moreover, the World Health Organization entered Misoprostol in the list of the essential drugs for obstetrical use and medical organisations such as the International Federation of Gynaecology and Obstetrics and the American College of Obstetrician and Gynaecologists recommended their use in pregnant women [2, 12–15].

In 2014 misoprostol was registered in Europe in form of a single controlled-release vaginal insert containing 200 µg, and approved for labour induction beyond 37 0/7 weeks' gestation [16]. A large phase III registration trial reported a favourable outcome with a similar rate in vaginal deliveries and CS in comparison with dinoprostone vaginal insert [17]. Misoprostol vaginal insert (MVI) use resulted in a reduced induction-to-delivery interval, reduced time to active labour, and decreased need for additional oxytocin. At the same time, uterine tachysystole requiring intervention was increased (13.3% vs. 4%) [17], whereas no difference in neonatal outcome could be observed. So far, no data are available about the comparison between MVI and MVT. The aim of the following study was therefore to compare MVI to MVT in terms of vaginal delivery within 24 h and maternal/fetal outcomes. Secondary outcome was the identification of predictors of vaginal birth within 24 h. Furthermore, this study aims to identify the predictive factors for the occurrence of uterine tachysystole associated with MVI use, since it is the only significant adverse outcome reported in the MVI group.

Methods

Between January 2012 and July 2016, a retrospective cohort study was conducted at the Department of Obstetrics and Gynaecology, University Hospital Bern – Inselspital (Switzerland). We included all consecutive women who had a labour induction > 36 0/7 weeks' gestation. Before May 2014, MVT was routinely used off-label for labour induction in this patient population. In May 2014, MVT was replaced with the novel, approved MVI. The analysis periods were set as follows: January 2012 to 30 April 2014 for the MVT cohort and 1 May 2014 to 31 July 2016 for the MVI cohort. Data were obtained from the patients' electronic medical records. Each patient signed an informed consent regarding data collection for scientific purpose. Exclusion criteria consisted in foetal malpresentation, previous CS or uterine scarring (e.g., previous caesarean section), < 36 + 0 weeks of gestation, premature rupture of the membranes less than 24-h before starting the induction, severe preeclampsia, body mass index (BMI) > 50, signs of maternal infections in peripheral blood samples, abnormal foetal heart rate tracings or signs of active labour at admission, and twin pregnancy. Patients received MVI (Misodel*, Ferring Inc., Saint-Prex, Switzerland) containing 200 µg misoprostol in a slow-release vaginal insert as a single application, left in place for a maximum of 24 h, or MVT with repetitive dosing every 4 h as indicated. MVT were prepared in the hospital's pharmacy by crushing Cytotec* (Pfizer Inc., New York, US) tablets containing 200 µg misoprostol and manufacturing custom-made vaginal tablets each containing 25 µg misoprostol. In each group, preparations were placed in the posterior vaginal fornix. Criteria for removing MVI and ceasing MVT administration were the onset of three or more contractions within 10 min, lasting for 45 s or longer, resulting in cervical change or leading to a cervical dilatation of 4 cm or more with any frequency of contractions, or after completion of the 24-h dosage period. If spontaneous rupture of the membranes occurred, antibiotic prophylaxis was started after 24 h or immediately if a vaginal group B streptococcal smear test was positive. In both groups, an interval of at least 30 min was set between the removal of the vaginal insert or the last administration of vaginal tablet and the start of intravenous oxytocin administration.

Baseline demographic data and patients' characteristics were prospectively collected including maternal age, BMI, parity, contractions and membrane rupture status, gestational age, Bishop score (evaluated at the time of labour induction), and ethnicity. Each patient underwent at least 30 min of cardiotocography assessment to record the foetal status and confirm that there was no uterine pattern of active labour before the induction. Time and mode of delivery (vaginal, CS, operative vaginal) were recorded. Primary outcome was the rate of vaginal delivery within 24 h. Secondary outcomes were the induction-to-vaginal delivery interval (IDI), rate of caesarean section and operative vaginal delivery, the proportion of women requiring predelivery oxytocin, and the rate of uterine tachysystole. Further outcomes included the rate of peridural anaesthesia or other pain relievers, uterine hyperstimulation syndrome, postpartaum haemorrhage, uterine rupture, and length of hospital stay (days). Uterine tachysystole was defined by any occurrence of five or more contractions within 10 min, averaged over three consecutive 10-min periods [18]. Uterine hyperstimulation syndrome was defined as uterine tachysytole with concurrent foetal heart rate decelerations or bradycardia [18]. Neonatal outcome included the rates of 5-min Apgar score < 7, umbilical artery/venous pH, and umbilical artery base excess – 12 mmol/L, presence of meconium and transfer to neonatal intensive care unit. Ethical approval for the study was obtained by the local institutional review board (Ethics Committee of the Canton of Bern, Switzerland).

Statistical analysis

The patients characteristics and the delivery outcomes of the two groups were compared using Student's t-test for continuous variables and chi-square test for dichotomous variables. Continuous values were expressed as mean ± standard deviation. Unpaired continuous data were analyzed using the Mann-Whitney test. Proportions were compared by the Fisher's exact test. A p value < 0.05 was considered to be statistically significant. P values with more then 3 decimals were reported as >/< 0.001. Age of the mother, BMI, ethnicity, parity, gestational age at delivery, Bishop score, indication for labour induction, and fetal weight were evaluated as predictors for vaginal delivery within 24 h and for tachysistole, in crude and fully logistic regression models (OR 95%). Data analysis was performed with GraphPad Prism version 5 for Mac (GraphPad Software, San Diego CA).

Results

During the study interval a total of 400 women were included, 200 consecutive women induced with MVI and 200 consecutive women induced with MVT. The clinical characteristics of the study population are summarized in Table 1. Both groups were homogenous with similar baseline characteristics, except for BMI. Vaginal delivery within 24 h occurred in 127 (63.5%) patients of the MVI group and 110 (55%) patients of the MVT group (p < 0.001). Induction-to-vaginal delivery interval was 1048 ± 814 min and 1510 ± 1043 min in the MVI and MVT group, respectively (p < 0.001) (Fig. 1). Uterine tachysystole was more frequent in the MVI group (36% n = 72 vs. 18% n = 36; p = 0.002). No

Table 1 Patients characteristics

	MVI n 200	MVT n 200	p-Value
Median Age (range)	32 (28-35)	32(28-36)	> 0.05
Mean Parity (±SD)	0.5 ± 0.7	0.6 ± 1	> 0.05
Median BMI (range)	22.8 (20.7-25.3)	24.2 (21.6-27.6)	< 0.001
Mean week of gestational age at delivery(±SD)	40 ± 1	39 ± 1	> 0.05
Ethnicity (%)			
Europe	149 (74.5)	153 (76.5)	> 0.05
Africa	27 (13.5)	25 (12.5)	> 0.05
America	5 (2.5)	4 (2.0)	> 0.05
Asia	17 (8.5)	18 (9.0)	> 0.05
Missing	2 (1.0)	0 (0.0)	> 0.05
Premature rupture of membrane (%)	19 (9.5)	12 (6)	> 0.05
Median Bishop's score (range)	2 (1-3)	2 (1-3)	1

Student's t-test was used for Age, parity, BMI, week of gestational age, and Bishop score; chi-square test was used for Etnicity and Premature rupture of Membrane
Abbreviations: *BMI* Body mass index, *MVI* Misoprostol vaginal insert, *MVT* Misoprostol vaginal tablets

significant differences were detected in the rate of epidural anaesthesia or other pain reliever use. CS rate (27% n = 54 vs. 20% n = 41, p = 0.58) and vaginal-operative deliveries (15.5% n = 31 vs. 15.5% n = 31, p = 0.77) were not significantly different between the groups. Postpartum haemorrhage occurrence was also similar in both groups (12.9% n = 25 vs. 9% n = 18, p = 0.33). No uterine rupture occurred. Neonatal outcomes (Apgar score, cord blood pH, transfer to neonatal intensive care unit) were not significantly different in both groups. Women in the MVI group had a significantly shorter length of hospital stay calculated in hours as compared with women in the MVT group (MVI 97.63 ± 32. vs MVT

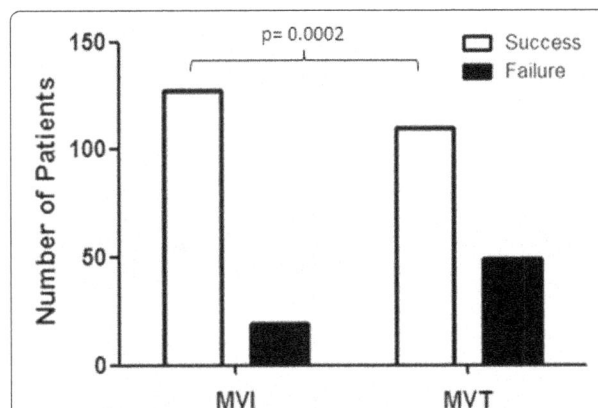

Fig. 1 Vaginal delivery within 24-h after induction of labour with MVI compared to MVT. Abbreviations: MVI = Misoprostol vaginal insert, MVT = Misoprostol vaginal tablets

118.5 ± 123; $p < 0.001$). Further deliveries outcomes are summarized in Table 2.

Since uterine tachysistole was significantly higher in MVI group, the predictors of uterine tachysystole among patients induced with MVI were interrogated and no significant association were found with the demographic and clinical parameters and therefore predictive power is lacking (Table 3). Bishop's score and parity were the strongest predictors of delivery within 24 h after adjusting for confounders in the same group (OR 0.90, CI 95% 0.85-0.96 $p < 0.001$) (Table 4).

Discussion

MVT was compared to other methods such as oxytocin, Dinoprostone and placebo in several clinical randomized trials in terms of efficacy (vaginal delivery within 24 h) and safety (perinatal or maternal outcomes) (8). Recently, MVI was compared to Dinoprostone vaginal insert, a prostaglandin E2 analog in a phase III trial reporting significantly reduced times to delivery (efficacy) and no evidence of differences in maternal or neonatal safety outcomes (safety) (17). Since this study, three studies have compared the vaginal insert to other induction methods in terms of delivery outcomes [19–21]. However, none of these studies have compared MVI to MVT.

Our study shows for the first time that labour induction with MVI has a significant higher rate of vaginal

Table 2 MVI vs MVT deliveries outcomes

	MVI n = 200	MVT n = 200	P value
Vaginal delivery within 24 h n°(%)	127 (63.5%)	110 (55%)	< 0.001
Induction to vaginal delivery interval minutes mean (±SD)	1048 ± 814	1510 ± 1043	< 0.001
Predelivery oxytocin n°(%)	6 (3)	11 (5.5)	> 0.05
Peridural anesthesia n°(%)	79 (39.5)	65 (32)	> 0.05
Pain reliviers (excl. PDA) n°(%)	132 (66)	143 (71.5)	> 0.05
Uterine Hyperstimulation n°(%)	13 (6.5)	13 (6.5)	> 0.05
Tachysistole n°(%)	72 (36)	36 (18)	0.002
Apgar < 7 n (%)	8 (4)	2 (1)	> 0.05
pH art < 7.15 n° (%)	36/149 (24)	25/161 (15)	> 0.05
Umbelical artery base excess mean ± SD	−3.7 ± 3	−4.1 ± 3	> 0.05
Neonatal birth weight mean ± SD	3428 ± 429	3389 ± 471	> 0.05
Meconium n°(%)	29 (14)	29 (14)	> 0.05
NICU n°(%)	14 (7)	20 (10)	> 0.05

Abbreviations: NICU Neonatal intensive care unit, MVI Misoprostol vaginal insert, MVT Misoprostol vaginal tablets

Table 3 Predictors of uterine tachysystole in MVI group

	Crude OR (95% CI)	p-Values	Adjusted OR (95% CI)	p-Values
Age of mother	0.71 (0.42-1.20)	0.19	0.69 (0.38-1.26)	0.23
BMI	0.99 (0.93-1.06)	0.81	0.99 (0.92-1.06)	0.73
Ethnicity		0.82		0.87
Europe	1.00 (reference)		1.00 (reference)	
Africa	1.49 (0.65-3.42)		1.45 (0.56-3.72)	
America	1.24 (0.20-7.68)		1.35 (0.17-8.84)	
Asia	1.02 (0.36-2.91)		1.03 (0.30-3.23)	
Parity	1.05 (0.72-1.54)	0.80	1.06 (0.68-1.65)	0.79
Gestations age	1.05 (0.84-1.31)	0.65	1.05 (0.77-1.44)	0.75
Bishop's score	1.01 (0.83-1.23)	0.92	1.02 (0.82-1.27)	0.86
over due date	1.00 (reference)		1.00 (reference)	
gestational diabetes mellitus	1.33 (0.57-3.12)		1.65 (0.54- 5.06)	
other	0.88 (0.44-1.73)		1.24 (0.49 -3.16)	
Fetus weight	1.23 (0.63-2.42)	0.54	1.23 (0.56-2.74)	0.60

Odds ratios (OR) and 95% CI for the occurrence of uterine tachysystole. Predictors from crude and fully adjusted logistic regression models. Age of the mother is taken in decades, and fetus weight was entered in kg

delivery within 24 h, and a shorter hospital stay compared to the labour induction with MVT. The two groups of patients were homogeneous for clinical and demographic characteristics, except for the BMI ($p < 0.001$). However, mean BMI values were lower than 25.00 Kg/m2 both in MVI and MVT groups. Since the overweight women with a BMI up to 25.00 kg/

Table 4 Predictors of vaginal deliveries within 24 h in MVI group

	Crude OR (95% CI)	p-Values	Adjusted OR (95% CI)	p-Values
Age of mother	0.97(0.83-1.12)	0.64	1.02 (0.87-1.20)	0.81
BMI	1.02 (1-1.04)	0.41	1.01 (0.99-1.03)	0.25
Ethnicity		0.72		0.51
Europe	1.00 (reference)		1.00 (reference)	
Africa	0.9 (0.7-1.15)		0.96 (0.73-1.23)	
America	1.06 (0.61-1.82)		1.12 (0.66-1.88)	
Asia	1.10 (0.81-1.50)		1.23 (0.90-1.69)	
Parity	0.81 (0.73-0.90)	< 0.001	0.84 (0.74-0.95)	0.004
Gestations age	0.95 (0.89-1.01)	0.12	1.02 (0.94-1.11)	0.66
Bishop's score	0.89 (0.84-0.94)	< 0.001	0.90 (0.85-0.96)	< 0.001
over due date	1.00 (reference)		1.00 (reference)	
gestational diabetes mellitus	1.37 (1.06-1.75)		1.43 (1.05-1.94)	0.55
other	1.22 (1-1.48)		1.14 (0.92 -1.41)	061
Fetus weight	0.91(0.75-1.11)	0.34	1.23 (0.56-2.74)	0.22

Odds ratios (OR) and 95% CI for the occurrence of vaginal delivery within 24 h. Predictors from crude and fully adjusted logistic regression models. Age of the mother is taken in decades, and fetus weight was entered in kg

m²are at increased risk of pregnancy complications at birth [22], we can speculatively justify the similar number of operative deliveries and CSs, and neonatal outcomes in the two groups despite the difference in BMI.

Furthermore, in MVI an increased incidence of uterine tachysystole was reported. However, this finding was not accompanied by an higher rate of operative deliveries, CS; similarly, neonatal outcomes do not differ among the groups. Interesting, we found that uterine tachysystole cannot be predicted by demographic or clinical factors.

In our study, adverse events such as CS, postpartum haemorrhage, meconium-stained amniotic fluid, Apgar score below 7, fetal acidosis (defined by arterial pH < 7. 15), and neonatal complications were similar in both groups. In line with previous studies, we detected a relatively high incidence of uterine tachysystole after Misoprostol use [8, 23, 24]. For example, Jozwiak et al. reported a 61% reduction of uterine hyperstimulation in the Foley catheter group compared to the use of 25 μg MVT and Hofmeyr et al. reported a lower incidence of tachysystole with similar results using vaginal / intracervical dinoprostone [8, 23]. Efficacy of misoprostol seems to be correlated with the dosage and therefore several studies focused on determining the optimal dosing regimen. In our study the dosages used in the MVT group was previously reported as the most effective for vaginal delivery success and is associated with the lowest rates of tachysystole [8]. Similarly, the efficacy and safety of MVI was evaluated with different dosages. For example, Wing et al. compared three different doses of MVI and determined that 200 μg was the most effective for the onset of active labour within 24-h but with the disadvantage of an increased rate of tachysystole (41.2%) compared to MVI 150 μg (25.6%) and MVI 100 μg (19.5%) [25]. In our study, the incidence of tachysytole was significantly higher than in the MVT group (36% vs. 18%). However, this higher incidence did not result in adverse maternal and/or neonatal outcomes. Further, the multivariate analysis displayed no maternal or fetal predictive factors for tachysytole. We hypothesize that the main reason for the higher incidence of uterine tachysytole are the pharmacokinetic properties of MVI such as the relatively long elimination half-time after removal of 40 min [16]. Thus, timely removal of the vaginal insert may reduce the incidence of tachysytole. Whether the inclusion of currently excluded patients with certain characteristics such as multiparty, low BMI, or rupture of membranes is warranted, needs to be evaluated in further prospective studies.

A general goal of clinical management during pregnancy is to avoid adverse maternal and fetal outcomes while avoiding unnecessary CS. For this reason, ACOG recommend in uneventful pregnancies inductions of labour at 41 0/7 weeks of gestations to reduce the number of elective CS and to improve perinatal outcomes [15]. However, several studies have shown an increased rate of failed induction and CS if women are induced with an unfavourable cervix [4–7]. In this context prostaglandins are effective agents for cervical ripening [8]. In our study, we observed that MVI did not reduce the CS rate but the time to delivery and therefore a significant reduction of hospital stay. Theoretically, the shorter hospital stay may be related to the higher rate of vaginal delivery within 24 h, however it is just a speculative assumption. If so, it might be beneficial for patients, particularly for those needing a rapid delivery such as late onset preeclampsia [26]. Although MVI (Misodel, 74.37 USD) might be more expensive compared to the MVT (Cytotec tablet, 0.26 USD), the reduced hospital stay outweighs this disadvantage. Furthermore, the litigation risks inherent to the use of misoprostol off-label can be avoided using the approved MVI preparation. A further important aspect is the women's preference regarding comfort and pain during induction of labour. As reported by Impey et al., women's expectation is to have a *safe and fast* labour with little pain [27]. Another study showed that 40% of women who experienced a labour induction expressed the desire to minimize the time duration of labour induction in case of the necessity of labour induction in the following pregnancy [28]. In this regard, MVI has the potential to increase patient satisfaction by decreasing the time to delivery interval. Limit of this study is its retrospective nature, and prospective future studies are needed to confirm our proof of concept.

Conclusions

MVI is able to induce higher rate of vaginal delivery within 24 h compared to MVT. A shorter hospital stay was also reported in the MVI group. The higher rate of tachysystole after MVI induction may represent the price to be paid for a quicklier time interval from induction to delivery. However, although more tachysystole events are reported after MVI induction, no differences in maternal and neonatal outcomes as well as in operative deliveries and CS are observed when comparing to MVT. Furthermore, no predictors of vaginal delivery within 24 h are identified in the MVI group, except for Bishop score and parity. It means that probably we need further prospective studies in order to identify which modifiable predictors can be used in the future to better select the patients to a more appropriate labour induction program.

Abbreviations
BMI: Body mass index; CS: Caesarean sections; IDI: Induction-to-vaginal delivery interval; MVI: Misoprostol vaginal insert; MVT: Misoprostol vaginal tablets

Funding
The study is supported in part by an unrestricted research grant from Ferring from December 4th 2015. The study sponsor had no insight into study design and methods, study conduction, result analysis and data interpretation, and manuscript writing.

Authors' contributions

Protocol/project development: DB, DS, LR. Data collection: SVW, APR. Data analysis: MLG, MM. Manuscript writing/editing: DB, DS, LR. Final revision: DB, DS. All authors read and approved of the final manuscript.

Competing interests

Ferring Pharmaceuticals funded the overall study (see Funding dection).

Author details

[1]Department of Obstetrics and Gynaecology, Inselspital, Bern University Hospital, University of Bern, Effingerstrasse 102, CH-3010 Bern, Switzerland. [2]Departments of Obstetrics, Gynaecology and Reproductive Sciences, Yale University School of Medicine, New Haven, USA.

References

1. Swamy GK. Current methods of labor induction. Semin Perinatol. 2012;36(5): 348–52. https://doi.org/10.1053/j.semperi.2012.04.018. Review
2. ACOG Committee on Practice. Bulletins-obstetrics. ACOG practice bulletin no. 107. Induction of labor. Obstet Gynecol. 2009;114(2 Pt 1):386–97.
3. Gülmezoglu AM, Crowther CA, Middleton P, Heatley E. Induction of labour for improving birth outcomes for women at or beyond term. Cochrane Database Syst Rev. 2012;6:CD004945. https://doi.org/10.1002/14651858. CD004945.pub3. Review
4. Vrouenraets FP, Roumen FJ, Dehing CJ, van der Akker ES, Aarts MJ, Scheve EJ. Bishop score and risk of cesarean delivery after induction of labor in nulliparous women. Obstet Gynecol. 2005;105:690–7.
5. Ennen CS, Bofill JA, Magann EF, Bass JD, Chauhan SP, Morrison JC. Risk factors for cesarean delivery in preterm, term, and post-term patients undergoing induction of labour with an unfavourable cervix. Gynecol Obstet Investig. 2009;67:113–7.
6. Pevnzer L, Rayburn WF, Rumney P, Wing DA. Factors predicting successful labor induction with dinoprostine and misoprostol vaginal inserts. Obstet Gynecol. 2009;114(2 Pt 1):261–7.
7. Ehrenthal DB, Jiang X, Strobino DM. Labour induction and the risk of cesarean delivery among nulliparous women at term. Obstet Gynecol. 2010; 116:35–42.
8. Hofmeyr GJ, Gülmezoglu AM, Pileggi C. Vaginal misoprostol for cervical ripening and induction of labour. Cochrane Database Syst Rev. 2010;10: CD000941. https://doi.org/10.1002/14651858.CD000941.pub2. Review
9. Aghideh FK, Mullin PM, Ingles S, Ouzounian JG, Opper N, Wilson ML, et al. A comparison of obstetrical outcomes with labor induction agents used at term. J Matern Fetal Neonatal Med. 2014;27(6):592–6. https://doi.org/10. 3109/14767058.2013.831066. Epub 2013 Aug 27
10. Krause E, Malorgio S, Kuhn A, Schmid C, Baumann M, Surbek D. Off-label use of misoprostol for labor induction: a nation-wide survey in Switzerland. Eur J Obstet Gynecol Reprod Biol. 2011;159(2):324–8. https://doi.org/10. 1016/j.ejogrb.2011.09.013. Epub 2011 Sep 28
11. Surbek DV, Bösiger H, Hösli I, Pavic N, Holzgreve W. A double-blind comparison of the safety and efficacy of intravaginal misoprostol and prostaglandin E2 to induce labor. Am J Obstet Gynecol. 1997;177:1018–23.
12. WHO Model list of essential medicines. 19th list, April 2015.
13. Tang J, Kapp N, Dragoman M, de Souza JP. WHO recommendations for misoprostol use for obstetric and gynecologic indications. Int J Gynaecol Obstet. 2013;121:186–9.
14. FIGO Guidelines (2012). Misoprostol Reccommended Dosages. https://www. figo.org/sites/default/files/uploads/project-publications/Miso/Misoprostol_ Recommended%20Dosages%202012.pdf.
15. American College of Obstetricians and Gynecologists (College); Society for Maternal-Fetal Medicine, Caughey AB, Cahill AG, Guise JM, Rouse DJ. Safe prevention of the primary cesarean delivery. Am J Obstet Gynecol. 2014;210: 179–93.
16. Powers BL, Wing DA, Carr D, Ewert K, Di Spirito M. Pharmacokinetic profiles of controlled-release hydrogen polymer vaginal inserts containing misoprostol. J Clin Pharmacol. 2008;48:26–34.
17. Wing DA, Brown R, Plante LA, Miller H, Rugarn O, Powers BL. Misoprostol vaginal insert and time to vaginal delivery: a randomized controlled trial. Obstet Gynecol. 2013;122(2 Pt 1):201–9. https://doi.org/10.1097/AOG. 0b013e31829a2dd6.
18. Heuser CC, Knight S, Esplin MS, Eller AG, Holmgren CM, Manuck TA, et al. Tachysystole in term labor: incidence, risk factors, outcomes, and effect on fetal heart tracings. Am J Obstet Gynecol. 2013;209(1):32.e1-32.e6. doi: https://doi.org/10.1016/j.ajog.2013.04.004. Epub 2013 Apr 6. Erratum in: Am J Obstet Gynecol. 2014;210(2):162.
19. Mayer RB, Oppelt P, Shebl O, Pömer J, Allerstorfer C, Weiss C. Initial clinical experience with a misoprostol vaginal insert in comparison with a dinoprostone insert for inducing labor. Eur J Obstet Gynecol Reprod Biol. 2016;200:89–93.
20. Dobert M, Brandstetter A, Henrich W, Rawnaq T, Hasselbeck H, Dobert TF, Hinkson L, Schwaerzler P. The misoprostol vaginal insert compared with oral misoprostol for labor induction in term pregnancies: a pair-matched casecontrol study. J Perinat Med. 2018;46(3):309–316. https://doi.org/10. 1515/jpm-2017-0049.
21. Gornisiewicz T, Jaworowski A, Zembala-Szczerba M, Babczyk D, Huras H. Analysis of intravaginal misoprostol 0.2 mg versus intracervical dinoprostone 0.5 mg doses for labor. Ginekol Pol. 2017;88(6):320–4.
22. Vinturache A, Moledina N, McDonald S, Slater D, Tough S. Pre-pregnancy body mass index (BMI) and delivery outcomes in a Canadian population. BMC Pregnancy Childbirth. 2014;14:422. https://doi.org/10.1186/s12884-014-0422-y.
23. Jozwiak M, ten Eikelder M, Oude Rengerink K, de Groot C, Feitsma H, Spaanderman M, et al. Foley catheter versus vaginal misoprostol: randomized controlled trial (PROBAAT-M study) and systematic review and meta-analysis of literature. Am J Perinatol. 2014;31(2):145–56. https://doi.org/ 10.1055/s-0033-1341573. Epub 2013 Apr 5
24. Rugarn O, Tipping D, Powers B, Wing DA. Induction of labour with retrievable prostaglandin vaginal inserts: outcomes following retrieval due to an intrapartum adverse event. BJOG. 2017;124(6):985–6. https://doi.org/ 10.1111/1471-0528.14406.
25. Wing DA, Miller H, Parker L, Powers BL, Rayburn WF. Misoprostol vaginal insert miso-Obs-204 investigators. Misoprostol vaginal insert for successful labor induction: a randomized controlled trial. Obstet Gynecol. 2011;117(3): 533–41. https://doi.org/10.1097/AOG.0b013e318209d669.
26. Lapaire O, Zanetti-Dällenbach R, Weber P, Hösli I, Holzgreve W, Surbek D. Labor induction in preeclampsia: is misoprostol more effective than dinoprostone? J Perinat Med. 2007;35:195–9.
27. Impey L. Maternal attitudes to amniotomy and labor duration: a survey in early pregnancy. Birth. 1999;26(4):211–4.
28. Shetty A, Burt R, Rice P, Templeton A. Women's perceptions, expectations and satisfaction with induced labour–a questionnaire-based study. Eur J Obstet Gynecol Reprod Biol. 2005;123(1):56–61.

Pregnancy outcomes in women with gestational diabetes mellitus diagnosed according to the WHO-2013 and WHO- 1999 diagnostic criteria: a multicentre retrospective cohort study

Eva A. R. Goedegebure[1†], Sarah H. Koning[2*†], Klaas Hoogenberg[3], Fleurisca J. Korteweg[4], Helen L. Lutgers[5], Mattheus J. M. Diekman[6], Eva Stekkinger[1], Paul P. van den Berg[7] and Joost J. Zwart[1]

Abstract

Background: The World Health Organization (WHO) adopted more stringent diagnostic criteria for GDM in 2013, to improve pregnancy outcomes. However, there is no global consensus on these new diagnostic criteria, because of limited evidence. The objective of the study was to evaluate maternal characteristics and pregnancy outcomes in two cohorts in the Netherlands applying different diagnostic criteria for GDM i.e. WHO-2013 and WHO-1999.

Methods: A multicenter retrospective study involving singleton GDM pregnancies in two regions, between 2011 and 2016. Women were diagnosed according to the WHO-2013 criteria in the Deventer region (WHO-2013-cohort) and according to the WHO-1999 criteria in the Groningen region (WHO-1999-cohort). After GDM diagnosis, all women were treated equally based on the national guideline. Maternal characteristics and pregnancy outcomes were compared between the two groups.

Results: In total 1386 women with GDM were included in the study. Women in the WHO-2013-cohort were older and had a higher pre-gestational body mass index. They were diagnosed earlier (24.9 [IQR 23.3–29.0] versus 27.7 [IQR 25.9–30.7] weeks, $p = < 0.001$) and less women were treated with additional insulin therapy (15.6% versus 43. 4%, $p = < 0.001$). Rate of spontaneous delivery was higher in the WHO-2013-cohort (73.1% versus 67.4%, $p = 0.032$). The percentage large-for-gestational-age (LGA) neonates (birth weight > 90th percentile, corrected for sex, ethnicity, parity, and gestational age) was lower in the WHO-2013- cohort, but not statistical significant (16.5% versus 18.5%, $p = 0.379$). There were no differences between the cohorts regarding stillbirth, birth trauma, low Apgar score, and preeclampsia.

Conclusions: Using the new WHO-2013 criteria resulted in an earlier GDM diagnosis, less women needed insulin treatment and more spontaneous deliveries occurred when compared to the cohort diagnosed with WHO-1999 criteria. No differences were found in adverse pregnancy outcomes.

Keywords: Gestational diabetes mellitus, GDM, WHO, Diagnostic criteria, Pregnancy outcomes

* Correspondence: s.h.koning@umcg.nl
†Equal contributors
[2]Department of Endocrinology, University of Groningen, University Medical Center Groningen, PO Box 30.001, 9700 RB Groningen, the Netherlands
Full list of author information is available at the end of the article

Background

Gestational diabetes mellitus (GDM) is defined as glucose intolerance detected during pregnancy [1]. The prevalence of GDM is increasing and affects between 1 and 14% of all pregnancies, caused by a global increase in the number of women with obesity around reproductive age and by more stringent diagnostic criteria for GDM [1–4]. Untreated GDM is associated with an increased rate of neonatal and obstetric complications [5–7]. Adverse pregnancy outcomes have been shown to improve with timely diagnosis and treatment of GDM [8].

In 2008, the international prospective Hyperglycemia and Adverse Pregnancy Outcomes (HAPO) study group demonstrated a continuous association between maternal hyperglycaemia and risk of adverse pregnancy outcomes, as birth weight greater than the 90th percentile, caesarean section, premature birth, birth injury, and preeclampsia [9]. Based on these findings and earlier observational studies, the International Association of Diabetes and Pregnancy Study Group (IADPSG) proposed more stringent diagnostic thresholds for GDM [10]. These new diagnostic criteria (fasting plasma glucose level ≥ 5.1 mmol/l and/or 1-h plasma glucose level ≥ 10.0 mmol/l and/or 2-h plasma glucose level ≥ 8.5 mmol/l) have been adopted by the American Diabetes Association in 2010, the World Health Organization (WHO) in 2013, and the International Federation of Gynaecology and Obstetrics in 2015 [1, 11, 12].

However, to date there is no global consensus on these new diagnostic criteria. A recent review on the current European situation showed a lack of consistency on GDM diagnosis [13]. The apparent reluctance to adopt the IADPSG criteria may result from studies showing an increase in prevalence of GDM and thus a higher burden to obstetric healthcare providers [4, 14], but most importantly from scepticism about the clinical benefit of lower diagnostic thresholds [14, 15].

Also in the Netherlands there is a debate regarding the diagnostic criteria for GDM. The Dutch Society of Obstetrics and Gynaecology guideline 2010 "Diabetes and Pregnancy" recommends screening for GDM in high-risk women using the 2-h 75-g oral glucose tolerance test (OGTT) using the older WHO-1999 criteria, utilizing a fasting blood glucose ≥7.0 and 2-h blood glucose of ≥7.8 mmol/l [16, 17]. Notwithstanding that, a few hospitals in the Netherlands already implemented the new WHO-2013 thresholds for diagnosis of GDM.

To verify the consequences of implementing these new WHO-2013 thresholds the following question need to be answered: What are the pregnancy outcomes of women diagnosed according the WHO-2013 criteria compared with women diagnosed according the older WHO-1999 criteria?

The objective of the current study was therefore to evaluate the maternal characteristics and obstetric and neonatal outcome in two typical population-based cohorts in the Netherlands which applied the two different diagnostic criteria for GDM i.e. WHO-2013 and WHO-1999.

Methods

Study population

A multicentre, retrospective cohort study was conducted involving three hospitals in the Netherlands (University Medical Center Groningen a tertiary care centre, Martini Hospital Groningen, and Deventer Hospital both secondary care centres). Both regions (Deventer region and Groningen region) are located in the relatively rural north-eastern part of the Netherlands. Part of the data of the Groningen region has been published previously [18, 19]. All pregnant women with diagnosis of GDM were eligible for inclusion in the study. Women with a twin pregnancy and women with pre-existing diabetes mellitus (DM) were excluded.

This study has been conducted in accordance with the guidelines of the Declaration of Helsinki and Good Clinical Practice. The patient data were retrospectively acquired from hospital records generated during care-as-usual. Statistical analysis was performed requiring patient anonymity in agreement with the ethics committee regulations [20]. According to the Dutch law on Medical Research with Human Subjects, this study has been exempted for approval by the local ethics committees.

Screening, diagnosis and treatment of GDM

Criteria for screening and diagnosis of GDM are summarized in Fig. 1 [16, 17]. After GDM diagnosis all women were treated based on the national guideline. First, all women received dietary counselling and instructions for self-monitoring of the blood glucose levels (SMBG). According to the guideline, insulin therapy was started if the blood glucose levels were repeatedly above the treatment targets (two blood glucose values above the treatment target at the same day) despite dietary treatment: fasting blood glucose level > 5.3 mmol/l and/or either a 1-h postprandial blood glucose level > 7.8 mmol/l, or 2-h postprandial blood glucose level > 6.7 mmol/l. Options for insulin therapy regimens were: ultra-short-acting insulin, once daily long-acting insulin, or a combination of both (basal-bolus). Metformin was occasionally prescribed in obese women (body mass index (BMI) > 30 kg/m^2) in the Deventer hospital (depending on glycaemic control). Based on SMBG women were advised to adjust diet or increase insulin- or metformin dose to maintain blood glucose levels within the target range.

Women were seen at the obstetric outpatient clinic regularly and foetal growth was evaluated by ultrasonography at least every 4 weeks. Moreover, all patients were

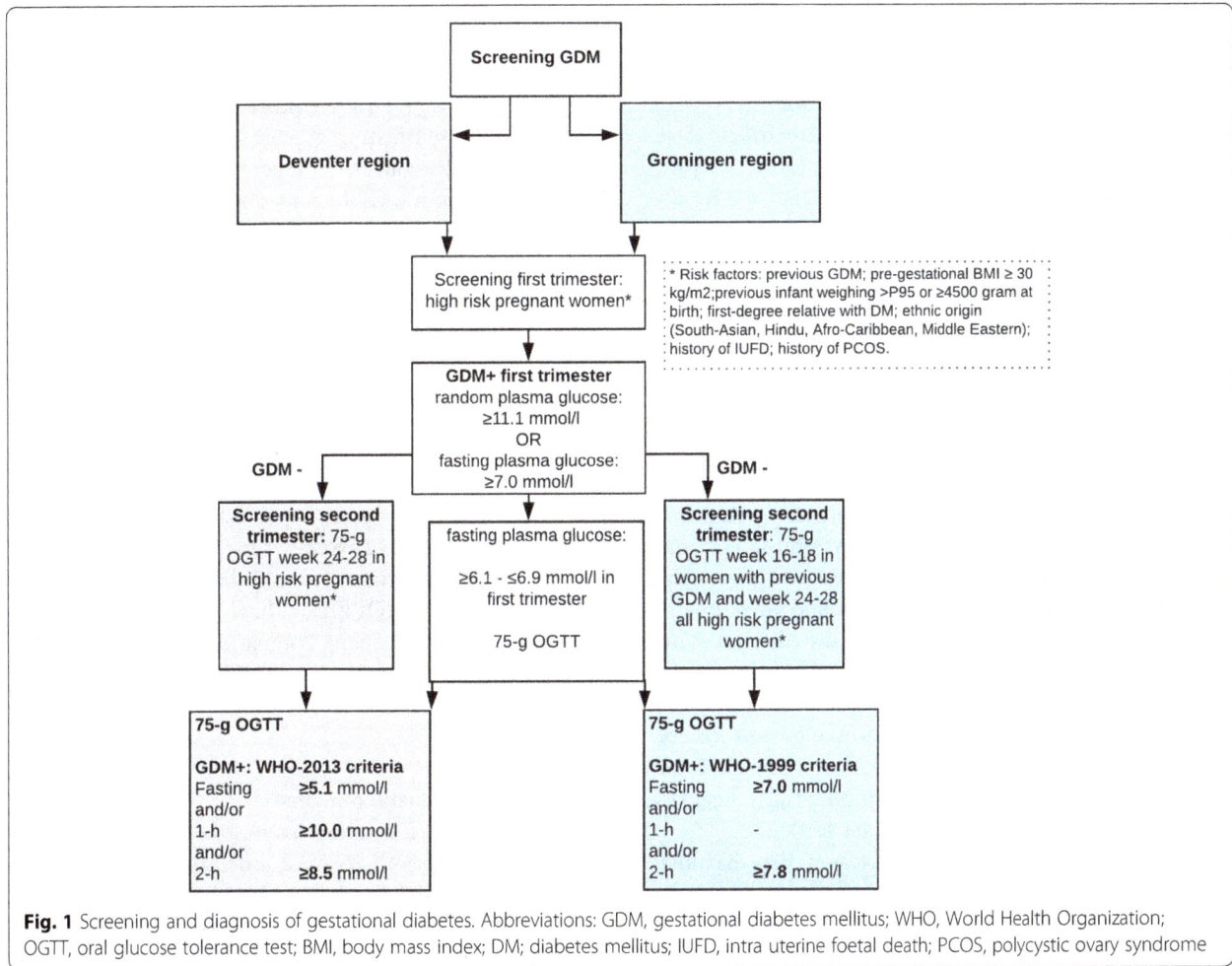

Fig. 1 Screening and diagnosis of gestational diabetes. Abbreviations: GDM, gestational diabetes mellitus; WHO, World Health Organization; OGTT, oral glucose tolerance test; BMI, body mass index; DM; diabetes mellitus; IUFD, intra uterine foetal death; PCOS, polycystic ovary syndrome

discussed every two to three weeks multidisciplinary. Based on similar guidelines in the two regions labour was induced between 38 and 39 weeks of gestation in women on insulin therapy or earlier on indication. In women with a diet, labour was induced between 38 and 40 weeks taking glycaemic control, estimated foetal weight and non-GDM related risk factors into consideration.

Outcomes and definitions

All electronic medical- and birth records were retrospectively reviewed and data between 2011 and 2016 were included in an anonymised database. Maternal characteristics were age, ethnicity (Caucasian, Asian, African American, Mediterranean or unknown), parity, pre-gestational BMI, risk factors for GDM, hypertensive disorders, results of 75-g OGTT, and treatment details. Chronic hypertension was defined as a systolic blood pressure (SBP) ≥140 mmHg and/or a diastolic blood pressure (DBP) ≥90 mmHg at booking before 20 weeks of gestation, or the use of blood-pressure lowering drugs before pregnancy.

Obstetric and neonatal outcomes

Obstetric outcomes collected were induction of labour, mode of delivery (spontaneous vaginal delivery, assisted vaginal delivery (vacuum extraction or forceps), intrapartum caesarean delivery or planned caesarean delivery), gestational age at birth, pregnancy-induced hypertension (PIH) and preeclampsia. PIH was defined as a SBP ≥140 mmHg and/or a DBP ≥90 mmHg, after 20 weeks of gestation in a previously normotensive woman. Preeclampsia was defined ad PIH plus the presence of proteinuria (≥300 mg/24-h) and also included women who had eclampsia and HELLP syndrome.

Neonatal outcomes were birth weight, large for gestational age (LGA; birth weight > 90th percentile, corrected for sex, ethnicity, parity, and gestational age) [21], small for gestational age (SGA; birth weight < 10th percentile, corrected for sex, ethnicity, parity, and gestational age) [21], preterm delivery (delivery before 37 weeks of gestation), 5 min Apgar score < 7, need for respiratory support, still birth/neonatal death, birth trauma (shoulder dystocia, fracture of humerus or clavicle, brachial plexus injury), neonatal hypoglycaemia, neonatal hyperbilirubinaemia, and admission to the neonatology department. Of note, neonates with extreme prematurity (delivery before 28 weeks of gestation, $n = 3$) were excluded prior to the analysis for the variable birth weight. Hyperbilirubinaemia was recorded if the neonate required treatment with phototherapy after birth. Neonatal hypoglycaemia (occurring > 2-h after birth) was defined as a blood glucose level < 2.6 mmol/l or treatment with glucose infusion [16]. Neonates born before 32 weeks ($n = 2$) of gestation with neonatal hypoglycaemia were excluded prior to the analysis as hypoglycaemia could well be caused by prematurity. Respiratory support was defined as the need for continuous positive airway pressure after birth or intubation.

Statistical analyses

Statistical analyses were carried out using statistical package IBM SPSS (version 23.0. Armonk, NY: IBM Corp). Continuous variables are presented as mean ± standard deviation (SD) or as median and inter quartile range (IQR) according to the normal distribution status. Categorical variables are presented as numbers and frequencies (%). Appropriate (non)parametric tests were used to compare differences between the groups for continuous variables (independent t-test or Mann-Whitney U-test in case of skewed distribution) and categorical variables (Chi-square or Fisher's exact test).

To examine the associations between the diagnostic groups and pregnancy outcomes, analyses were performed using logistic regression models in which the ORs and 95% CIs for the WHO-2013 group were calculated using the WHO-1999 group as reference group. Results were presented as unadjusted models and multivariable-adjusted models, with the multivariable-adjusted models adjusted for maternal age, prepregnancy BMI, ethnicity and parity. Only for the variables with sufficient statistical power multivariable-adjusted models were performed. The model analysing the association between the diagnostic groups and LGA-neonates was adjusted for maternal age and prepregnancy BMI. P-value < 0.05 was considered statistically significant.

Results

Maternal characteristics are summarized in Table 1. A total of 1386 women with GDM were included in the study, 437 in the WHO-2013-cohort and 949 in the WHO-1999-cohort. In the WHO-2013-cohort, 49.4% of the women had GDM according to both the WHO-1999 criteria and WHO-2013 criteria. In the WHO-1999-cohort, 24.7% of the GDM women would not have had GDM according to the WHO-2013 criteria.

In total, 1341 women (96.4%) were diagnosed by OGTT and 45 (3.6%) women were already diagnosed in first trimester by a random or fasting glucose level. The median fasting glucose level was higher in the WHO-2013-cohort and the 2-h glucose level was lower, compared to the WHO-1999-cohort. GDM diagnosis was based on elevated fasting glucose level only in 40.2% in the WHO-2013-cohort, compared with 0.8% in the WHO-1999-cohort. GDM was diagnosed based on elevated 2-h value in 10.9% in the WHO-2013-cohort and in 95.4% in the WHO-1999-cohort. Women in the WHO-2013-cohort were diagnosed earlier in pregnancy (24.9 [IQR 23.3–29.0] vs. 27.7 [IQR 25.9–30.7] weeks) and less women had their OGTT performed based on symptoms or signs in third trimester (15.1% vs. 28.5%) instead of screening based on predefined GDM risk-factors. Of the 270 women in the WHO-1999-cohort diagnosed with GDM based on signs suggestive of GDM, 127 (47.0%) retrospectively appeared to have risk factors for GDM. Of these, 12 women tested negative on a first OGTT in the 2nd trimester and 115 women were not screened. In the WHO-2013-cohort 15.6% of the women received insulin treatment compared with 43.4% in the WHO-1999-cohort. In the WHO-2013-cohort, 14 (3.2%) women were treated with metformin.

Obstetric and neonatal outcome

Table 2 summarizes the obstetric outcomes. In the WHO-2013-cohort there were more spontaneous deliveries (73.1% vs. 67.4%, adjusted OR 1.52 (1.15–2.01)), less planned caesarean deliveries (7.8% vs. 11.7%, OR 0.64 (0.43–0.96)). Median gestational age at birth was higher for women in the WHO-2013-cohort (39.0 vs. 38.3 weeks, $p = < 0.001$) and women in the WHO-2013-cohort were less like to have induced labour (59.3% vs. 63.9%, adjusted OR 0.76 (0.59–0.98). There were no differences between the groups with respect to assisted vaginal delivery and intrapartum caesarean delivery. Prevalence of PIH was higher in the WHO-2013-cohort, although no differences were seen between the two groups regarding incidence of preeclampsia.

Table 3 shows the neonatal outcomes. The percentage of LGA neonates (corrected for sex, ethnicity, parity, and gestational age) was lower in the WHO-2013-cohort (16.5% vs. 18.5%, adjusted OR 0.90 (0.66–1.25)), but this was not statistical significant. Birth weight was accordingly higher (3512 vs. 3399 g, $p = < 0.001$). Neonatal hypoglycaemia was more often diagnosed in offspring of the WHO-2013-cohort (9.6% vs. 4.2%, adjusted OR 2.48 (1.52–4.05)). There were no significant differences seen between the two groups with respect to neonatal hyperbilirubinaemia, preterm delivery, birth weight in categories, SGA, 5 min Apgar score < 7, need for respiratory support, birth trauma, still birth/neonatal death, and admission to the neonatology department.

Table 1 Maternal characteristics of women diagnosed with gestational diabetes mellitus

Characteristics	Cohort		
	WHO-2013	WHO-1999	P-value*
N	437	949	
Age (years)	34.7 ± 5.1	32.1 ± 5.1	< 0.001
Ethnicity, n (%)			< 0.001
Caucasian	357 (81.7)	741 (78.1)	
Asian	9 (2.1)	72 (7.6)	
African-American	2 (0.5)	39 (4.1)	
Mediterranean	64 (14.6)	69 (7.3)	
Unknown	5 (1.1)	28 (3.0)	
Parity, n (%)			0.232
0	158 (36.2)	386 (40.7)	
1–2	242 (55.5)	499 (52.6)	
> 2	36 (8.3)	64 (6.7)	
First degree relative with DM, n (%)	82 (18.8)	376 (41.1)	< 0.001
History of PCOS, n (%)	10 (2.3)	50 (5.3)	0.011
History of GDM, n (%)	44 (10.1)	103 (10.9)	0.650
Previous infant weighing ≥4500 g at birth, n (%)	42 (9.6)	97 (10.2)	0.716
History of IUFD, n (%)	4 (0.9)	20 (2.1)	0.113
Pre-gestational BMI (kg/m^2)	29.7 [26.0–34.4]	27.7 [24.2–31.8]	< 0.001
Pre-gestational BMI, n (%)			< 0.001
< 25 kg/m^2	88 (20.8)	291 (31.5)	
25–29.9 kg/m^2	129 (30.4)	288 (31.2)	
≥ 30 kg/m^2	207 (48.8)	344 (37.3)	
Chronic hypertension, n (%)	8 (1.8)	43 (4.5)	0.013
Indication for OGTT, n (%)			< 0.001
Screening based on risk factors	362 (82.8)	650 (68.5)	
Diagnostic test based on symptoms/signs	66 (15.1)	270 (28.5)	
Unknown	9 (2.1)	29 (3.1)	
Diagnosis based on OGTT, n (%)‡	422 (96.6)	919 (96.8)	0.791
Gestational age at time of OGTT (weeks)	24.9 [23.3–29.0]	27.7 [25.9–30.7]	< 0.001
Gestational age at time of OGTT screening only (weeks)	24.4 [22.6–26.9]	27.3 [25.1–28.7]	< 0.001
Gestational age at time of OGTT diagnostic 3rd trimester only (weeks)	33.1 [28.7–35.3]	30.4 [27.7–33.6]	0.001
75-g OGTT			
Fasting glucose level (mmol/l)	5.3 [5.1–5.6]	5.0 [4.6–5.5]	< 0.001
1-h glucose level (mmol/l)	9.6 [8.0–10.5]	–	NA
2-h glucose level (mmol/l)	7.7 [6.6–9.0]	8.6 [8.1–9.4]	< 0.001
Diagnosis based on elevated fasting glucose level only, n (%)	170 (40.2)	8 (0.9)	< 0.001
Diagnosis based on elevated 2-h glucose level only, n (%)	46 (10.9)	877 (95.4)	< 0.001
Insulin treatment, n (%)	68 (15.6)	412 (43.4)	< 0.001
Metformin treatment, n (%)	14 (3.2)	–	NA

Abbreviations: WHO World health Organization, *BMI* body mass index, *DM* diabetes mellitus, *IUFD* intrauterine foetal death, *PCOS* polycystic ovary syndrome, *OGTT* oral glucose tolerance test, *NA* not applicable. Data are expressed as mean ± SD, median [IQR], or proportion of n (%)
*P-values were based on Student's unpaired *t*-test (non-skewed continuous variables), Mann-Whitney U-Test (skewed continuous variables) or chi-square test (categorical variables)
‡Total number of women diagnosed with a 75-g OGTT. The other women (*n* = 45) were diagnosed with a random or fasting glucose level in first trimester of their pregnancy. Data with respect to first degree relative with DM 35 (3.7%) (WHO-1999-cohort), BMI 13 (3.0%) (WHO-2013-cohort) and 26 (2.7%) (WHO-1999-cohort), gestational age at time of OGTT 15 (1.6%) (WHO-1999-cohort), are missing

Table 2 Obstetric outcomes of women diagnosed with gestational diabetes mellitus

Outcome variable	Cohort		P-value*	OR**	Adjusted OR**
	WHO-2013	WHO-1999			
N	437	949			
Induction of labour, n (%)	256 (59.3)	606 (63.9)	0.102	0.82 (0.65–1.04)	0.76 (0.59–0.98)
Delivery type, n (%)					
Spontaneous vaginal delivery	318 (73.1)	638 (67.4)	0.032	1.32 (1.02–1.70)	1.52 (1.15–2.01)
Assisted vaginal delivery	35 (8.0)	79 (8.3)	0.712	0.93 (0.61–1.40)	NA
Intrapartum caesarean delivery	48 (11.0)	121 (12.8)	0.365	0.85 (0.60–1.21)	NA
Planned caesarean delivery	34 (7.8)	111 (11.7)	0.029	0.64 (0.43–0.96)	NA
Gestational age at birth (weeks)	39.0 [38.3–39.6]	38.3 [38.0–39.0]	< 0.001	NA	NA
Pregnancy-induced hypertension, n (%)	50 (11.5)	61 (6.4)	0.001	1.89 (1.28–2.80)	1.71 (1.11–2.63)
Preeclampsia, n (%)	12 (2.8)	30 (3.2)	0.683	0.87 (0.44–1.71)	NA

Abbreviations: WHO World health Organization, *OR* odds ratios, *NA* not applicable. Data are expressed as mean ± SD, or proportion of n (%)
*P-values were based on Student's unpaired t-test (non-skewed continuous variables), or chi-square test (categorical variables)
**OR, 95% confidence intervals were derived from logistic regression models using the WHO-1999 group as reference group. Multivariable adjustment included maternal age, pre-gestational body mass index, ethnicity and parity. When the statistical power of a variable was not sufficient or the outcome variable was continuous 'NA' was reported

Discussion

This multicentre, retrospective cohort study shows the pregnancy outcomes in two cohorts applying different diagnostic criteria for GDM i.e. WHO-2013 and WHO-1999. Women in the WHO-2013-cohort had a higher pre-gestational BMI and more often PIH. However, they were diagnosed earlier, less often needed insulin therapy and had a higher percentage of spontaneous deliveries. No other differences in adverse obstetric and neonatal outcomes were seen between the two cohorts.

A number of previous international studies have addressed the effects of introduction of the WHO-2013

Table 3 Neonatal outcomes of women diagnosed with gestational diabetes mellitus

Outcome variable	Cohort		P-value*	OR**	Adjusted OR**
	WHO-2013	WHO-1999			
N	437	949			
Preterm delivery, n (%)	27 (6.2)	60 (6.3)	0.934	0.98 (0.61–1.57)	NA
Birth weight (g)	3512 ± 459	3399 ± 532	< 0.001	NA	NA
Birth weight, n (%)			0.136	NA	NA
Infants < 4000 g	384 (87.9)	831 (87.8)			
Infants 4000–4499 g	42 (9.6)	104 (11.0)			
Infants ≥4500 g	11 (2.5)	11 (1.2)			
Large for gestational age, n (%) ‡	72 (16.5)	176 (18.5)	0.379	0.87 (0.65–1.18)	0.90 (0.66–1.25)
Small for gestational age, n (%) ‡	14 (3.2)	37 (3.9)	0.538	0.82 (0.44–1.54)	NA
5 min Apgar < 7, n (%)	7 (1.6)	32 (3.4)	0.068	0.47 (0.21–1.08)	NA
Respiratory support, n (%)	14 (3.2)	37 (3.9)	0.519	0.81 (0.44–1.52)	NA
Birth trauma, n (%)	15 (3.4)	30 (3.2)	0.791	1.09 (0.58–2.05)	NA
Hypoglycaemia, n (%)	42 (9.6)	40 (4.2)	< 0.001	2.41 (1.54–3.78)	2.48 (1.52–4.05)
Hyperbilirubinaemia, n (%)	4 (0.9)	24 (2.5)	0.062	0.36 (0.12–1.03)	NA
Still birth/neonatal death, n (%)	1 (0.2)	2 (0.2)	1.000	NA	NA
Admission to the neonatology department, n (%)	54 (12.4)	139 (14.6)	0.272	0.83 (0.59–1.16)	0.79 (0.55–1.14)

Abbreviations: WHO World health Organization, *OR* odds ratios, *NA* not applicable. Data are expressed as mean ± SD, or proportion of n (%)
*P-values were based on Student's unpaired t-test (non-skewed continuous variables), or chi-square test (categorical variables)
**OR, 95% confidence intervals were derived from logistic regression models using the WHO-1999 group as reference group. Multivariable adjustment included maternal age, pre-gestational body mass index, ethnicity and parity. Large for gestational age was adjusted for maternal age and pre-gestational body mass index. Only for the variables with sufficient statistical power multivariable adjustment was performed. When the statistical power was not sufficient or the outcome variable was continuous 'NA' was reported
‡Corrected for sex, ethnicity, parity, and gestational age

criteria on pregnancy outcomes [22–27]. They retrospectively studied pregnancy outcomes in women previously classified as non-GDM with other diagnostic criteria and newly defined as GDM with the WHO-2013 criteria [22–27]. These studies suggested that women newly diagnosed with the WHO-2013 criteria if untreated were at increased risk for adverse pregnancy outcomes, including PIH, preeclampsia, neonatal intensive care admission, caesarean section, shoulder dystocia, macrosomia and LGA neonates, compared to non-GDM women [22–27]. In contrast to the aforementioned studies, women in our study both diagnosed with WHO-2013 or WHO-1999 criteria were treated similarly according to our national guideline. Two comparable studies with regard to treatment and comparison of two diagnostic approaches (Carpenter-Coustan criteria compared with the WHO-2013 criteria) showed that the percentage of LGA neonates was lower in the WHO-2013-cohort [28, 29]. In addition, one study also showed a reduction in caesarean deliveries, PIH, and assisted delivery after implementation of the WHO-2013 criteria [29].

In terms of the likelihood of having an LGA neonate, we found no significant differences between women diagnosed having GDM on the WHO-2013 criteria and women diagnosed having GDM on the WHO-1999 criteria. However, the percentage LGA neonates was lower in the WHO-2013-cohort. The reduction of LGA neonates is an important treatment target in GDM, since LGA is associated with short- and long term complications for the neonate. There are several potential explanations for the lower rates of LGA neonates in the WHO-2013-cohort found in our study and others [28, 29]. Firstly, the WHO-2013 criteria included a new group of women: 40.2% of the women were only diagnosed based on the fasting glucose cut-off value compared to 0.8% in the WHO-1999-cohort. By applying the more strict WHO-2013 criteria the prevalence of GDM increases, including presumably more mild cases of GDM, resulting in a lower percentage of LGA neonates. Several other studies have demonstrated that implementation of the WHO-2013 increases the prevalence of GDM [4, 14]. Moreover, a lower percentage of women in our WHO-2013-cohort (15.6%) required additional insulin therapy compared with the WHO-1999-cohort (43.4%).

Secondly, women in the WHO-2013-cohort were screened and diagnosed with GDM earlier (WHO-2013-cohort: median ~ 25 weeks, WHO-1999-cohort: median ~ 28 weeks), so that group had earlier dietary or insulin intervention. More women in the WHO-1999-cohort were diagnosed based on signs suggestive of GDM (e.g. polyhydramnios/foetal macrosomia). Therefore the WHO-1999-cohort may include women with a more advanced stage of GDM leading to higher rates of LGA. Nevertheless, approximately 50% of all women

diagnosed with GDM based on signs suggestive of GDM, retrospectively had a risk factor for GDM that justified 2nd trimester screening in the first place. However, even when we only considered women who were diagnosed based on 2nd trimester screening because of GDM risk factors, gestational age at diagnoses remained different between the groups. The earlier screening and diagnosis of GDM in the WHO-2013-cohort could have led to earlier treatment and therefore to a better outcome. Landon et al. also demonstrated that offering early treatment to women with modest degrees of hyperglycaemia in pregnancy results in reduction of foetal overgrowth [30].

The only obstetric parameters which differed between the two cohorts were the higher incidence of planned caesarean section and induction of labour in the WHO-1999-cohort. This may be due to difference in clinical obstetric practice between both regions. But may also be due to differences related to GDM including more estimated macrosomia on ultrasound, worse glycaemic control indicated by significantly more insulin therapy.

An increase in neonatal hypoglycaemia was seen in the WHO-2013-cohort. This can be explained by an active screening policy in all neonates in the hospital that used the WHO-2013 criteria unlike the "WHO-1999 hospitals", that screened neonates by indication. This finding suggests that roughly 50% neonatal hypoglycaemia might be missed without active screening, potentially leading to long-term adverse outcomes. Moreover, in the WHO-2013-cohort a higher percentage of women were diagnosed with PIH. In the WHO-1999-cohort more women were diagnosed with chronic hypertension in first trimester of their pregnancy. This finding suggests that the difference in PIH between the WHO-2013-cohort and WHO-1999-cohort also can be explained by an earlier diagnosis of chronic hypertension in first trimester in the WHO-1999 cohort.

This study gives no information on differences in incidence of GDM between the two diagnostic approaches. In the WHO-2013-cohort, 50.6% of the women were positive for GDM according the WHO-2013 criteria only and 49.4% had GDM according to both the WHO-2013 criteria and WHO-1999 criteria. Both cohorts differed in some clinical characteristics: women in the WHO-2013 cohort were older, had a higher pre-gestational BMI and were more often diagnosed on the fasting glucose level compared with the WHO-1999-cohort. These factors are associated with a less favourable metabolic profile. Although the WHO-2013-cohort seemingly consisted of a group of women with milder glucose intolerance, they appeared to have a worse metabolic profile. It seems that the WHO-2013 criteria have a better ability to select women with a worse metabolic profile.

The main strength of this study is that it evaluates the pregnancy outcomes of women with GDM diagnosed by the old and new WHO-criteria in a real-life clinical setting. Moreover, after GDM diagnosis all women were treated equally based on the national guideline. Several potential limitations of this study should be noted. First, this study was conducted in three different hospitals in two regions of the Netherlands. It is possible that the study populations and obstetric management between the hospitals were different. One centre is a tertiary care centre and two are larger secondary care centres and this might have led to a selection bias. However, the only important difference between secondary care centres and tertiary care centres in the Netherlands is the referral function for deliveries under 32 weeks of gestational age for neonatal purposes. In all other aspects, population and care is comparable. Secondly, the study was limited by its retrospective study design and this resulted in missing data for some variables in the electronic medical- and birth records. Thirdly, the sample size was limited to find significant differences between the groups for relatively rare pregnancy outcomes, such as birth trauma, still birth/neonatal death, and preeclampsia. Due to the lack of statistical power for some pregnancy outcomes it was not possible to adjust these outcomes for possible confounding factors. Finally, this study gives no information on differences in incidence of GDM between the two diagnostic approaches since the exact number of pregnant women in the two populations is not known. The national guideline advocate targeted testing for GDM, and therefore we do not have data on universal testing.

Conclusions

In summary, this study demonstrated that application of the WHO-2013 criteria was associated with a reduced need for insulin treatment and more spontaneous deliveries. Although an earlier diagnosis of GDM might contribute to these differences, milder GDM by selection is proposed to play a major role. No differences were found in adverse pregnancy outcomes between the two diagnostic approaches.

This study contributes to the current debate regarding the value of implementation of new WHO-2013 diagnostic criteria for GDM but cannot provide a definitive answer. The data of well conducted population-based randomised studies (and meta-analyses) directly comparing the two diagnostic approaches are necessary to determine whether treatment of women with mild GDM is beneficial and cost-effective. Moreover, there is more information needed whether women with a 2-h glucose value between ≥7.8 - ≤8.4 mmol/l can be safely left untreated.

Abbreviations

BMI: Body mass index; DBP: Diastolic blood pressure; DM: Diabetes mellitus; GDM: Gestational diabetes mellitus; HAPO: Hyperglycemia and Adverse Pregnancy Outcomes; IADPSG: International Association of the Diabetes and Pregnancy Study Groups; IQR: Inter quartile range; LGA: Large for gestational age; OGTT: Oral glucose tolerance test; PIH: Pregnancy-induced hypertension; SBP: Systolic blood pressure; SD: Standard deviation; SGA: Small for gestational age; SMBG: Self-monitoring of the blood glucose levels; WHO: World Health Organization

Funding

Novo Nordisk Netherlands provided an unrestricted research grant for studying the WHO-1999-cohort. The study sponsor was not involved in the designs of the study; the collection, analysis and interpretation of data; writing the report; or the decision to submit the report for publication.

Authors' contributions

EARG, SHK collected and analyzed the data and wrote most of the manuscript under supervision. JJZ, PPB conceived and designed the study and participated in the planning of the project, interpretation of data and writing process and reviewing the manuscript. KH, FJK, HLL, MJMD, and ES made intellectual contributions to the manuscript and have read and approved the final version.

Competing interests

The authors declare that they have no competing interests. Novo Nordisk Netherlands provided an unrestricted research grant for studying the WHO-1999-cohort (SHK and BHRW). The study sponsor was not involved in the designs of the study; the collection, analysis and interpretation of data; writing the report; or the decision to submit the report for publication.

Author details

[1]Department of Obstetrics and Gynaecology, Deventer Hospital, Deventer, the Netherlands. [2]Department of Endocrinology, University of Groningen, University Medical Center Groningen, PO Box 30.001, 9700 RB Groningen, the Netherlands. [3]Department of Internal Medicine, Martini Hospital, Groningen, the Netherlands. [4]Department of Obstetrics and Gynaecology, Martini Hospital, Groningen, the Netherlands. [5]Department of Internal Medicine, Medical Center Leeuwarden, Leeuwarden, the Netherlands. [6]Department of Internal Medicine, Deventer Hospital, Deventer, the Netherlands. [7]Department of Obstetrics and Gynaecology, University of Groningen, University Medical Center Groningen, Groningen, the Netherlands.

References

1. American Diabetes Association. Diagnosis and classification of diabetes mellitus. Diabetes Care. 2014;37(suppl 1):s81–90.
2. Hunt KJ, Schuller KL. The increasing prevalence of diabetes in pregnancy. Obstet Gynecol Clin N Am. 2007;34:173–99.
3. Ferrara A. Increasing prevalence of gestational diabetes mellitus: a public health perspective. Diabetes Care. 2007;30(suppl 2):s141–6.

4. Moses RG, Morris GJ, Petocz P, San Gil F, Garg D. The impact of potential new diagnostic criteria on the prevalence of gestational diabetes mellitus in Australia. Med J Aust. 2011;194:338.

5. Yang X, Hsu-Hage B, Zhang H, Zhang C, Zhang Y, Zhang C. Women with impaired glucose tolerance during pregnancy have significantly poor pregnancy outcomes. Diabetes Care. 2002;25:1619–24.

6. Langer O, Yogev Y, Most O, Xenakis EMJ. Gestational diabetes: the consequences of not treating. Obstet Gynecol. 2005;192:989–97.

7. Sermer M, Naylor CD, Gare DJ, Kenshole AB, Ritchie J, Farine D, et al. Impact of increasing carbohydrate intolerance on maternal-fetal outcomes in 3637 women without gestational diabetes: the Toronto tri-hospital gestational diabetes project. Obstet Gynecol. 1995;173:146–56.

8. Brown J, Alwan NA, West J, Brown S, Mckinlay CJ, Farrar D, Crowther CA. Lifestyle interventions for the treatment of women with gestational diabetes. Cochrane Database Syst Rev. 2017;5:cd01197.

9. Hapo Study Cooperative Research Group. Hyperglycemia and adverse pregnancy outcomes. N Engl J Med. 2008;358:1991–2002.

10. International association of diabetes and pregnancy study groups consensus panel. International association of diabetes and pregnancy study groups recommendations on the diagnosis and classification of hyperglycemia in pregnancy. Diabetes Care. 2010;33:676–82.

11. World Health Organization. Diagnostic criteria and classification of hyperglycemia first detected in pregnancy. 2013.http://apps.who.int/iris/bitstream/10665/85975/1/who_nmh_mnd_13.2_eng.pdf. Accessed 2 Jun 2017.

12. Hod M, Kapur A, Sacks DA, Hadar E, Agarwal M, Di Renzo GC, et al. The international federation of gynecology and obstetrics (figo) initiative on gestational diabetes mellitus: a pragmatic guide for diagnosis, management, and care. Int J Gynaecol Obstet. 2015;131(suppl 3):s173–211.

13. Benhalima K, Damm P, Van Assche A, Mathieu C, Devlieger R, Mahmood T, et al. Screening for gestational diabetes in europe: where do we stand and how to move forward?: a scientific paper commissioned by the european board & college of obstetrics and gynaecology (ebcog). Eur J Obstet Gynecol Reprod Biol. 2016;201:192–6.

14. Cundy T, Ackermann E, Ryan EA. Gestational diabetes: new criteria may triple the prevalence but effect on outcomes is unclear. BMJ. 2014;348:g1567.

15. Visser GHA, De Valk HW. Is the evidence strong enough to change the diagnostic criteria for gestational diabetes now? Obstet Gynecol. 2013;208:260–4.

16. The Dutch Society Of Obestetrics And Gynaecology. Diabetes mellitus and pregnancy. Clinical guideline version 2.0. 2010. http://www.nvog-documenten.nl/index.php?pagina=/richtlijn/item/pagina.php&richtlijn_id=863. Accessed 2 Jun 2017.

17. World Health Organization. Definition and classification of diabetes mellitus and its complications. In: Report of a who consultation. Part 1: diagnosis and classification of diabetes mellitus. Geneva: WHO; 1999. Department of noncommunicable disease surveillance.

18. Koning SH, Hoogenberg K, Scheuneman KA, Baas MG, Korteweg FJ, Sollie KM, et al. Neonatal and obstetric outcomes in diet- and insulin-treated women with gestational diabetes mellitus: a retrospective study. BMC Endocr Disord. 2016;16:52.

19. Koning SH, Scheuneman KA, Lutgers H, Korteweg FJ, Van Den Berg G, Sollie KM, et al. Risk stratification for healthcare planning in women with gestational diabetes mellitus. Neth J Med. 2016;74:262–9.

20. University Medical Center Groningen. Research Code University Medical Center Groningen. 2013. *https://www.umcg.nl/sitecollectiondocuments/english/researchcode/umcg-researchcode,%20basic%20principles%202013.pdf.* Accessed 2 June 2017.

21. Visser GH, Eilers PH, Elferink-Stinkens PM, Merkus HM, Wit JM. New dutch reference curves for birthweight by gestational age. Early Hum Dev. 2009;85:737–44.

22. Laafira A, White SW, Griffin CJ, Graham D. Impact of the new iadpsg gestational diabetes diagnostic criteria on pregnancy outcomes in Western Australia. Aust N Z J Obstet Gynaecol. 2016;56:36–41.

23. Benhalima K, Hanssens M, Devlieger R, Verhaeghe J, Mathieu C. Analysis of pregnancy outcomes using the new iadpsg recommendation compared with the carpenter and coustan criteria in an area with a low prevalence of gestational diabetes. Int J Endocrinol. 2013;2013:248121.

24. Meek C, Lewis HB, Patient C, Murphy HR, Simmons D. Diagnosis of gestational diabetes mellitus: falling through the net. Diabetologia. 2015;58:2003–12.

25. O'sullivan E, Avalos G, O'reilly M, Dennedy M, Gaffney G, Dunne F, et al. Atlantic diabetes in pregnancy (dip): the prevalence and outcomes of gestational diabetes mellitus using new diagnostic criteria. Diabetologia. 2011;54:1670–5.

26. Lapolla A, Dalfrà M, Ragazzi E, De Cata A, Fedele D. New international association of the diabetes and pregnancy study groups (iadpsg) recommendations for diagnosing gestational diabetes compared with former criteria: a retrospective study on pregnancy outcome. Diabet Med. 2011;28:1074–7.

27. Ethridge JK Jr, Catalano PM, Waters TP. Perinatal outcomes associated with the diagnosis of gestational diabetes made by the international association of the diabetes and pregnancy study groups criteria. Obstet Gynecol. 2014;124:571–8.

28. Hung T. The effects of implementing the international association of diabetes and pregnancy study groups criteria for diagnosing gestational diabetes on maternal and neonatal outcomes. PLoS One. 2015;10:e0122261.

29. Duran A, Saenz S, Torrejon MJ, Bordiu E, Del Valle L, Galindo M, et al. Introduction of iadpsg criteria for the screening and diagnosis of gestational diabetes mellitus results in improved pregnancy outcomes at a lower cost in a large cohort of pregnant women: the st. Carlos gestational diabetes study. Diabetes Care. 2014;37:2442–50.

30. Landon MB, Spong CY, Thom E, Carpenter MW, Ramin SM, Casey B, et al. A multicenter, randomized trial of treatment for mild gestational diabetes. N Engl J Med. 2009;361:1339–48.

Delayed interval delivery of the second twin in a woman with altered markers of inflammation

George Daskalakis[1], Panagiotis Fotinopoulos[1]* ⓘ, Vasilios Pergialiotis[2], Mariana Theodora[1], Panagiotis Antsaklis[1], Michail Sindos[1], Nikolaos Papantoniou[2] and Dimitrios Loutradis[1]

Abstract

Background: Delayed interval intertwin delivery rates are expected to rise during the next years as potent and targeted tocolytic agents are employed and antenatal surveillance methods become more sophisticated and specific in predicting the critical delivery timepoint of optimal perinatal outcome.

Case presentation: We present a case of delayed intertwin delivery after delivery of the first twin due to premature prelabor rupture of the membranes. Maternal serum White Blood Cells and C-Reactive Protein levels remained high until delivery of the second twin (34 days after the first was delivered), although maternal temperature remained constant. The mother underwent close antenatal surveillance and she was hospitalized. She had an uncomplicated delivery of the second twin at 29^{+2} weeks by cesarean section due to an abnormal Non-Stress Test.

Conclusion: We strongly suggest future evaluation of maternal serum inflammatory markers among these rare cases as these could predict intraamniotic infection.

Keywords: Intertwin , Delayed , Delivery , Monitoring , Inflammation

Background

The rate of multiple pregnancies over the last three decades has increased dramatically due to extended implementation of Artificial Reproduction Techniques (ART) [1]. The rate of twin pregnancies in the U.S. has climbed to 33.2 per 1.000 births in 2009 (increased by 76% since 1980) [2] . Higher order pregnancies remained constant from 2001 until a steep rise of 4% (153.5 per 100,000 births) in 2009 [2]. About 50% of live births in twins are preterm (< 37 weeks of gestational age), whereas higher order pregnancies are almost entirely born premature preterm. Furthermore it seems that ART twin pregnancies (regardless as to whether they are In Vitro Fertilization or not) have a tendency to be born prematurely than the naturally conceived ones [3] .

Although preterm deliveries seem to rise the last 20years, an unexpected inverse variance with birth weight is also noted, leading to the assumption that fetal growth is improved, possibly due to better antenatal surveillance [4]. Perinatal outcome is negatively affected by low and very low birth weight. Therefore, all efforts by means of improved antenatal surveillance and therapeutic tocolysis should be focused on controlling prolongation of the pregnancy. Twin pregnancy that is complicated by very preterm delivery of the first fetus is a challenge in modern obstetrics and, to date, evidence regarding the optimal time of delivery of the second twin is lacking. Although, clinical chorioamnionitis (including fever, uterine tenderness and presence of contractions) is an absolute indication for delivery, to date, there is no consensus regarding the method of antenatal surveillance of twin pregnancies that are complicated with expulsion of the first fetus in the second, or early third trimester. In the present study we report a case of

* Correspondence: fotinopoulos@hotmail.com
[1]1st Department of Obstetrics and Gynecology, Athens Medical School, Alexandra General Hospital, 9 Aristeidou Street , 17563 P. Faliro, Athens, Greece
Full list of author information is available at the end of the article

delayed interval delivery of the second twin 34 days following delivery of the first.

Case presentation

A thirty four years-old G2P1 woman was admitted in the high risk pregnancy unit of our The First Dpt of Obstetrics and Gynecology at 23^{+4} weeks of twin gestation due to premature prelabor rupture of the membranes (*PPROM*). The twins were dichorionic according to the first trimester ultrasound scan. The patient reported the presence of increased "vaginal discharge" during the last week. Nitrazine tape test was positive showing amniotic fluid leakage. She had an uncomplicated previous singleton term vaginal delivery 3 years ago. Her personal medical history revealed the presence of hypothyroidism that was treated with thyroxine 175 mcg twice a day, an appendicectomy 12 years ago and cervical cryotherapy for Human Papilloma Virus (HPV) 1 year ago.

During physical examination, she was normotensive, afebrile and the cervix was not dilated or effaced. Laboratory examinations at admission were obtained and revealed the presence of mild leucocytosis ($12,300/\mu$l) and an elevated C- Reactive Protein (CRP) (40.98 mg/L with upper normal laboratory limit of 1.0 mg/L), while both dipstick urine examination and urinary cultures were normal. The patient received amoxicillin and metronidazole regimen eight hourly for 10 days and betamethasone 12 mg intramuscularly with a repeated dose at 24 h. Ultrasound examination revealed the presence of two embryos with positive cardiac function that weighted 535 and 606 g. The first of them had an amniotic fluid index (*AFI*) of 5 cm and the second an AFI of 14 cm. The patient's cervical length was 28 mm and funneling was not noted. Ultrasonographic and laboratory assessment was performed every 3 days. Three days later WBCs were raised ($14,200/\mu$l) whereas CRP value declined at 2.90 mg/L.

One week following admission (24^{+4}) the patient experienced blood stained brownish vaginal secretions and the vaginal examination revealed a Bishop score of 8. She was transferred to the labor ward where she delivered a female that weighted 550 g. Manual extraction of the placenta failed and the umbilical cord was ligated just above the level of the external cervical os. The vagina was rinsed with antiseptic solution (povidone iodine, Betadine®) and she remained in the labor ward under close surveillance of vital signs and fetal heart rate for the next 4 h. No signs of active labor were noticed. After informed consent and detailed counselling about the possible benefits and complications, the woman opted for delayed delivery of the second twin.

The next day the delivered twin died from respiratory distress syndrome. Blood samples were obtained from the patient that once again revealed raised white blood cells (WBCs) ($12,400/\mu$l) and increased CRP (13.14 mg/L). The patient remained in the high-risk pregnancy department and 5 days later she had a new blood and urine examination along with urine cultures that revealed elevated WBCs ($13.900/\mu$l), an a steep rise in CRP (31.78 mg/L) along with the presence of enterobacteriae spp. An expert in infectious diseases was advised and the patient received cefuroxime 750 mg eight hourly for 7 days. The surveillance protocol involved close laboratory assessment (WBC and CRP levels three times a week), ultrasonographic evaluation twice a week, vital signs clinical assessment (arterial pressure, heart rate, temperature) and electronic fetal monitoring (non stress test, NST) twice a day . The fluctuations of CRP and WBC values during the patient's hospitalization are shown in the Fig. 1. She remained afebrile with no clinical evidence of chorioamnionitis. A repeated dose of steroids was administered to the patient during her 26th and 27th day of hospitalization (28th week of gestation).

The second female fetus was finally delivered 34 days after the first fetus (29^{+2}) with cesarean section due to an abnormal NST. The neonate weighed 1150 g and had an Apgar score of 7 at the first minute and 9 at 5 minutes. It remained in the Neonatal Intensive Care Unit (NICU) for about 4 weeks.

Discussion

Prematurity and very low birth weight pose great risks for the neonate due to inability of its organs to adapt. Respiratory Distress Syndrome (RDS), sepsis, necrotizing enterocolitis, intraventricular hemorrhage and periventricular leucomalacia) are common complications that are attributed to prematurity. In a previous study, tocolytics, antenatal steroids and surfactant administration within the first 2 hours following delivery were the most important predictors of neonatal survival for twins born between 22 and 26 weeks of gestational age [5]. The advancement of gestational age is very important in extremely premature neonates (less than 27 weeks of gestational age) as each day improves survival rates and decrease the duration of hospitalization in the NICU [6] . In singleton, neonatal survival following delivery at 24, 25, and 26 weeks is estimated to be 31.2, 59.1, and 75.3%, respectively [7]. In multiple gestations, the mortality rate reaches 32% from 23 to 25 weeks' gestational age, compared to 19.2% from 26 to 27 weeks' gestational age and 11.1% in all gestational age [8].

In multiple gestations with preterm delivery of the first baby, the second is usually delivered within a short time frame. Occasionally, however, uterine contractions stop and the cervix reconstitutes.The condition is referred to as Delayed Interval Delivery (DID) of the second twin. Due to the rarity of DID, standard protocols for the management of these patients don't exist.

Contraindication for delayed delivery are fetal distress, congenital abnormalities, preterm rupture of membranes of the remaining fetus, chorioamnionitis, monoamniotic or monochorionic pregnancies, and severe vaginal blood loss. The aseptic ligation of the umbilical cord stump close to the placenta reduces the risk of developing infection due to maceration and is practiced in these cases. Some authors routinely perform cervical cerclage immediately after the first delivery while others don't recommend it. Arabin and van Eyck (2009) suggest that cerclage should be best avoided due to concerns of chorioamnionitis. On the contrary, Zhang et al. (2003) support cerclage, because it can minimize fetal membranes' exposure to vaginal bacteria and acidity, prolonging delay interval.

Numerous studies were published during the last decade addressing the case of delayed interval delivery of the second twin. One of the largest series was recorded from a population based study in the U.S. [9] .The authors concluded that when fetal expulsion of the first twin occurred between 22 and 23 weeks the prolongation of the intertwin interval could decrease perinatal mortality of the second twin. Interestingly, however, this beneficial effect persisted up to 3 weeks following delivery of the first twin. When the interval was prolonged more than 4 weeks the incidence of a Small for Gestational Age (SGA) second twin was also increased. Although 5 min Apgar scores less than 7 significantly decreased, they were not accompanied by a subsequent reduction in rates of respiratory distress syndrome. Arabin et al. confirmed these results stating that although the prolongation of the interval led to decreased perinatal mortality and morbidity of the second twin it was followed by an increase in the prevalence of SGA neonates [10]. The same authors extended their study in triplet gestations and found that regardless the interval between the first and second fetus, the third triplet was delivered at a maximum interval of 2 days, following delivery of the second triplet.

Farkouh et al. observed in pregnancies with delivery of the first twin during the 22th week of gestation that the concurrent placement of cerclage increased the intertwin delivery interval compared to pregnancies with delivery of the first twin after removal of an elective cerclage (≥49 vs ≤26 days) [11] . The same authors concluded that even modest intervals of delivery could improve neonatal morbidity and mortality. However, we must underline the fact that all women in their series received routine antibiotic and tocolytic therapy and amniocentesis of the remaining twin was offered prior to cerclage placement to preclude intraamniotic infection. Furthermore, all pregnant women were informed that although the procedure could increase the intertwin delivery interval, the fetal outcome and the occurrence of maternal morbidity could not be excluded.

Zhang et al. retrospectively analyzed 7 cases that were offered cervical cerclage after delivery of the first twin and found that the procedure did not increase the risk for intrauterine infection [12]. Recent systematic review by Feys et al., shows clear evidence of lower mortality risk of the second twin with DID [13] .

In our case, the leading twin after PPROM and amniotic fluid leakage was finally delivered by normal labor. We chose not to perform an episiotomy during its delivery. Maternal laboratory examinations were initially suggestive of the presence of infection, however there was no clinical evidence, as uterine tenderness and fever were absent. The mother was informed regarding the potential existence of chorioamnionitis and was offered the chance to perform amniocentesis to preclude infection; however she declined the operation and wished to continue her pregnancy with conservative treatment. WBCs and CRP were routinely assessed every 3 days, or once a day when a steep rise was observed (Fig. 1).

WBCs fluctuated between higher normal limits (12,000/µl) and 24,700/µl, whereas CRP was continuously at least 2-fold higher than higher normal laboratory limit (although the fluctuation of its levels could not be clinically interpreted). During delivery the vagina was cleansed with antiseptic solution and a high umbilical cord ligation was performed (above the level of the external cervical os). Given the presence of biochemical signs of infection we chose to avoid cervical cerclage and tocolytic therapy. The patient remained hospitalized. In a retrospective evaluation of 73 women with PPROM investigators found that maternal CRP levels were not effective in predicting chorioamnionitis [14]. However, an increased CRP could potentially predict future chorioamnionitis development. In another study, maternal CRP levels of more than 20 mg/L were found predictive of funisitis among singleton pregnancies [15]. In their systematic review Van de Laar et al. conclude that although CRP was found to be a moderate predictor of chorioamnionitis, its use isn't yet supported [16]. Popowski et al. noted that maternal WBC count has a poor predictive value, and is only considered highly specific when the threshold of 16,000/µl is exceeded [17]. Park et al. suggested that the evaluation of maternal WBC and CRP levels, along with parity and gestational age could be used as a predictive model of intraamniotic infection in singletons with PPROM [18]. The area under the curve of the model was particularly high (0.848 (95% CI 0.788–0.908) and its sensitivity and specificity reached values of 81 and 75% respectively. Our case differs from the aforementioned studies, as the latter are focused in singleton pregnancies, therefore not taking into account the potential confounders that may lead to extrauterine infection after the live birth of the first twin.

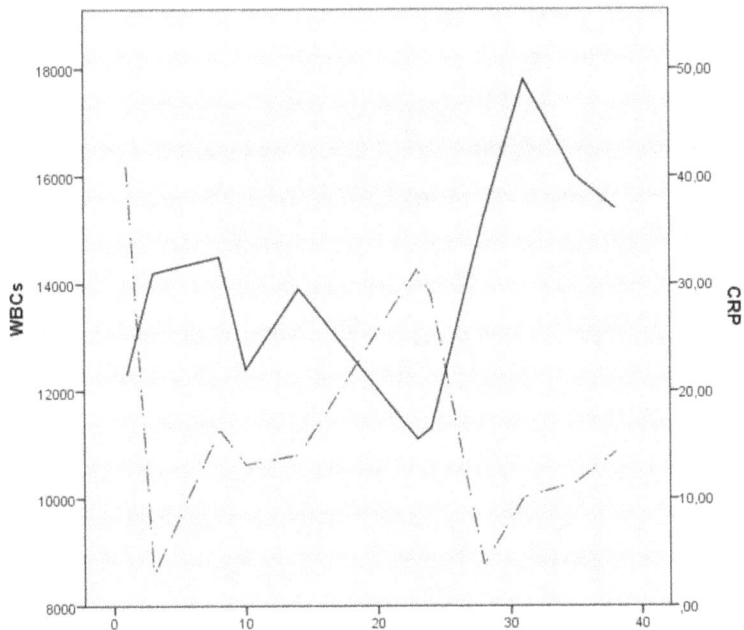

Fig. 1 Time-trends in WBC (cells/ mm³, solid line) and CRP (mg/L, dotted line) values during hospitalization. Delayed interval delivery of the second twin represents a clinical challenge. Subclinical chorioamnionitis cannot be excluded and its impact on the pregnancy course and perinatal outcome remains unknown. WBCs and CRP may provide evidence of deterioration of the patients` pregnancy course. Future studies are needed to investigate the predictive accuracy of these indices.

Conclusions

Delayed interval intertwin delivery rates are expected to increase during the next years as antenatal surveillance becomes more intensive and new tocolytic agents become more popular. Elective cerclage may be considered in twin pregnancies with delivery of the first twin before 23 weeks of gestation. However, this approach should be taken into account in women with no signs of infection. Although we strongly suggest routine performance of amniocentesis for the evaluation of the amniotic fluid for inflammatory markers and routine cultures, a number of patients may still deny this invasive technique. Close antenatal surveillance of both mother and fetus is strongly suggested among these special cases. Given the fact that subclinical chorioamnionitis cannot be precluded, and its effects on the pregnancy course remain undetermined in cases of delayed interval delivery of the second twin, laboratory assessment of markers of inflammation could be potentially considered in these special cases. White blood cells WBCs and CRP have been widely adopted to trace down infections in internal medicine and to follow the course of infectious diseases. Their actual predictive value in delayed delivery of the second twin remains uninvestigated. Our case report presents such a case and may be used as a reference for future studies in this field. These should specifically investigate the sensitivity and specificity of blood biomarkers in predicting chorioamnionitis and fetal infection to help reduce perinatal maternal and neonatal morbidity and mortality.

Abbreviations
AFI: Amniotic fluid index; ART: Artificial reproduction techniques; CRP: C-reactive protein; DID: Delayed interval delivery; NICU: Neonatal intensive care unit; NST: Non stress test; *PPROM*: Premature prelabor rupture of the membranes; RDS: Respiratory distress syndrome; SGA: Small for gestational age; WBC: White blood cells

Authors' contributions
All authors made substantial contributions during the acquisition and interpretation of data, and during the writing process. Furthermore, all authors gave their final approval for the present version and agreed to be accountable for all aspects of the work in ensuring that questions related to the accuracy or integrity of any part of the work are appropriately investigated and resolved. Specifically, DG conceived of the study, and participated in its design, writing and coordination. Also, participated in the clinical assessment of the patient and the clinical and therapeutical decisions during hospital stay of the patient. FP helped to draft the manuscript and revised the manuscript. PV helped to draft the manuscript and revised the manuscript. TM participated in the clinical assessment of the patient and the clinical and therapeutical decisions during her admission, wrote and revised the manuscript. AP helped to draft the manuscript and revised the manuscript. SM participated in the clinical assessment of the patient and the clinical and therapeutical decisions during her admission, wrote and revised the manuscript. PN provided supervision and clinical evidence during the critical intertwin delivery period, wrote and revised the manuscript. LD provided supervision and clinical evidence during the critical intertwin delivery period, wrote and revised the manuscript.

Authors' information
DG is associate Professor of Obstetrics and Gynecology in Athens Medical School and Head of Fetal-Maternal and High-Risk Pregnancy Unit in the 1st Department of Obstetrics and Gynecology, Athens Medical School, Alexandra General Hospital.
FP is Academic fellow in Fetal-Maternal and High-Risk Pregnancy Unit in the 1st Department of Obstetrics and Gynecology, Athens Medical School, Alexandra General Hospital.
PV is Academic fellow in the 3rd Department of Obstetrics and Gynecology, Athens Medical School, Attikon General Hospital.
TM is lecturer in Fetal-Maternal and High-Risk Pregnancy Unit in the 1st Department of Obstetrics and Gynecology, Athens Medical School, Alexandra General Hospital.
AP is Academic fellow in Fetal-Maternal and High-Risk Pregnancy Unit in the 1st Department of Obstetrics and Gynecology, Athens Medical School, Alexandra General Hospital.
SM is Consultant in Fetal-Maternal and High-Risk Pregnancy Unit in the 1st Department of Obstetrics and Gynecology, Athens Medical School, Alexandra General Hospital.
PN is Professor of Obstetrics and Gynecology in Athens Medical School and Director in the 3rd Department of Obstetrics and Gynecology, Athens Medical School, Attikon General Hospital.
LD is Professor of Obstetrics and Gynecology in Athens Medical School and Director in the 1st Department of Obstetrics and Gynecology, Athens Medical School, Alexandra General Hospital.

Competing interests
The authors declare that they have no competing interests.

Author details
[1]1st Department of Obstetrics and Gynecology, Athens Medical School , Alexandra General Hospital, 9 Aristeidou Street , 17563 P. Faliro, Athens, Greece. [2]3rd Department of Obstetrics and Gynecology, Athens Medical School, Attikon General Hospital, Athens, Greece.

References
1. Callahan TL, Hall JE, Ettner SL, Christiansen CL, Greene MF, Crowley WF Jr. The economic impact of multiple-gestation pregnancies and the contribution of assisted-reproduction techniques to their incidence. N Engl J Med. 1994;331:244–9. http://www.nejm.org/doi/full/10.1056/NEJM199407283310407. Accessed 7/2017.
2. Martin JA, Hamilton BE, Ventura SJ, et al. Births: final data for 2009. Natl Vital Stat Rep 2011;60:1–70. https://www.cdc.gov/nchs/data/nvsr/nvsr60/nvsr60_01.pdf. Accessed 7/2017.
3. Verstraelen H, Goetgeluk S, Derom C, et al. Preterm birth in twins after subfertility treatment: population based cohort study. BMJ 2005;331:1173. http://www.bmj.com/content/331/7526/1173.long. Accessed 7/2017.
4. Gielen M, van Beijsterveldt CE, Derom C, et al. Secular trends in gestational age and birthweight in twins. Hum Reprod 2010;25:2346–2353. https://academic.oup.com/humrep/article/25/9/2346/2915542. Accessed 7/2017.
5. Fellman V, Hellstrom-Westas L, Norman M, et al. One-year survival of extremely preterm infants after active perinatal care in Sweden. JAMA 2009;

301:2225–33. http://jamanetwork.com/journals/jama/fullarticle/184015. Accessed 7/2017.
6. Markestad T, Kaaresen PI, Ronnestad A, et al. Early death, morbidity, and need of treatment among extremely premature infants. Pediatrics 2005;115: 1289–98. http://pediatrics.aappublications.org/content/115/5/1289.long?sso=1&sso_redirect_count=1&nfstatus=401&nftoken=00000000-0000-0000-0000-000000000000&nfstatusdescription=ERROR%3a+No+local+token. Accessed 7/2017.
7. P.-Y. Ancel, F. Goffinet, P. Kuhn et al., Survival and morbidity of preterm children born at 22 through 34 weeks' gestation in France in 2011: results of the EPIPAGE-2 cohort study, JAMA Pediatr, vol. 169, no. 3, pp. 230–238, 2011. http://jamanetwork.com/journals/jamapediatrics/fullarticle/2091623. Accessed 7/2017.
8. Yeo KT, Lee QY, Quek WS et al., Trends in morbidity and mortality of extremely preterm multiple gestation newborns, Pediatrics 2015 Aug;136(2): 263–271. http://pediatrics.aappublications.org/content/136/2/263.long. Accessed 7/2017.
9. Oyelese Y, Ananth CV, Smulian JC, Vintzileos AM. Delayed interval delivery in twin pregnancies in the United States: impact on perinatal mortality and morbidity. Am J Obstet Gynecol 2005;192:439–444. http://www.ajog.org/article/S0002-9378(04)00839-7/fulltext. Accessed 7/2017.
10. Arabin B, van Eyck J. Delayed-interval delivery in twin and triplet pregnancies: 17 years of experience in 1 perinatal center. Am J Obstet Gynecol 2009;200:154 e1–154 e8. http://www.ajog.org/article/S0002-9378(08)00982-4/fulltext. Accessed 7/2017.
11. Farkouh LJ, Sabin ED, Heyborne KD, Lindsay LG, Porreco RP. Delayed-interval delivery: extended series from a single maternal-fetal medicine practice. Am J Obstet Gynecol 2000;183:1499–503. http://www.ajog.org/article/S0002-9378(00)68860-9/fulltext. Accessed 7/2017.
12. Zhang J, Johnson CD, Hoffman M. Cervical cerclage in delayed interval delivery in a multifetal pregnancy: a review of seven case series. Eur J Obstet Gynecol Reprod Biol 2003;108:126–30. http://www.ejog.org/article/S0301-2115(02)00479-7/fulltext. Accessed 7/2017.
13. Feys S, Jacquemyn Y. Delayed-interval delivery can save the second twin: evidence from a systematic review. Facts Views Vis Obgyn. 2016;8(4):223–31. https://www.ncbi.nlm.nih.gov/pmc/articles/PMC5303700/. Accessed 7/2017.
14. Smith EJ, Muller CL, Sartorius JA, White DR, Maslow AS. C-reactive protein as a predictor of chorioamnionitis. J Am Osteopath Assoc 2012;112:660–664. http://jaoa.org/article.aspx?articleid=2094391. Accessed 7/2017.
15. Perrone G, Anceschi MM, Capri O, et al. Maternal C-reactive protein at hospital admission is a simple predictor of funisitis in preterm premature rupture of membranes. Gynecol Obstet Investig 2012;74:95–99. https://www.karger.com/Article/Abstract/337717. Accessed 7/2017.
16. Van de Laar R, van der Ham DP, Oei SG, Willekes C, Weiner CP, Mol BW. Accuracy of C-reactive protein determination in predicting chorioamnionitis and neonatal infection in pregnant women with premature rupture of membranes: a systematic review. Eur J Obstet Gynecol Reprod Biol 2009; 147:124–129. https://www.ejog.org/article/S0301-2115(02)00479-7/fulltext. Accessed 7/2017.
17. Popowski T, Goffinet F, Batteux F, Maillard F, Kayem G. [Prediction of maternofetal infection in preterm premature rupture of membranes: serum maternal markers]. Gynecol Obstet Fertil 2011;39:302–308. https://www.ncbi.nlm.nih.gov/pubmed/21515086. Accessed 7/2017.
18. Park KH, Kim SN, Oh KJ, Lee SY, Jeong EH, Ryu A. Noninvasive prediction of intra-amniotic infection and/or inflammation in preterm premature rupture of membranes. Reprod Sci 2012;19:658–665. http://journals.sagepub.com/doi/abs/10.1177/1933719111432869?url_ver=Z39.88-2003&rfr_id=ori%3Arid%3Acrossref.org&rfr_dat=cr_pub%3Dpubmed&. Accessed 7/2017.

10

Signs and symptoms of disordered eating in pregnancy: a Delphi consensus study

Amy Jean Bannatyne[1,2]* ⓘ, Roger Hughes[3], Peta Stapleton[1], Bruce Watt[1] and Kristen MacKenzie-Shalders[2]

Abstract

Background: This study aimed to establish consensus on the expression and distinction of disordered eating in pregnancy to improve awareness across various health professions and inform the development of a pregnancy-specific assessment instrument.

Methods: A three-round modified Delphi method was used with two independent panels. International clinicians and researchers with extensive knowledge on and/or clinical experience with eating disorders formed the first panel and were recruited using structured selection criteria. Women who identified with a lived experience of disordered eating in pregnancy formed the second panel and were recruited via expressions of interest from study advertising on pregnancy forums and social media platforms. A systematic search of academic and grey literature produced 200 sources which were used to pre-populate the Round I questionnaire. Additional items were included in Round II based on panel feedback in Round I. Consensus was defined as 75% agreement on an item.

Results: Of the 102 items presented to the 26 professional panel members and 15 consumer panel members, 75 reached consensus across both panels. Both panels clearly identified signs and symptoms of disordered eating in pregnancy and endorsed a number of clinical features practitioners should consider when delineating disordered eating symptomatically from normative pregnancy experiences.

Conclusion: A list of signs and symptoms in consensus was identified. The areas of collective agreement may be used to guide clinicians in clinical practice, aid the development of psychometric tools to detect/assess pregnancy-specific disordered eating, in addition to serving as starting point for the development of a core outcome set to measure disordered eating in pregnancy.

Keywords: Disordered eating, Eating disorders, Pregnancy, Antenatal, Definition, Distinction, Delphi

Background

Disordered eating has typically been defined as a range of unhealthy eating behaviours and cognitions that negatively impact an individual's emotional, social, and physical well-being [1, 2]. The distinction between disordered eating and a threshold eating disorder (ED) is often the degree of severity and frequency of symptomatology, with disordered eating occurring at a lesser frequency and/or lower level of severity [2]. Much work has been done to understand the symptomatology of disordered eating in a non-pregnant context; however, the presentation and manifestation of disordered eating in pregnancy is less clear. The focus of this Delphi study was to improve clarity around the signs and symptoms of disordered eating in pregnancy, and how these can be differentiated from normative pregnancy-related changes. Such findings may assist in improving the identification of disordered eating in pregnancy.

Disordered eating in pregnancy has been linked to numerous negative consequences, such as miscarriage, prematurity, low birth weight, increased need for caesarean section, and other obstetric and postpartum difficulties [3, 4]. Adjusting to the morphological, endocrinological, and psychological changes in pregnancy, combined with the age-related vulnerability of developing disordered eating during a woman's prime childbearing years [5–8], places pregnancy as a period of increased risk for the onset, resurgence, or exacerbation of disordered eating

* Correspondence: abannaty@bond.edu.au
[1]School of Psychology, Bond University, 14 University Drive, Robina, QLD 4229, Australia
[2]Faculty of Health Sciences and Medicine, Bond University, 14 University Drive, Robina, QLD 4229, Australia
Full list of author information is available at the end of the article

symptomatology, even for women with no history of such symptoms [9–19].

Over the past two decades, studies have estimated the prevalence of disordered eating in pregnancy is between 0.6 and 27.8% [12, 17, 20–23]. It is plausible, however, that existing rates under- or over- estimate the prevalence of such symptoms due to the clinical overlap between symptoms disordered eating and the experience of pregnancy, and the absence of pregnancy-specific disordered eating psychometric instruments [12]. In addition to representing a persistent pattern of disturbance, disordered eating can also represent changes in eating and exercise patterns due to developmental stages (e.g., pregnancy, early childhood, and advancing age), other mental health conditions (e.g., major depressive disorder), or certain life events (e.g., moving away from home, relationship breakdown). In these circumstances, the changes in an individual's eating and/or exercise patterns are typically transient and/or not accompanied by significant psychological or physical distress [2].

In relation to pregnancy, most women report disturbances in normal eating patterns [18], usually in the form of food cravings, increases or decreases in appetite, changes to dietary preferences, inconsistent eating patterns, food aversions, and nausea and vomiting [24, 25]. Despite these behaviours being normal within the context of pregnancy due to hormonal fluctuations, changes in sensory perception, and maternal and/or fetal nutritional needs [26], many of these pregnancy-appropriate changes overlap with, and could possibly mask, disordered eating symptomatology [12]. For example, 'eating for two' could be confused with binge eating, persistent pregnancy sickness could be explained by purging, and changes in dietary preferences and/ or reduced appetite could be equated to dietary restriction. A further barrier for identification of disordered eating in pregnancy is introduced when volitional stigma is considered, with research suggesting women experiencing disordered eating in pregnancy are reluctant to disclose their symptoms due to fear of stigma [27–30]. Frontline antenatal practitioners (e.g., midwives/nurses, obstetricians, and general practitioners [GPs]), in addition to other allied health professionals in contact with women during pregnancy (e.g., psychologists, dietitians) may therefore struggle to identify disordered eating in pregnant women, particularly when symptoms fluctuate between alleviation and exacerbation depending on the course and stage of pregnancy [31]. In many instances, clinicians also lack the required training for such identification [7].

The aim of the present Delphi study was to obtain subject matter expert consensus on the expression and distinction of disordered eating in pregnancy to improve awareness and understanding of such symptoms across various health professions (e.g., obstetrics, midwifery/nursing, general practice, psychology, dietetics, exercise physiology, and physiotherapy) and at a community level, in addition to informing the development a pregnancy-specific assessment instrument that may assist in facilitating early identification.

Methods

The present study used a modified Delphi method [32–34]; a formal methodology used in a range of fields and settings to facilitate consensus discussions among a group of experts when accepted knowledge about a topic/issue/definition is absent or limited [35]. In a broad sense, the Delphi method involves several iterative questionnaires (rounds) to canvass and organise the opinions of an anonymous group of individual experts (panellists). The panel moderator provides structured feedback in between each round to elicit ongoing reflection, usually summaries of the quantitative results and qualitative themes from the previous rounds. This multi-stage procedure continues until a certain level of consensus is reached [33] or, in more recent years, a 'stop' criterion is met [36]. The process used is shown in Fig. 1.

Participants (Panellists)

Two independent Delphi panels were recruited to ensure diverse opinions could be generated and all perspectives considered. International clinicians and researchers with expertise in the field of disordered eating, particularly in relation to pregnancy and/or women's health (i.e., professionals) formed one panel. The other panel consisted of women who identified with a lived experience of disordered eating in pregnancy (i.e., consumers). Panel recruitment and data collection was approved by the Bond University Human Research Ethics Committee (#15278) in Australia.

Professionals in the current study met one of the following criteria: (a) established interest and expertise in the treatment of disordered eating, preferably within the context of the perinatal period, and/or women's health; (b) distinguished contribution to the field of EDs as evidenced by (i) Fellowship status by the Academy for Eating Disorders (AED), (ii) Associate Professor or Professor in the field of EDs and/or women's health, (iii) more than 10 years experience working in the field of EDs and/or women's health, or (iv) publication of peer-reviewed journal article(s) and/or book(s) focused on EDs/disordered eating and/or women's health in the perinatal period. Researchers were identified through authorship of relevant articles during a systematic review of literature, and clinicians were identified via online searches, membership of special interest groups, and professional network suggestions. AED Fellows with relevant clinical or research interests, as listed on the AED website, were also contacted. Potential professional panel members were invited to participate in the study via an email that outlined the rationale and purpose of the study, how the results would be used, and the procedure of a Delphi study. It was also noted the study would be carried out in English. Of the

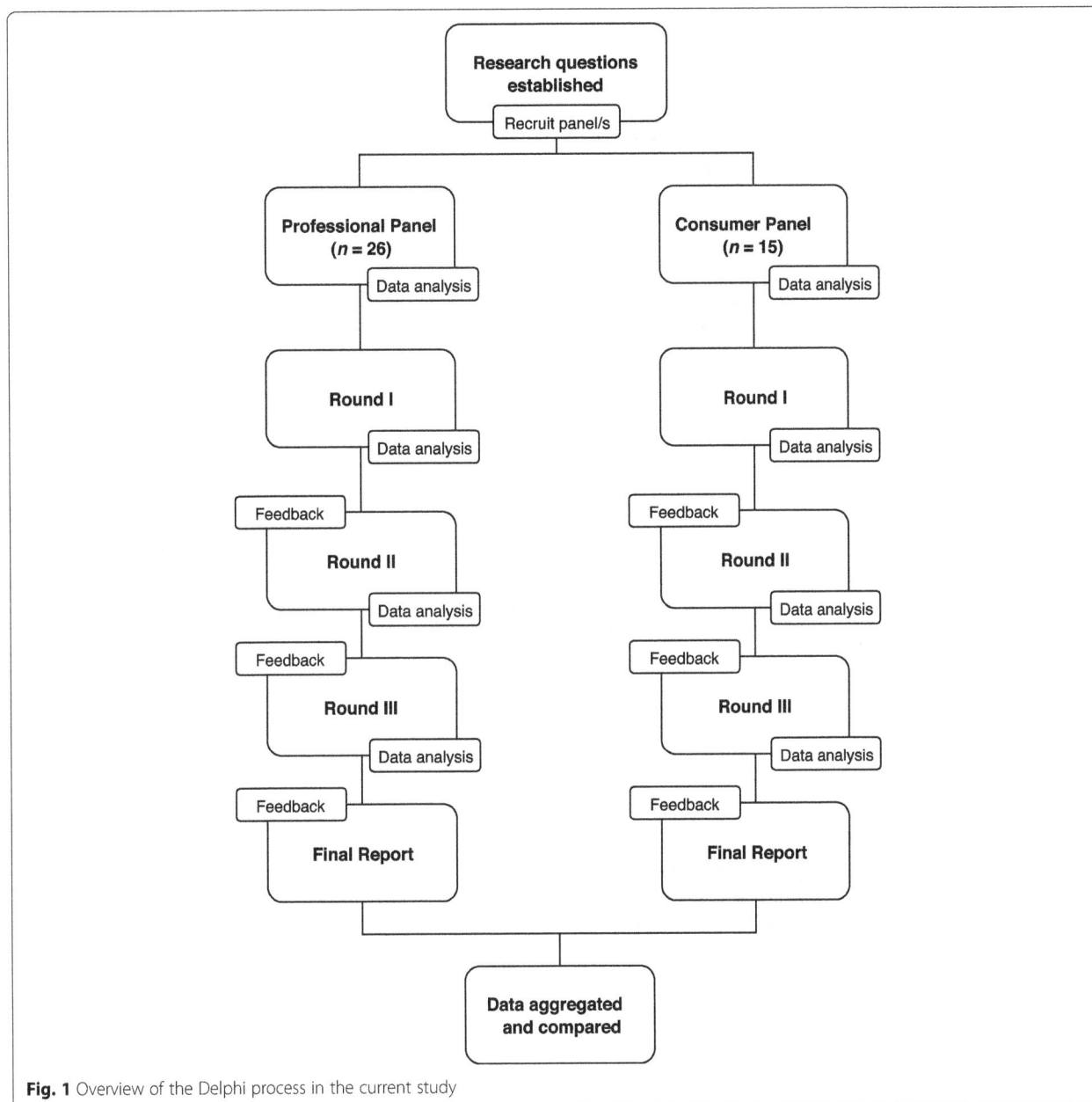

Fig. 1 Overview of the Delphi process in the current study

80 emails sent, there was a 44% response rate, which is similar to other published Delphi studies on the topic of EDs [37–39].

Unlike recruitment for the professional panel, it was not possible to employ purposive invitation-based sampling for the consumer panel due to ethical reasons. As such, expression of interest recruitment was utilised, similar to other Delphi studies [40]. This was achieved by posting advertisements on online pregnancy and parenting forums (e.g., BubHub, Raising Children Network, Essential Baby, and Huggies), in addition to targeted advertising on social media platforms (e.g., Facebook, Twitter). Women who identified with an experience of disordered eating in pregnancy, and were interested in participating in the study,

were asked to contact the primary researcher and briefly detail their experience. This primarily occurred via email. As one of the main aims of the Delphi process was to clarify the symptomatology of disordered eating in pregnancy, the inclusion criteria for the consumer panel were broad. During the pre-screening process, if a woman described eating-, body image-, or exercise-related behaviours, attitudes, or thoughts that were distressing or caused functional impairment during pregnancy, an invitation to participate was offered. Women who disclosed a medical condition that may have produced such symptoms (e.g., hyperemesis gravidarum) were not invited to participate. Women were invited to participate regardless of symptoms being active or inactive at the time of recruitment.

Of the 22 consumers who were invited to participate, there was an 86.4% participation rate.

Procedure

Data were collected across three questionnaire rounds between March and November 2016 using a secure, online survey platform (Qualtrics). Professional and consumer panellists were given four to 5 weeks to complete each questionnaire round, with reminder emails sent twice during each questionnaire completion period. In a systematic review of 100 Delphi studies, Diamond et al. [41] revealed the median threshold for determining consensus was 75% (range: 50 to 97%). As such, consensus in the current study was defined as at least 75% agreement (i.e., ratings of *important* and *very important*, or *agree* and *strongly agree*) on an individual item. All items were rated at least twice (i.e., in Rounds I and II) prior to the decision to include (≥ 75% agreement), re-rate in Round III (50–74% agreement) or remove (< 50% agreement). Items suggested at the end of Round I were automatically rated in Rounds II and III to obtain two rounds of data. Items were evaluated independently in each panel, and then compared at the end of the study.

Round I

Consistent with a modified Delphi method, a comprehensive literature search of both academic and grey literature was conducted between October and December 2015 to inform the content of the initial questionnaire. Key search terms were used to locate relevant websites, journal articles, reports, clinical guidelines, books (including diagnostic criteria), booklets, and training manuals. Consistent with Bond et al. [42], the grey literature search was conducted using Google Australia, Google UK, Google USA, and Google Books, while the academic literature search was performed using PubMed and PsycINFO databases. The key search terms used were: (eating disorders OR disordered eating) in pregnancy; (manage* OR support* OR treat*) (disordered eating OR eating disorders) in pregnancy; (defining OR symptoms of) disordered eating in pregnancy; (screening OR assessment OR identification) of (disordered eating OR eating disorders) in (pregnancy OR antenatal OR perinatal OR maternity care).

The first 50 items in each search were retrieved and reviewed for relevance, after duplicate sources were removed [42–44]. To minimise the influence of searching algorithms on Google, as recommended by Bond et al. [42], several steps were undertaken: (a) the history in Google's search settings was routinely cleared to minimise the influence of previous searches, (b) care was taken to ensure the primary researcher was not logged into any Google-related accounts (e.g., Gmail) that may utilise demographic details to target searches or information; (c) location features that may bias information presented were disabled and the 'any country' function on Google's searches was de-selected to ensure only local pages in each search region were shown. Sources were included if they were in English, related to EDs/disordered eating specifically in the context of pregnancy, and addressed the key areas under consideration. Pertinent information from each source was categorised thematically according to the areas of investigation in a spreadsheet by the primary researcher. When a search hit generated a website landing page with multiple hyperlinks, all links were reviewed. Overall, 200 sources were used to develop the Round I questionnaire (see Table 1).

The primary researcher met with each member of the research team on several occasions to finalise the Round I questionnaire, which resulted in three main sections. Each section included a brief summary of existing literature to contextualise the items that followed. The purpose of these summaries was not to prime panellists in responding, but to present a rationale for why rating of such items was necessary. Throughout the study, panellists were encouraged to draw upon their own experiences when responding to each item. In section one, panellists were asked to indicate the extent to which they agreed that an item reflected a sign or symptom of disordered eating in pregnancy on a 5-point Likert scale (1 = *strongly disagree* to 5 = *strongly agree*). A total of 61 symptoms were presented to both panels for rating in Round I. In section two, panellists were asked to indicate how important certain factors were in distinguishing disordered eating from pregnancy-appropriate symptomatology (foci items) on a 5-point Likert scale (1 = *not important* to 5 = *very important*). A total of 32 foci items were presented to both panels for rating in Round I. Assessment patterns and

Table 1 Summary of Sources that Contributed to the Development of the Round I Questionnaire

Source type	Number included	Example/s
Websites (general educational materials, pamphlets, news articles, forums)	72	https://www.thewomens.org.au/health-information/pregnancy-and-birth/mental-health-pregnancy/eating-disorders-in-after-pregnancy/http://www.cci.health.wa.gov.au/docs/ACF383.pdf
Empirical journal articles	84	Easter et al. (2013) [12], Tierney et al. (2013) [59]
Clinical guidelines or reports	18	National Eating Disorders Collaboration (2015) [16]
Conference proceedings	3	Burton (2014) [60]
Theses	6	Tremblay (2015) [61]
Books	17	American Psychiatric Association (2013) [1] Franko (2006) [62]

methods were assessed in section three; the results of this section are presented in Bannatyne et al. [45].

To allow rich data to emerge for subsequent questionnaire round development, open-ended questions were included in the Round I questionnaire to facilitate and elicit feedback and suggestions for additional items in each section. Round II and III also included open-ended text boxes; however, use of these was limited to panellists contextualising responses (if required) or providing feedback to the panel moderator if there was difficulty answering a question. Prior to administration, the final version of the Round I questionnaire was piloted on 10 colleagues unconnected to the study (5 academic researchers and 5 clinicians) to ensure adequate face and content validity.

Round II

Responses from the Round I questionnaire were pooled and analysed in SPSS Version 23 using measures of central tendency (mean and mode), dispersion (standard deviation), and frequency. Panel comments elicited from the open-ended text boxes were downloaded and transferred into a Word processing document and analysed using thematic analysis. Common themes were identified and grouped together, and cross-coded by two independent researchers to ensure accuracy. These comments were then translated into new quantitative items to be included in Round II, provided the ideas had not been included in the Round I questionnaire and were relevant to the scope of the project. It should be noted that although the professional and consumer panel were recruited concurrently, there was a delay in receiving the Round I responses of four consumer panel members due to technology difficulties. To prevent significant attrition from the professional panel, the decision was made to send out the Round II questionnaire for the professional panel, while waiting for the consumer responses to be returned. The outcome of this decision was that Round I item suggestions from the professional panel (8 new symptom items, 1 new foci item) could be incorporated into the Round II questionnaire of both the professional and consumer panel; however, the Round I item suggestions from the consumer panel (20 new symptom items, 1 new foci item) could only be incorporated into the Round II questionnaire of the consumer panel (i.e., the professional panel did not rate new items suggested by the consumer panel). This also meant that items ratings were evaluated independently in each panel. In other words, the two panels operated independently of each other until the end of the study when items that reached consensus in both panels were compared.

Administration of the Round II questionnaire was identical in terms of instruction and format to the Round I questionnaire; however, the Round II questionnaire included a summary of the group results from Round I at the beginning of each section. This summary included both central tendency scores for each item and a summary of qualitative feedback. Items that reached the 75% consensus agreement threshold were highlighted for panellists using bolding and asterisks.

Round III

A similar collation and analysis process was performed on the data from Round II. Administration of the Round III questionnaire followed the same format as the Round II questionnaire. No new symptom or foci items were introduced in Round III; however, panellists were asked to determine the broad frequency at which symptoms might be considered 'disordered' in pregnancy. These symptoms were framed as "a significant influence of body weight and shape on self-evaluation in the presence of any compensatory behaviour aiming to prevent/reduce pregnancy-related weight gain AND/OR the presence of binge eating episodes/behaviours that occur and are followed by feelings of guilt or shame". Frequency response options included *once per month, once per fortnight, once per week,* and *twice per week*. Panellists were asked to select one response. The purpose of this question was to identify a broad proxy that may assist clinicians to distinguish disordered eating from normative pregnancy experiences.

Results
Panel demographics
Professional panel
A total of 32 experts were recruited, with 26 completing all three rounds (81.3% retention rate). Overall, the final sample consisted of 23 women and three men from geographically diverse areas, with an average of 19.08 years ($SD = 11.56$) respective professional experience and 14.42 years ($SD = 10.97$) specialisation in the field of EDs/disordered eating. Seven panel members also identified as AED Fellows, a status that recognises distinguished contributions in the area of EDs. See Table 2 for additional panel details.

Consumer panel
A total of 19 women were recruited, with 15 completing all three rounds (79.0% retention rate). The age of the final sample ranged from 23 to 43 years ($M = 45.62$ years, $SD = 12.08$), with the majority of Caucasian ethnicity (86.6%). Of the final sample, five women were pregnant at the time of recruitment (31.2%), one had recently given birth within the past 6 months (6.3%), one had given birth within the past year (6.3%), seven had given birth within the past 2 years (43.8%), and one had given birth within the past 3 years (6.3%). In exploring the pregnancy that disordered eating was experienced in, 10 women (66.7%) reported an experience of disordered

Table 2 Additional demographic details for the professional panel (*N* = 26)

Demographic variable	n (%)
Residing country	
Australia	12 (46.2%)
United States	6 (23.1%)
United Kingdom	4 (15.4%)
Canada	2 (7.7%)
Sweden	2 (7.7%)
Highest level of education	
Doctorate / PhD	19 (73.1%)
Masters Degree	4 (15.4%)
Postgraduate Degree (unspecified)	2 (7.7%)
Undergraduate Degree	1 (3.8%)
Professional field	
Psychology / Psychiatry	21 (80.1%)
Dietetics	4 (15.4%)
Obstetrics	2 (7.7%)
Midwifery	1 (3.8%)
Professional activities	
Researcher also involved in clinical practice	11 (42.3%)
Clinician with no research activities	8 (30.8%)
Researcher with no current clinical practice	4 (15.4%)
Clinician with some research involvement	2 (7.7%)
Other	1 (3.8%)

eating in only one pregnancy, with 70% noting this was experienced in their first pregnancy (*n* = 7). Five women (33.3%) reported experiences of disordered eating in multiple pregnancies, including their first pregnancy. For most of the panel, disordered eating was experienced during a planned pregnancy (80.0%). Of the five women who were pregnant during the study, all had given birth previously and all reported experiencing disordered eating in their previous and current pregnancy.

Section 1: Signs and symptoms of disordered eating in pregnancy

Overall, 48 of the 69 potential attributes rated across both panels reached the consensus agreement criterion, including behavioural (22 of 27), physical (3 of 14), cognitive (13 of 16), and affective (10 of 12) symptomatology. An additional 20 items were generated and rated only by the consumer panel, with 19 reaching the consensus threshold. See Table 3 for a list of all the symptom attributes. Both panels endorsed a similar number of behavioural, cognitive, and affective symptom attributes; however, the professional panel endorsed a greater number of physical symptom attributes compared to the consumer panel (10 vs 3, respectively). Cohen's kappa (κ) was performed to determine endorsement agreement between the two panels. Results differed depending on the symptom category under consideration, with poor agreement on physical symptoms (κ = .165) but very strong agreement on behavioural symptoms (κ = .867). Overall, agreement on all symptoms was modest (κ = .467).

Section 2: Distinguishing disordered eating from pregnancy-appropriate symptoms

Overall, 27 of the 33 indicators rated across both panels to distinguish symptoms of disordered eating from pregnancy-appropriate symptomatology reached the consensus agreement criterion. One additional foci item was generated and rated only by the consumer panel, reaching consensus. Endorsement agreement between the panels was very strong (κ = 1.00). In general, there was agreement across both panels that practitioners could clarify the clinical overlap using a blend of clinical judgment, functional analysis, observation of informational discrepancies, assessment of impact and impairment, and consideration of patient and familial historical factors. The list of foci item ratings can be found in Table 4, while key quantitative and qualitative factors for clinicians to consider are shown in Table 5.

In terms of the broad threshold at which behaviours would be considered 'disordered', the most commonly endorsed response by the professional panel was weekly frequency, closely followed by fortnightly and monthly frequency. Over half the consumer panel indicated symptoms would only need to occur at least once per month to be considered problematic (see Fig. 2).

Discussion

The present study utilised responses from professionals (clinical experts and experienced ED clinicians and researchers) and consumers (women with lived experience) to identify the signs and symptoms of disordered eating in pregnancy. Overall, the Delphi process allowed consensus to be reached between professionals and consumers on these topics.

In clarifying the manifestation of disordered eating in pregnancy, a range of behavioural, physical, cognitive, and affective signs and symptoms were identified. There was a modest level of consistency across the panels (47 symptoms meeting consensus in both panels), and generally a high level of consensus on items (31 with a consensus rate greater than 85% across both panels, 21 with a consensus rate greater than 90% across both panels). Notably, two cognitive and two affective symptoms reached 100% consensus across both panels. Cognitive symptoms were perceived to be particularly concerning by both panels given the affective distress these symptoms can produce for a woman. Such distress may have detrimental and lasting impacts on an unborn child,

Table 3 Panel ratings for the potential symptom attributes of disordered eating in pregnancy

	Panel	Mean (SD)	Mode	% of panel agreement	Consensus
Behavioural symptom items					
Dietary consumption that does not support a healthy pregnancy	P	4.88 (.33)	5.00	100%	Yes
	C	4.67 (1.05)	5.00	93.3%	Yes
Dieting behaviours (e.g., calorie counting)	P	4.15 (.68)	4.00	92.3%	Yes
	C	4.13 (1.41)	5.00	80.0%	Yes
Inflexibility and rigidity with diet (i.e., strict consumption of diet foods only)	P	4.88 (.33)	5.00	100%	Yes
	C	4.07 (1.03)	4.00	86.7%	Yes
Fasting and/or skipping meals	P	4.88 (.33)	5.00	100%	Yes
	C	4.53 (1.06)	5.00	93.3%	Yes
Use of meal replacements (when not advised by a health professional)	P	4.54 (.81)	5.00	88.5%	Yes
	C	4.40 (1.40)	5.00	86.7%	Yes
Repeated weighing	P	3.85 (.78)	4.00	76.9%	Yes
	C	4.67 (1.05)	5.00	93.3%	Yes
Refusing to eat outside of one's home	P	4.65 (.56)	5.00	96.2%	Yes
	C	4.33 (1.23)	5.00	86.7%	Yes
Eating in secret	P	4.73 (.45)	5.00	100%	Yes
	C	4.60 (1.06)	5.00	93.3%	Yes
Eating an objectively large amount of food	P	3.85 (.54)	4.00	76.9%	Yes
	C	3.93 (1.03)	4.00	80.0%	Yes
Eating for "two"	P	2.46 (.76)	2.00	7.7%	No
	C	3.33 (.72)	3.00	33.3%	No
Eating when not physically hungry	P	3.08 (.56)	3.00	19.2%	No
	C	4.13 (.52)	4.00	93.3%	Yes
Using food to cope with/soothe strong emotions, or reward oneself	P	3.92 (.63)	4.00	84.6%	Yes
	C	4.07 (1.10)	4.00	80.0%	Yes
Eating rapidly and until uncomfortably full	P	4.31 (.62)	4.00	92.3%	Yes
	C	4.13 (1.13)	5.00	80.0%	Yes
Self-induced vomiting	P	4.85 (.46)	5.00	96.2%	Yes
	C	4.53 (1.13)	5.00	86.7%	Yes
Obsessively exercising for the purpose of controlling weight and shape	P	4.15 (.54)	4.00	92.3%	Yes
	C	4.60 (1.06)	5.00	93.3%	Yes
Exercising against medical recommendations	P	4.92 (.27)	5.00	100%	Yes
	C	4.60 (1.06)	5.00	93.3%	Yes
Exercising in secret	P	4.88 (.33)	5.00	100%	Yes
	C	4.80 (.56)	5.00	93.3%	Yes
Refusing to purchase maternity clothing	P	2.96 (.82)	3.00	15.4%	No
	C	2.93 (1.22)	2.00	33.3%	No
Wearing specific clothing to conceal pregnancy	P	2.88 (.71)	3.00	15.4%	No
	C	3.67 (1.05)	4.00	68.8%	No
Misuse of gestational diabetes medication	P	4.96 (.20)	5.00	100%	Yes
	C	4.80 (.78)	5.00	93.3%	Yes
Use of laxatives or enemas to reduce gestational weight gain/induce weight loss	P	4.92 (.27)	5.00	100%	Yes
	C	4.80 (.78)	5.00	93.3%	Yes
Use of appetite suppressants or "diet pills"	P	4.88 (.43)	5.00	96.2%	Yes

Table 3 Panel ratings for the potential symptom attributes of disordered eating in pregnancy *(Continued)*

	Panel	Mean (SD)	Mode	% of panel agreement	Consensus
Use of natural supplements (e.g., tea detox)	C	4.80 (.78)	5.00	93.3%	Yes
	P	4.81 (.49)	5.00	96.2%	Yes
Body checking behaviours	C	4.67 (.82)	5.00	93.3%	Yes
	P	4.00 (.49)	4.00	88.5%	Yes
Self-harm	C	4.80 (.41)	5.00	100%	Yes
	P	4.85 (.37)	5.00	100%	Yes
Not consuming enough food during pregnancy to produce milk or sustain breastfeeding, resulting in weight loss and/or binge eating behaviours [a]	C	4.40 (.91)	5.00	86.7%	Yes
	P	4.87 (.34)	5.00	100%	Yes
	C	4.60 (.63)	5.00	93.3%	Yes
Spending an excessive amount of time (i.e., multiple hours per week) researching about the most effective ways to reduce pregnancy weight gain and/or ways to lose weight after birth	P	–	–	–	–
	C	4.93 (.26)	5.00	100%	Yes
Searching for or seeking information about disordered eating in pregnancy	P	–	–	–	–
	C	4.53 (.92)	5.00	86.7%	Yes
Using the pregnancy as a 'valid' excuse/reason to avoid feared foods and/or not violate dietary rules	P	–	–	–	–
	C	4.53 (.52)	5.00	100%	Yes
Obsessively recording anticipated and achieved weight gain and calculating calorie intake and exercise output to ensure only the absolute minimum weight gain (and feeling distressed if anything interferes with this)	P	–	–	–	–
	C	5.00 (.00)	5.00	100%	Yes
Preferring to ensure the nausea and ignore physical hunger signals due to fear of weight gain or changes to shape	P	–	–	–	–
	C	5.00 (.00)	5.00	100%	Yes
Going to bed hungry at the end of the day and thinking about food, but not allowing oneself to eat to subside this hunger	P	–	–	–	–
	C	4.93 (.26)	5.00	100%	Yes
Excessively reassuring doctors/midwives that low weight during pregnancy OR lack of weight gain is nothing to be concerned about by reporting vague eating habits (e.g., "I eat heaps")	P	–	–	–	–
	C	4.80 (.78)	5.00	93.3%	Yes
Requesting early discharge from hospital because of the food that might be served and feeling anxious is this early discharge does not or cannot occur	P	–	–	–	–
	C	4.73 (.59)	5.00	93.3%	Yes
Frequent 'fat talk' (i.e., if a pregnant woman talks a lot about how 'fat' she looks or is)	P	–	–	–	–
	C	4.40 (.91)	5.00	86.7%	Yes
Chewing and spitting out large amounts of food, particularly forbidden foods	P	–	–	–	–
	C	4.93 (.26)	5.00	100%	Yes
Physical symptom items					
Low body weight	P	3.96 (.53)	4.00	96.2%	Yes
	C	3.80 (.56)	4.00	73.3%	No
Losing weight while pregnant	P	4.73 (.60)	5.00	92.3%	Yes
	C	3.80 (.68)	4.00	80.0%	Yes
Inadequate gestational weight gain	P	4.77 (.65)	5.00	96.2%	Yes
	C	4.46 (.64)	5.00	93.3%	Yes
Excessive gestational weight gain	P	3.88 (.65)	4.00	80.8%	Yes
	C	3.80 (.68)	4.00	66.7%	No
Rapid gestational weight gain	P	3.92 (.56)	4.00	80.8%	Yes
	C	3.60 (.83)	4.00	66.7%	No

Table 3 Panel ratings for the potential symptom attributes of disordered eating in pregnancy *(Continued)*

	Panel	Mean (*SD*)	Mode	% of panel agreement	Consensus
Dizziness and/or fatigue	P	3.54 (.76)	3.00	46.2%	No
	C	2.93 (.80)	3.00	13.3%	No
Feeling nauseated most of the time	P	2.08 (.85)	2.00	7.7%	No
	C	2.67 (1.18)	3.00	20.0%	No
Severe morning sickness that does not stop after the first trimester (hyperemesis gravidarum)	P	4.31 (.84)	5.00	84.6%	Yes
	C	2.00 (1.36)	1.00	20.0%	No
Dehydration	P	4.58 (.58)	5.00	96.2%	Yes
	C	3.27 (.80)	3.00	33.3%	No
Abdominal bloating	P	3.04 (.60)	3.00	11.5%	No
	C	2.93 (.80)	3.00	13.3%	No
Gastrointestinal discomfort	P	3.00 (.63)	3.00	19.2%	No
	C	2.47 (.99)	2.00	13.3%	No
Unborn baby is small/underdeveloped for gestational age [a]	P	3.96 (.48)	4.00	87.0%	Yes
	C	3.47 (.74)	3.00	33.3%	No
Asymmetrical or slow foetal growth [a]	P	3.96 (.48)	4.00	87.0%	Yes
	C	3.53 (.74)	3.00	40.0%	No
The woman's blood tests show electrolyte imbalances (e.g., low potassium) [a]	P	4.31 (.84)	5.00	84.6%	Yes
	C	4.13 (.74)	4.00	80.0%	Yes
Cognitive symptom items					
Overvaluation of body shape and weight	P	4.42 (.50)	4.00	100%	Yes
	C	4.93 (.26)	5.00	100%	Yes
Perceptual disturbance (e.g., perceiving self to be overweight for pregnancy stage, when objectively not)	P	4.42 (.50)	4.00	100%	Yes
	C	4.87 (.35)	5.00	100%	Yes
Poor body image	P	4.12 (.52)	4.00	92.3%	Yes
	C	4.47 (.99)	5.00	80.0%	Yes
Low self-esteem	P	3.77 (.65)	4.00	73.0%	No
	C	4.20 (.56)	4.00	93.3%	Yes
Rumination about gestational weight gain	P	4.04 (.53)	4.00	88.5%	Yes
	C	4.87 (.35)	5.00	100%	Yes
Rumination about health of baby	P	3.08 (.63)	3.00	15.4%	No
	C	3.07 (.80)	3.00	20.0%	No
Fixation on post-partum weight loss	P	4.12 (.52)	4.00	92.3%	Yes
	C	4.80 (.56)	5.00	93.3%	Yes
Self critical thoughts and fear of criticism	P	3.31 (.79)	3.00	42.3%	No
	C	4.20 (.56)	4.00	93.3%	Yes
Comparing personal eating habits to others	P	3.77 (.59)	4.00	76.9%	Yes
	C	3.87 (.74)	4.00	80.0%	Yes
Need for pregnancy to be "perfect"	P	3.88 (.71)	4.00	76.9%	Yes
	C	4.20 (.78)	4.00	93.3%	Yes
Desire for baby to be "small" or "petite"	P	4.73 (.53)	5.00	96.2%	Yes
	C	4.20 (1.08)	5.00	80.0%	Yes
Suicidal thoughts/ideation	P	4.62 (.94)	5.00	88.5%	Yes
	C	4.40 (.83)	5.00	80.0%	Yes
	P	4.74 (.45)	5.00	100%	Yes

Table 3 Panel ratings for the potential symptom attributes of disordered eating in pregnancy *(Continued)*

	Panel	Mean (SD)	Mode	% of panel agreement	Consensus
Frequent comparison of weight and shape, with pregnant and non-pregnant women [a]	C	4.67 (.62)	5.00	93.3%	Yes
Belief that vomiting will not adversely impact the fetus/baby because "all pregnant women vomit" [a]	P	4.78 (.52)	5.00	96.0%	Yes
	C	4.60 (.74)	5.00	86.7%	Yes
Obsessive thoughts during pregnancy that relate to food (e.g., fear of food contamination, "clean eating" to avoid pesticides) [a]	P	4.74 (.45)	5.00	100%	Yes
	C	4.47 (.83)	5.00	93.3%	Yes
Obsessive thoughts regarding health and normality of pregnancy [a]	P	3.96 (.64)	4.00	87.0%	Yes
	C	4.07 (.85)	4.00	80.0%	Yes
Thoughts during pregnancy about using breastfeeding as a purgatory method and/or prolonging breastfeeding for weight loss	P	–	–	–	–
	C	4.73 (.80)	5.00	93.3%	Yes
Agonising and debating the absolute necessity of every food item consumed and/or bargaining with oneself	P	–	–	–	–
	C	4.93 (.26)	5.00	100%	Yes
Urges and thoughts of wanting to vomit to relieve physical or psychological tension	P	–	–	–	–
	C	2.93 (1.22)	2.00	33.3%	No
Thoughts that one does not deserve to eat, and having to justify food consumption 'for the baby'	P	–	–	–	–
	C	5.00 (.00)	5.00	100%	Yes
Thoughts of wanting to be 'just bump' (i.e., weight gain is only acceptable in 'pregnancy-appropriate' areas such as the stomach, but not the arms/thighs etc)	P	–	–	–	–
	C	4.33 (.82)	4.00, 5.00	93.3%	Yes
Thoughts of returning to a restrictive diet once the baby is no longer dependent on mother's body (e.g., to grow in the womb, for breastfeeding, etc)	P	–	–	–	–
	C	4.60 (.74)	5.00	86.7%	Yes
Preoccupation with diets, weight management information, and the lack of weight gained by other pregnant individuals and/or admiration for how rapidly these individuals 'snap back' to their pre-pregnancy body weight and shape	P	–	–	–	–
	C	4.93 (.26)	5.00	100%	Yes
Affective symptom items					
Distress regarding changing shape + fear of fatness	P	4.27 (.45)	4.00	100%	Yes
	C	4.53 (1.06)	5.00	86.7%	Yes
Distress or guilt after eating "unhealthy" or "bad" foods	P	4.19 (.49)	4.00	96.2%	Yes
	C	4.53 (.83)	5.00	93.3%	Yes
Mood disturbance	P	3.92 (.80)	4.00	84.6%	Yes
	C	3.13 (.99)	3.00	33.3%	No
Anxiety about certain foods/food groups	P	4.08 (.56)	4.00	84.6%	Yes
	C	4.67 (.49)	5.00	100%	Yes
Feeling "out of control" of one's body	P	4.27 (.45)	4.00	100%	Yes
	C	4.60 (.91)	5.00	86.7%	Yes
Feeling a "loss of control" over eating	P	4.77 (.59)	5.00	92.3%	Yes
	C	4.53 (1.06)	5.00	93.3%	Yes
Guilt after eating (any food)	P	4.35 (.49)	4.00	100%	Yes
	C	4.73 (.46)	5.00	100%	Yes
Feelings of shame + disgust about body	P	4.92 (.27)	5.00	100%	Yes
	C	4.80 (.41)	5.00	100%	Yes
Sensitivity to comments regarding weight, shape, or appearance	P	4.04 (.60)	4.00	92.3%	Yes
	C	4.20 (.94)	5.00	80.0%	Yes

Table 3 Panel ratings for the potential symptom attributes of disordered eating in pregnancy *(Continued)*

	Panel	Mean (*SD*)	Mode	% of panel agreement	Consensus
Emotional detachment from pregnancy	P	4.46 (.86)	5.00	84.6%	Yes
	C	4.27 (.82)	4.00	80.0%	Yes
Social isolation	P	4.31 (.97)	5.00	84.6%	Yes
	C	4.47 (.74)	5.00	86.7%	Yes
Interpersonal mistrust	P	3.73 (.72)	4.00	76.9%	Yes
	C	3.73 (.88)	4.00	73.3%	No
Feeling relieved or thankful for pregnancy serving as a valid explanation to avoid certain foods or eating very little	P	–	–	–	–
	C	4.87 (.35)	5.00	100%	Yes
Distress in relation to increased appetite during pregnancy	P	–	–	–	–
	C	4.87 (.35)	5.00	100%	Yes
Feeling resentful toward the baby for needing constant food and nutrients to grow in the womb, followed by significant guilt and shame for feeling resentful	P	–	–	–	–
	C	4.60 (1.12)	5.00	93.3%	Yes

P professional panel (*N* = 26), *C* consumer panel (*N* = 15) Items were rated on a 5-point Likert scale (1 = *strongly disagree* to 5 = *strongly agree*)
[a]additional item suggested by professional panel in Round I

depending on the timing of cortisol exposure [46]. Differences in panel agreement were, however, evident for a subset of symptom attributes. In particular, the professional panel endorsed a greater number of physical symptom attributes than the consumer panel (10 vs. 3, respectively). This difference likely reflects the medical knowledge and experiences of the professional panel. As such, it may not have been appropriate to ask the consumer panel to rate such items [34].

While many of the endorsed symptoms were consistent with those likely observed in a non-pregnant context, a number of unique pregnancy-specific symptoms were endorsed across both panels including overvaluation of the offspring's weight and shape (e.g., desire for the baby to be "small" or "petite"), rationalisation of self-induced vomiting as pregnancy-appropriate, and emotional detachment from the pregnancy. Behaviours often normalised outside of pregnancy, such as the use of natural supplements (e.g., tea detoxes) for weight loss, were also considered to be reflective of disordered eating in pregnancy and cause for concern if disclosed to clinicians practicing in this area.

Collectively, the findings suggest that practitioners working with pregnant women should be cognisant of two main factors. First, that an absence of physical or behavioural symptomatology alone does not necessarily imply a woman is unaffected by disordered eating concerns during pregnancy. Previous researchers have also suggested that while observable disordered eating behaviours often reduce during pregnancy, high levels of weight and shape concern, which cannot be easily observed and may not be disclosed freely, often persist [12, 21, 47, 48]. Second, that disordered eating in pregnancy reflects a spectrum of behaviours that do not

necessarily result in physical weight or shape changes, and that particular exploration of binge eating behaviours and cognitions may be justified. Such notion supports previous work [4, 10, 11, 17]. Together these findings seem reasonable; yet, antenatal practitioners report a lack of knowledge and confidence in identifying disordered eating symptomatology [7, 29]. Furthermore, ED literature suggests that community understanding of the spectrum of disordered eating is poor, with binge eating and/or non-purgatory weight control behaviours often perceived as normative or benign [49]. To assist clinicians working in this area, the signs, symptoms, and delineating factors revealed in this study could be used as a starting point to aid identification. Results of the current study may also encourage and assist in the development of training resources to increase frontline antenatal practitioners' (e.g., obstetricians, GPs, midwives, and nurses) and other allied health professionals' (e.g., dietitians, psychologists, exercise physiologists, and physiotherapists) awareness, knowledge, and understanding of the expression and manifestation of disordered eating in pregnancy.

Furthermore, emphasising the finding that disordered eating is multifaceted experience is essential, not only for practitioner awareness in potential screening and detection efforts, but also when educating women who may have limited knowledge or insight in relation to disordered eating symptoms. Historically, presentations of disordered eating in pregnancy have often been labelled 'pregorexia' in popular media, a term describing an excessive fear of pregnancy-related weight gain and engagement in various compensatory behaviours to avoid weight or shape changes that are characteristic of a healthy pregnancy [50–52]. Given the general population is increasingly reliant on popular

Table 4 Panel ratings for potential factors relevant in distinguishing disordered eating in pregnancy from pregnancy-appropriate symptomatology

Distinguishing foci	Panel	Mean (SD)	Mode	% of panel agreement	Consensus
Severity of behaviours	P	4.88 (.43)	5.00	96.2%	Yes
	C	4.80 (.41)	5.00	100%	Yes
Severity of cognitions	P	4.88 (.43)	5.00	96.2%	Yes
	C	5.00 (.00)	5.00	100%	Yes
Frequency of behaviours	P	4.85 (.46)	5.00	96.2%	Yes
	C	4.87 (.35)	5.00	100%	Yes
Frequency of cognitions	P	4.85 (.46)	5.00	96.2%	Yes
	C	5.00 (.00)	5.00	100%	Yes
Dietary behaviours in excess to recommended guidelines	P	4.46 (.71)	5.00	88.5%	Yes
	C	4.13 (.64)	4.00	86.7%	Yes
Dietary behaviours in deficit to recommended guidelines	P	4.73 (.60)	5.00	92.3%	Yes
	C	4.33 (.62)	4.00	93.3%	Yes
Exercise behaviours in excess to recommended guidelines	P	4.35 (.75)	5.00	84.6%	Yes
	C	4.33 (.49)	4.00	100%	Yes
Exercise behaviours in deficit to recommended guidelines	P	3.19 (.90)	3.00	34.6%	No
	C	3.33 (1.11)	3.00	40.0%	No
Appropriateness of gestational weight gain	P	3.96 (.45)	4.00	88.5%	Yes
	C	4.20 (.56)	4.00	93.3%	Yes
Health risk or distress to fetus	P	4.88 (.43)	5.00	96.2%	Yes
	C	5.00 (.00)	5.00	100%	Yes
Health risk or distress to mother	P	4.85 (.54)	5.00	92.3%	Yes
	C	5.00 (.00)	5.00	100%	Yes
Distress of (or worry by) family	P	3.92 (.48)	4.00	92.3%	Yes
	C	4.13 (.92)	4 /5.00	80.0%	Yes
History of pregnancy complications (e.g., miscarriage, premature labour)	P	3.96 (.48)	4.00	84.6%	Yes
	C	4.67 (.72)	5.00	86.7%	Yes
Level of physical impairment or impact	P	4.04 (.66)	4.00	88.5%	Yes
	C	4.93 (.26)	5.00	100%	Yes
Level of psychological impairment or impact (e.g., affective state of mother)	P	4.31 (.66)	4.00	92.3%	Yes
	C	5.00 (.00)	5.00	100%	Yes
Level of social impairment or impact	P	4.12 (.59)	4.00	88.5%	Yes
	C	4.93 (.26)	5.00	100%	Yes
Level of relational impairment or impact	P	4.04 (.59)	4.00	84.6%	Yes
	C	4.93 (.26)	5.00	100%	Yes
Degree of flexibility with dietary rules	P	4.58 (.58)	5.00	96.2%	Yes
	C	4.47 (.52)	4.00	100%	Yes
Level of insight and/or denial	P	4.81 (.49)	5.00	96.2%	Yes
	C	4.40 (.83)	5.00	93.3%	Yes
Discrepancy between self-reported functioning and medical observations	P	4.81 (.49)	5.00	96.2%	Yes
	C	5.00 (.00)	5.00	100%	Yes
Discrepancy between the woman's report and partner/family reports	P	4.73 (.53)	5.00	96.2%	Yes
	C	4.73 (.46)	5.00	100%	Yes
Available coping strategies (e.g., emotion regulation skills)	P	4.00 (.63)	4.00	88.5%	Yes

Table 4 Panel ratings for potential factors relevant in distinguishing disordered eating in pregnancy from pregnancy-appropriate symptomatology (Continued)

Distinguishing foci	Panel	Mean (SD)	Mode	% of panel agreement	Consensus
	C	4.80 (.41)	5.00	100%	Yes
Available social support	P	4.92 (.69)	4.00	92.3%	Yes
	C	4.73 (.46)	5.00	100%	Yes
History of any psychiatric condition	P	4.08 (.69)	4.00	88.5%	Yes
	C	5.00 (.00)	5.00	100%	Yes
History of an eating disorder	P	4.85 (.46)	5.00	96.2%	Yes
	C	5.00 (.00)	5.00	100%	Yes
History of subclinical disordered eating behaviours	P	4.85 (.46)	5.00	96.2%	Yes
	C	4.93 (.26)	5.00	100%	Yes
Family history of an eating disorder	P	4.00 (.57)	4.00	92.3%	Yes
	C	4.20 (.56)	4.00	93.3%	Yes
Younger age (< 30 years)	P	2.88 (.59)	3.00	7.7%	No
	C	1.40 (1.06)	1.00	6.7%	No
Older age (> 30 years)	P	2.85 (.54)	3.00	3.8%	No
	C	1.53 (1.25)	1.00	13.3%	No
Ethnicity	P	2.73 (.67)	3.00	0.0%	No
	C	1.60 (1.12)	1.00	6.7%	No
Primigravidity (first pregnancy)	P	2.96 (.44)	3.00	7.7%	No
	C	2.20 (1.52)	1.00	20.0%	No
Multigravidity (subsequent pregnancies)	P	2.88 (.52)	3.00	3.8%	No
	C	2.13 (1.41)	1.00	20.0%	No
Ability to return to "normal eating" and regain feelings of control (w/out being restrictive) after bouts of pregnancy-related appetite changes [a]	P	4.52 (.47)	5.00	86.9%	Yes
	C	4.73 (.53)	5.00	100%	Yes
Intent behind the behaviour (e.g., restricting one's food intake is only problematic if the intention is to minimise weight gain or lose weight during pregnancy, as opposed to restricting due to nausea)	P	–	–	–	–
	C	4.93 (.26)	5.00	100%	Yes

P professional panel (N = 26). C consumer panel (N = 15) Items were rated on a 5-point Likert scale (1 = not important to 5 = very important)
[a] additional item suggested by professional panel in Round I

media sources to obtain important information regarding their health and wellbeing [53, 54], it is plausible that women experiencing symptoms inconsistent with the explanation of pregorexia may dismiss or downplay their symptoms. Health professionals interacting with pregnant women must be aware of the potential inaccuracies popular media presentations of disordered eating may result in and the need for appropriate psychoeducation to foster awareness and insight. It is also vital that popular media outlets disseminate accurate depictions of disordered eating in pregnancy to the general population to increase awareness and reduce stigma around such symptoms, which may not be visible to a woman's social support network.

Arguably, one of the most challenging aspects of identifying disordered eating in pregnancy is distinguishing clinical features from normative pregnancy experiences [12]. While results of the current study do not entirely clarify this nuanced distinction, there was a strong level of agreement across both panels on various quantitative and qualitative factors (outlined in Table 5) that might assist practitioners evaluate concerning symptoms. Practically, information needed to assess these factors could be gathered in routine history taking, followed by more specific questioning, particularly when symptoms are explicit. When symptoms are more subtle or ambiguous, the professional panel noted implementation of clinical judgment would be required. This may include normative comparison of behaviours to clinical guidelines; evaluation of functional impairment across multiple domains; and assessment of insight/denial via observed behavioural discrepancies. In terms of the frequency at which symptoms may be considered problematic, our findings revealed the consumer panel considered symptoms of relatively low frequency (once per month) to be distressing, compared to professional panel who considered

Table 5 Questions to consider when evaluating potential symptoms of disordered eating in pregnancy

- How often is the symptom/s occurring, and with what intensity?
- What is the context and/or intent of the symptom? (e.g., *is a woman's dietary restriction to reduce nausea or minimise gestational weight gain?*)
- Does the symptom deviate from clinical recommendations during pregnancy (e.g., deficits in dietary intake, excess in exercise behaviours)?
- Is the woman's weight in a healthy range relative to pregnancy stage? Could the symptom negatively impact gestational weight gain?
- Is there an actual or anticipated health risk or distress to the mother and/or unborn child?
- Does a woman's family express concern about the symptom/s?
- Does the woman have a history of pregnancy complications (e.g., miscarriage, premature labour)?
- Is the symptom/s causing physical, psychological, social, and/or relational impairment/difficulty for the woman?
- Does the woman have insight into the presence and impact of the symptom/s?
- Is the woman open to addressing the concern?
- Is there a discrepancy between a woman's self-reported functioning and the results of medical tests/observations?
- Is there a discrepancy between a woman's report of functioning and partner/family reports of functioning?
- Does the woman have a history of mental health conditions, particularly eating disorders/disordered eating?
- Is there a history of disordered eating in the woman's family?

Note. The features in this table are reflective of the distinguishing foci that reached consensus across both panels

weekly frequency to be concerning. Further research is, however, required to explore/confirm this finding.

Although the current study has provided a preliminary expert-derived template for understanding and distinguishing disordered eating from pregnancy-appropriate symptomatology, there are a few limitations worth noting. First, it is acknowledged that the list of symptom attributes and delineating foci generated in the current study is not exhaustive and further discussion in this area is required. Second, as the Delphi methodology does not allow panelists to discuss topics directly with each other, it is possible that rich information often elicited from intellectual discourse with one's peers may have been missed [33]. This could have been achieved through the implementation of a consultation meeting [55]; however, the anonymity of the panels likely prevented power-imbalances and group think that may have developed via direct contact [56, 57]. Third, although the professional panel did consist of various professions, it was difficult to recruit certain professionals, namely obstetricians, and male panellists for balanced viewpoint. There are several possible explanations for this. One likely explanation is that the schedules and unpredictable workload of obstetricians have precluded participation in a study over a six-month period; however, flexible completion options were offered to all participants. Possibly, potential panellists from the field of obstetrics may not have identified with the label 'expert' due to the limited knowledge of disordered eating in pregnancy. This has been revealed in previous research and may be indicative of a greater educational issue in the field [7, 29]. Future discourse in this area would benefit from a more diverse sample of professionals of both sexes who work directly with disordered eating in an antenatal setting.

Limitations of the consumer panel should also be noted. Although the value of recruiting consumers alongside professionals has been emphasised in recent literature [34], it is possible the broad criteria for selecting consumers may have affected results, particularly given a structured criteria was employed when selecting the professional panel. This may partially explain the modest agreement between the two panels for the overall questionnaire ($\kappa = .529$); however, strong agreement was demonstrated on sections that did not rely heavily on technical knowledge, potentially suggesting that some of the discrepancies between panels (e.g., physical symptoms) were more representative of

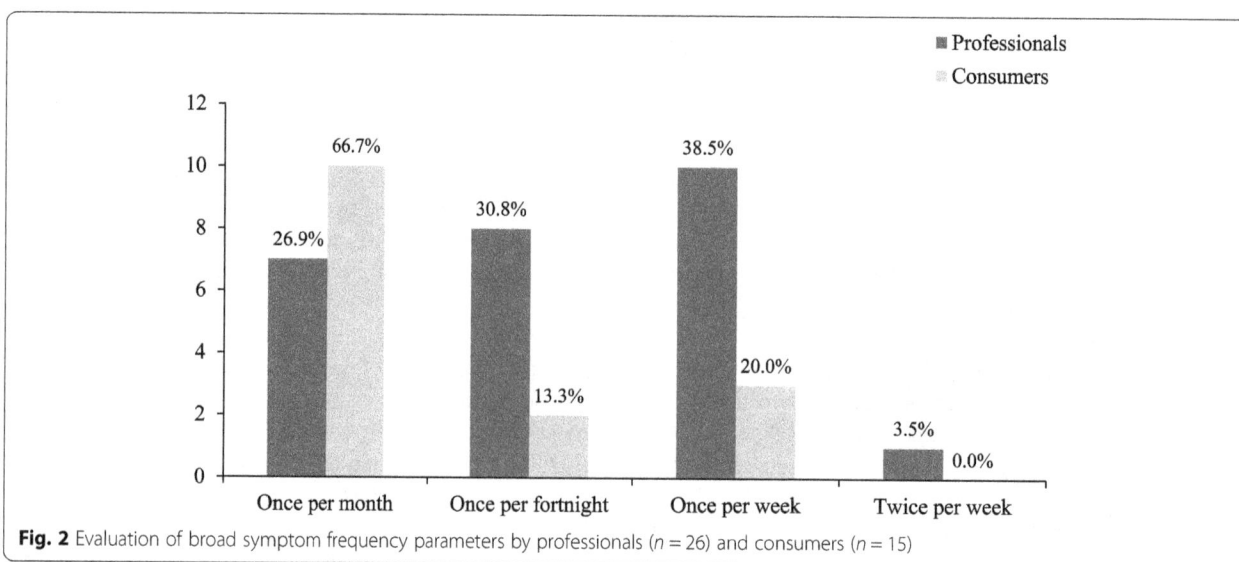

Fig. 2 Evaluation of broad symptom frequency parameters by professionals ($n = 26$) and consumers ($n = 15$)

knowledge, rather than attitudinal differences. If ratings for the physical symptoms were removed, there was good agreement between the panels (κ = .672). Future research may wish to develop more specific consumer recruitment criteria based on the findings of this study, while also ensuring all viewpoints are considered. The timing discrepancy in administering the Delphi questionnaire rounds between the two panels was also undesirable, as this meant new items suggested by the consumer panel at the end of Round I could not be incorporated into the Round II questionnaire for the professional panel. Furthermore, this discrepancy precluded the possibility of evaluating items across both panels during the study. As such, the only outcome was to compare the findings of the two independent panels at the end of the study. Future research may benefit from combining consumers and professionals into a single panel (provided questions are appropriate and do not rely on specialist knowledge), or at least ensure concurrent administration of both panels to facilitate feedback and item evaluation across both panels during the Delphi process.

Conclusions

To conclude, the areas of collective agreement in this study could guide clinicians in identifying and delineating disordered eating from pregnancy-appropriate symptomatology. It is hoped that results of this study will assist the development of psychometric tools to detect/assess pregnancy-specific disordered eating, in addition to serving as starting point for the development of a core outcome set to measure disordered eating in pregnancy [58]. This could encourage a unified research approach when measuring disordered eating symptomatology in the perinatal context and present opportunities for antenatal clinicians to provide appropriate care and support when concerning symptoms are identified.

Abbreviations
AED: Academy for eating disorders; ED: Eating disorder; GPs: General practitioners; UK: United Kingdom; USA: United States of America

Acknowledgments
The authors wish to express their sincerest gratitude to all the panel members who generously contributed their time and expertise to this study. The authors gratefully acknowledge the following members of the professional panel, who have consented to be recognised for their contributions: Ms. Jacqueline Byrne, Ms. Amanda Davis, Dr. Justine Ebenreuter, Dr. Melissa Freizinger, Dr. Christine Furber, Dr. Anthea Fursland, Ms. Kelly Gall, Dr. Marcia Herrin, Professor Angelica Lindén Hirschberg, Associate Professor Mimi Israël, Emeritus Professor Michael Levine, Ms. Shelly Read, Associate Professor Elizabeth Rieger, Professor Helen Skouteris, Dr. Stephanie Tierney, Ms. Natalie Watson, Associate Professor Jennifer Wildes, and Associate Professor Stephanie Zerwas. To protect the privacy of the consumer panel members, no individual names have been listed. We are, however, indebted to all the consumers who participated in this study, demonstrating great honesty and courage in sharing their opinions and pregnancy experiences with us. The authors also wish to thank Dr. Elizabeth J Edwards for her support and invaluable feedback during the drafting of this manuscript, in addition to Dr. Pamela Pilkington and Dr. Bassel H. Al Wattar for their helpful feedback during the peer review process.

Funding
A Research Training Program Scholarship funded by the Australian Government Department of Education and Training supported this research (AB).

Authors' contributions
AB and RH conceived the study. AB, RH, PS, BW, and KMS contributed to the design and structure of the study. AB coordinated the study, carried out data collection, performed all relevant statistical analyses, and synthesised the findings. RH, PS, BW, and KMS cross-analysed the data. AB drafted and revised the manuscript. RH, PS, and BW provided critical feedback for revision. All authors read and approved the final manuscript.

Competing interests
The authors declare that they have no competing interests.

Author details
[1]School of Psychology, Bond University, 14 University Drive, Robina, QLD 4229, Australia. [2]Faculty of Health Sciences and Medicine, Bond University, 14 University Drive, Robina, QLD 4229, Australia. [3]School of Medicine, University of Tasmania, 17 Liverpool Street, Hobart, TAS 7001, Australia.

References
1. American Psychiatric Association. Diagnostic and statistical manual of mental disorders. 5th ed. Arlington: American Psychiatric Publishing; 2015.
2. National Eating Disorders Collaboration: Disordered eating and dieting. (2017). http://www.nedc.com.au/disordered-eating. Accessed 26 Jul 2017.
3. Linna MS, Raevuori A, Haukka J, Suvisaari JM, Suokas JT, Gissler M. Reproductive health outcomes in eating disorder. Int J Eat Disord. 2014;46:826–33.
4. Watson HJ, Torgersen L, Zerwas S, Reichborn-Kjennerud T, Knoph C, Stoltenberg C, et al. Eating disorders, pregnancy, and the postpartum period: findings from the Norwegian mother and child cohort study (MoBa). Nor Epidemiol. 2014;24:51–62.
5. Abebe DS, Lien L, von Soest T. The development of bulimic symptoms from adolescence to young adulthood in females and males: a population-based longitudinal cohort study. Int J Eat Disord. 2012;45:737–45.
6. Hsu LG. The gender gap in eating disorders: why are the eating disorders more common among women? Clin Psychol Rev. 1989;9:393–407.
7. Leddy MA, Jones C, Morgan MA, Schulkin J. Eating disorders and obstetric-gynecologic care. J Women's Health. 2009;18:1395–401.
8. Stice E, Marti CN, Rohde P. Prevalence, incidence, impairment, and course of the proposed dsm-5 eating disorder diagnoses in an 8-year prospective community study of young women. J Abnorm Psychol. 2013;122:445–57.
9. Andersen AE, Ryan GL. Eating disorders in the obstetric and gynecologic patient population. Obstet Gynecol. 2009;114:1353–67.
10. Knoph Berg C, Torgersen L, Von Holle A, Harmer RM, Bulik CM, Reichborn-Kjennerud T. Factors associated with binge eating disorder in pregnancy. Int J Eat Disord. 2011;44:124–33.
11. Bulik CM, Von Holle A, Hamer R, Knoph Berg C, Torgersen L, Magnus P, Stoltenberg C, Siega-Riz A, Sullivan P, Reichborn-Kjennerud T. Patterns of remission, continuation and incidence of broadly defined eating disorders

during early pregnancy in the Norwegian mother and child cohort study (MoBa). Psychol Med. 2007;37:1109–18.

12. Easter A, Bye A, Taborelli E, Corfield F, Schmidt U, Treasure J, Micali N. Recognising the symptoms: how common are eating disorders in pregnancy? Eur Eat Disord Rev. 2013;21:340–4.

13. Harris AA. Prenatal advice for caring for women with eating disorders during the perinatal period. J Midwifery Womens Health. 2010;55:579–86.

14. Hawkins LK, Gottlieb B. Screening for eating disorders in pregnancy: how uniform screening during a high risk period could minimise under-recognition. J Women's Health. 2013;22:390–2.

15. Knoph C, Von Holle A, Zerwas S, Torgersen L, Tambs K, Stoltenberg C, Bulik CM, Reichborn-Kjennerud T. Course and predictors of maternal eating disorders in the postpartum period. Int J Eat Disord. 2013;46:355–68.

16. National Eating Disorders Collaboration. Pregnancy and eating disorders. A professional's guide to assessment and referral. Crows Nest: NEDC; 2015.

17. Soares RM, Nunes MA, Schmidt MA, Giacomelle A, Manzolli P, Camey S, et al. Inappropriate eating behaviours during pregnancy: prevalence and associated factors among pregnant women attending primary care in southern Brazil. Int J Eat Disord. 2009;42:387–93.

18. Tiller J, Treasure J. Eating disorders precipitated by pregnancy. Eur Eat Disord Rev. 1998;6:178–87.

19. Ward VB. Eating disorders in pregnancy. BMJ. 2008;336:93–6.

20. Broussard B. Psychological and behavioural traits associated with eating disorders and pregnancy: a pilot study. J Midwifery Womens Health. 2012;57:61–6.

21. Micali N, Treasure J, Simonoff E. Eating disorders symptoms in pregnancy: a longitudinal study of women with recent and past eating disorders and obesity. J Psychosom Res. 2007;63:297–303.

22. Pettersson CB, Zandian M, Clinton D. Eating disorder symptoms pre- and postpartum. Arch Womens Ment Health. 2016;19:675–80.

23. Turton P, Hughes P, Bolton H, Sedgwick P. Incidence and demographic correlates of eating disorder symptoms in a pregnant population. Int J Eat Disord. 1999;26:448–52.

24. Dickens G, Trethowan WH. Cravings and aversions during pregnancy. J Psychosom Res. 1971;15:259–68.

25. Fairburn CG, Stein A, Jones R. Eating habits and eating disorders during pregnancy. Psychosom Med. 1992;54:665–72.

26. Orloff NC, Hormes JM. Pickles and ice cream! Food cravings in pregnancy: hypotheses, preliminary evidence, and directions for future research. Front Psychol. 2014;5:1–15.

27. Franko DL, Walton BE. Pregnancy and eating disorders: a review and clinical implications. Int J Eat Disord. 1993;13:41–7.

28. Franko DL, Spurrell EB. Detection and management of eating disorders during pregnancy. Obstet Gynecol. 2000;95:942–6.

29. Morgan JF. Eating disorders and gynecology: knowledge and attitudes among clinicians. Acta Obstet Gynecol Scand. 1999;78:233–9.

30. Newton MS, Chizawsky LL. Treating vulnerable populations: the case of eating disorders during pregnancy. J Psychosom Obstet Gyn. 2006;27:5–7.

31. Easter A. Understanding eating disorders in the antenatal and postnatal periods. Perspect. 2015;26:14–5.

32. Linstone HA, Turoff M. Introduction. In: Linstone HA, Turoff M, editors. The Delphi method: techniques and applications. Reading: Addison-Wesley Publishing Company; 1975. p. 3–12.

33. Hasson F, Keeney S, McKenna H. Research guidelines for the Delphi survey technique. J Adv Nurs. 2000;32:1008–15.

34. Jorm AF. Using the Delphi expert consensus method in mental health research. Aust N Z J Psychiatry. 2015;49:87–897.

35. Sumison T. The Delphi technique: an adaptive research tool. Br J Occup Ther. 1998;61:153–6.

36. Holey EA, Feeley JL, Dixon J, Whittaker VJ. An exploration of the use of simple statistics to measure consensus and stability in Delphi studies. BMC Med Res Methodol. 2007;7:52.

37. Mittnacht AM, Bulik CM. Best nutrition counseling practices for the treatment of anorexia nervosa: a Delphi study. Int J Eat Disord. 2015;48:111–22.

38. MacFarlane L, Owens G, Del Pozo Cruz B. Identifying the features of an exercise addiction: a Delphi study. J Behav Addict. 2016;5:474–84.

39. Noetel M, Dawson L, Hay P, Touyz S. The assessment and treatment of unhealthy exercise in adolescents with anorexia nervosa: a Delphi study to synthesize clinical knowledge. Int J Eat Disord. 2017;50:378–88.

40. Ross AM, Kelly CM, Jorm AF. Re-development of mental health first aid guidelines for non-suicidal self-injury: a Delphi study. BMC Psychiatry. 2014;14:236.

41. Diamond IR, Grant RC, Feldman BM, Pencharz PB, Ling SC, Moore AM, Wales PW. Defining consensus: a systematic review recommends methodologic criteria for reporting Delphi studies. J Clin Epidemiol. 2014;67:401–9.

42. Bond KS, Jorm AF, Kelly CM, Kitchener BA, Morris SL, Mason RJ. Considerations when providing mental health first aid to an LGBTIQ person: a Delphi study. Adv Ment Health. 2017;15:183–97.

43. Kelly CM, Jorm AF, Kitchener BA, Langlands RL. Development of mental health first aid guidelines for suicidal ideation and behaviour: a Delphi study. BMC Psychiatry. 2008;8:17.

44. Langlands RL, Jorm AF, Kelly CM, Kitchener BA. First aid for depression: a Delphi consensus study with consumers, carers and clinicians. J Affect Disord. 2008;105:157–66.

45. Bannatyne AJ, Hughes R, Stapleton P, Watt B, MacKenzie-Shalders K. Consensus on the assessment of disordered eating in pregnancy: an international Delphi study. Arch Womens Ment Health. 2017; [Epub ahead of print]

46. Davis EP, Sandman CA. The timing of prenatal exposure to maternal cortisol and psychological stress is association with human infant cognitive development. Child Dev. 2010;81:131–48.

47. Blais MA, Becker AE, Burwell RA, Flores AT, Nussbaum KM, Greenwood DN, et al. Pregnancy: outcome and impact on symptomatology in a cohort of eating-disordered women. Int J Eat Disord. 2000;27:140–9.

48. Crow SJ, Agras WS, Crosby R, Halmi K, Mitchell JE. Eating disorder symptoms in pregnancy: a prospective study. Int J Eat Disord. 2008;41:277–9.

49. Mond JM, Hay PJ, Rodgers B, Owen C. Self-recognition of disordered eating among women with bulimic-type eating disorders: a community-based study. Int J Eat Disord. 2006;39:747–53.

50. Mathieu J. What is pregorexia? J Am Diet Assoc. 2009;21:976–9.

51. Wallace K: 'Pregorexia': Extreme dieting while pregnant. (2013). http://edition.cnn.com/2013/11/20/living/pregnant-dieting-pregorexia-moms/ . Accessed 24 Jul 2017.

52. Hall-Flavin DK: Is pregorexia for real?. (2015). http://www.mayoclinic.org/healthy-lifestyle/pregnancy-week-by-week/expert-answers/pregorexia/faq-20058356. Accessed 24 Jul 2017.

53. Hogue MCB, Doran E, Henry DA. A prompt to the web: the media and health information seeking behaviour. PLoS One. 2012;7:34314.

54. Fox S, Duggan M. Health online 2013. Washington, DC: Pew Research Center's Internet & American Life Project; 2013.

55. Graefe A, Armstrong JS. Comparing face-to-face meetings, nominal groups, Delphi and prediction markets on an estimation task. Int J Forecasting. 2016;27:183–95.

56. Hsu CC, Sandford BA. The Delphi technique: making sense of consensus. Pract Assess Res Eval. 2007;12:1–8.

57. Williams M, Haverkamp BE. Identifying critical competencies for psychotherapeutic practice with eating disordered clients: a Delphi study. Eat Disord. 2010;18:91–109.

58. Duffy JMN, Rolph R, Gale C, Hirsch M, Khan KS, McManus RK. Core outcome sets in women's and newborn health: a systematic review. BJOG. 2017;124:1481–9.

59. Tierney S, McGlone C, Furber C. What can qualitative studies tell us about the experiences of women who are pregnant that have an eating disorder? Midwifery. 2013;29:542–49.

60. Burton T. Walking a tightrope: women's experiences of having an eating disorder while pregnant. Aust Nurs Midwifery J. 2014;21:45.

61. Tremblay KA. Eating and psychological distress during pregnancy: The use of ecological momentary assessment (doctoral dissertation). 2015. Retrieved from ProQuest Dissertations and Theses Database (UMI No. 3732671).

62. Franko DL. Eating disorders in pregnancy and the postpartum. In: Hendrick V, editor, Psychiatric disorders in pregnancy and the postpartum. Totowa: Humana Press; 2006. pp. 179–196.

11

Macular choroidal thickness in highly myopic women during pregnancy and postpartum: a longitudinal study

Wei Chen[1†], Li Li[1†], Hongyuan Zhang[2], Yan Li[1], Xu Chen[2] and Yue Zhang[1*]

Abstract

Background: High myopia, a cause of serious visual impairment, is a significant global public health concern. We investigate longitudinal changes in macular choroidal thickness (CT) during pregnancy and 6-months postpartum in women with high myopia (HM).

Methods: A prospective longitudinal study was conducted in HM-pregnant women during the course of pregnancy ($n = 42$ eyes, 42 patients) and 6 months postpartum ($n = 40$ eyes, 40 patients, two cases lost).Macular CT was measured via enhanced-depth imaging (EDI)-optical coherence tomography (OCT) (EDI-OCT). Intraocular pressure (IOP), axial length (AL), refractive error, mean arterial pressure (MAP), mean ocular perfusion pressure (MOPP), and body mass index (BMI) were also measured.

Results: Macular CTs of HM pregnant women (214.3 ± 52.3 μm) had increased significantly during the third trimester of pregnancy compared with postpartum women (192.7 ± 51.9 μm, $p = 0.014$). No significant differences in AL, refractive error, or MAP were found between pregnant and postpartum groups ($p > 0.05$ for all parameters).During pregnancy, macular CT was negatively correlated with AL (first trimester: $p = 0.010$; second trimester: $p = 0.013$; and third trimester: $p = 0.008$) and positively correlated with refractive error (first trimester: $p = 0.038$; second trimester: $p = 0.024$; and third trimester: $p = 0.010$). No correlations between macular CT and age, IOP, MOPP, MAP, or BMI were found.

Conclusions: Our study revealed the presence of a significantly thicker choroid during the third trimester of pregnancy compared with 6-mo postpartum in HM women. Macular CT positively correlated with refractive error and negatively correlated with AL during pregnancy, but did not correlate with gestational age, MOPP, IOP, MAP, or BMI.

Keywords: Macular CT, Highly myopic pregnancy, Enhanced depth imaging optical coherence tomography, Postpartum

Background

As the worldwide prevalence of myopia increases, the proportion of patients with high myopia (HM) is now as high as ~ 4% in the adult Asian population [1]. Thus, the possibility exists that there will be an increase in pregnant women with HM in China. HM, which is defined as a myopic refractive error of > 6 diopters (D) or an axial length (AL) of > 26.5 mm, is accompanied by characteristic pathological changes, including chorioretinal myopic atrophy, i.e., thinning of the choroid and retina [2]. This debilitating condition results in photoreceptor cell death and is accompanied by an irreversible and progressive loss of central visual function. HM pregnant women often discuss ocular changes as their first healthy problem with their obstetricians, therefore, awareness of these fundus changes is important to better care for HM pregnant patients.

Enhanced depth imaging (EDI)-optical coherence tomography (OCT) (EDI-OCT) is a recently developed technique that provides high-quality images of the choroid [3]. Thus, EDI-OCT measurements of choroidal thickness (CT) is useful for observing choroidal changes in HM pregnant women. Using EDI-OCT, Kara et al. demonstrated that subfoveal CT increases in pregnant women compared with age-matched non-pregnant women, but provided no longitudinal data [4]. However, Takahashi et

* Correspondence: zmoon1976@sina.com
†Wei Chen and Li Li contributed equally to this work.
1Clinical College of Ophthalmology, Tianjin Medical University, No.4, Gansu Road, Tianjin City, People's Republic of China
Full list of author information is available at the end of the article

al. demonstrated that CTs did not differ significantly between pregnant and non-pregnant women [5]. While several studies have focused on measuring CT in HM persons or pregnant women [4, 6], none have done so in HM women during pregnancy. Thus, the goal of our study was to know the morphological changes of choroid during the course of pregnancy in HM women longitudinally.

During pregnancy, the maternal cardiovascular system undergoes profound adaptive hemodynamic changes, including increased cardiac output and stroke volume, and reduced blood pressure and peripheral vascular resistance [7]. Vascular blood flow relies on perfusion pressure (PP), and mean ocular perfusion pressure (MOPP) is considered as the driving force of ocular blood flow [8]. Considering the highly vascular nature of the choroid, we hypothesized that MOPP and intraocular pressure (IOP) are major factors associated with CT in HM pregnancy, and that correlations exist between CT and MOPP and between CT and IOP during pregnancy. Thus, we also sought to determine the key factors associated with CT during pregnancy. Furthermore, since studies of refractive error changes are conflicting in their findings, we also chose to investigate such changes during HM pregnancy [9, 10].

We investigated the longitudinal changes in CT in HM women during pregnancy and 6 months postpartum via EDI-OCT, and evaluated the relationships between macular CT and age, AL, refractive error, IOP, mean arterial pressure (MAP), MOPP, and body mass index (BMI).

Methods

Subjects

Recruitment and follow-up were conducted between June 2013 and June 2015 at Tianjin Central Hospital of Gynecology Obstetrics and Tianjin Eye Hospital, Tianjin, China. Although patients with bilateral HM were enrolled in the study, only the eye with higher myopia was studied. Tianjin Central Hospital of Gynecology Obstetrics is a major child birth hospital in Tianjin, China, overseeing delivery of > 10,000 babies annually. Written consent from each patient was obtained at recruitment. The study followed the tenets of the Declaration of Helsinki and was approved by the local ethics committee.

A total of 42 HM pregnant women ($n = 42$ eyes) were recruited during their first antenatal visit (11 weeks gestation). Inclusion criteria for the study comprised healthy patients with eyes of AL > 26.5 mm (biometric definition, as previously suggested [11]), refractive error > 6 D, no apparent macular abnormalities (e.g., choroidal neovascularization or macular holes), and aged 25–35 years. Exclusion criteria comprised pregnancy-induced complications (e.g., pre-eclampsia), previous ocular surgery, use of immunosuppressive drugs, glaucoma, retinal detachment, or eyes with poorly visualizable chorioscleral interfaces measured by EDI-OCT.

Patients were scheduled for four examinations each during gestation weeks 11–12 (first trimester group), gestation weeks 22–24 (second trimester group), gestation weeks 32–34 (third trimester group), and postpartum month ~ 6 (postpartum group). As two cases were lost to follow-up at 6-months postpartum, the postpartum group comprised 40 patients ($n = 40$ eyes).

Examinations

All participants underwent full ophthalmic examinations (including assessment of visual acuity (VA), refractive error, and IOP, AL measurements, and optic nerve head evaluation with a 90-D lens.

IOP was measured by noncontact tonometry (TX-20 model) (Canon, Tokyo, Japan) at the time of OCT imaging, and the average of three measurements was used for analysis. Spherical equivalents (SE) of refractive error were measured by autorefractometry (RK-3) (Canon, Tokyo, Japan) and ALs, by interferometry (IOL-Master) (Carl Zeiss Meditec, Dublin, CA, USA). Again, the average of three measurements was used for analysis.

Standard protocol blood pressure (BP) measurements were taken on the upper right arm using the automatic Omron HEM 705CP sphygmomanometer (Omron Healthcare Inc., Lake Forest, IL, USA) following a 5-min rest period [12]. Three separate measurements were averaged for analysis. Measurements were performed with the patient in a seated, resting position just before EDI-OCT imaging. MOPP was calculated according to the following equation: MOPP = (2/3 × MAP - IOP) [13], where MAP = diastolic BP + 1/3 × (systolic BP- diastolic BP) [14].

Body weight and height (bare feet) were measured to an accuracy of 0.1 kg and 0.1 cm, respectively, using an adjusted weighing machine and a height measuring instrument. Both measurements were taken separately and measured twice. If the first two measurements differed by 1.0 cm (height) or 200 g (weight), a third measurement was taken and included in the average calculation. BMI was calculated as weight divided by height squared (kg/m^2).

The scan protocol of the Cirrus OCT (Carl Zeiss Meditec, Jena, Germany) generates a cube of data through a 9-mm line around the macula via its HD 5-line raster mode [15]. Using the caliper system provided by the software, CT was measured from the outer surface of the hyper-reflective retinal pigment epithelium (RPE) line to the hyper-reflective line of the inner scleral border. CTs at the fovea, and 3 mm superiorly, inferiorly, temporally, and nasally to the fovea were measured between 9:00 a.m. and 12:00 p.m. on test days. The mean overall CT was obtained by calculating average values of CTs at all locations and was recorded as macular CT. Two independent observers manually measured each CT. Measurements obtained from two observers were averaged for analysis.

Statistical analyses

Statistical analyses were performed using version 17.0 SPSS software (SPSS, Inc., Chicago, IL, USA). All data are reported as mean ± standard deviation (SD), with a 95% confidence interval (CI). An unpaired t-test was used to compare variables between various groups (with normal distribution); the Mann–Whitney U-test was used to compare variables between various groups (without normal distribution). To examine the association between macular CT variables and age, AL, refractive error, IOP, MOPP, MAP, and BMI, the multiple regression analysis were calculated. A $p < 0.05$ was considered statistically significant.

Results

Demographics and clinical features

Significant differences were seen in age (all $p < 0.05$, postpartum group compared with the first, and second trimesters groups), IOP and BMI (both $p < 0.01$, postpartum group compared with the third trimester group), MOPP and macular CT (both $p < 0.05$, postpartum group compared with the third trimester), while no significant differences in AL, refractive error, or MAP were found between pregnant, and postpartum groups (all values of $p > 0.05$) (Table 1).

IOPs were significantly lower in the third trimester group compared to first trimester ($p = 0.02$), and postpartum ($p = 0.004$) groups, but not when compared to the second trimester ($p > 0.05$) group. There were no significant differences in IOPs observed between any other two groups (all $p > 0.05$) (Fig. 1).

MOPPs increased throughout pregnancy, and was significantly higher in the third trimester group than in the postpartum ($p = 0.035$) groups, while no differences were found in the first ($p > 0.05$) and second trimester ($p > 0.05$) groups. There were no significant difference in MOPPs between any other two groups (all $p > 0.05$) (Fig. 2).

BMIs were significantly higher in the third trimester group than in the first, second, postpartumgroups (all $p < 0.001$), while no significant differences were found between any other two groups (all $p > 0.05$).

Macular CT

Macular CTs increased significantly in the third trimester group compared to the postpartum ($p = 0.014$) groups, while no significant differences were observed in the first and second trimester groups (both $p > 0.05$); There were no significant differences in macular CT between any other two groups (all $p > 0.05$) (Fig. 3).

Correlation of macular CT with other variables

In studying the correlation between macular CT and measured variables, we found a significantly negative correlation with AL: ($p = 0.01$ in the first trimester; $p = 0.013$ in the second trimester; and $p = 0.008$ in the third trimester), while there was a strong positive correlation with refractive error: ($p = 0.038$ in the first trimester; $p = 0.024$ in the second trimester; and $p = 0.01$ in the third trimester). However, no significant correlations were found between macular CT and age, IOP, MOPP, MAP, or BMI during pregnancy (all $p > 0.05$) (Table 2).

Discussion

CT is a significant indicator of fundus lesions in HM [16]. In the present study, we found that macular CTs in the third trimester of pregnancy reached their

Table 1 Demographics and Clinical Characteristics of the patients throughout pregnancy and 6-months postpartum

Variables	Groups			
	First trimester ($n = 42$)	Second trimester ($n = 42$)	Third trimester ($n = 42$)	Postpartum ($n = 40$)
Mean Age (years)	28.5 ± 1.7	28.9 ± 1.7	29.3 ± 1.6	29.7 ± 1.7[a]
AL (mm)	27.6 ± 0.7	27.6 ± 0.7	27.6 ± 0.7	27.6 ± 0.7
Refractive error (D)	−9.7 ± 1.4	− 9.7 ± 1.4	−9.8 ± 1.4	− 9.6 ± 1.4
IOP (mmHg)	15.4 ± 2.8	15.0 ± 2.4	14.4 ± 2.8	15.8 ± 2.8[b]
MOPP (mmHg)	38.8 ± 3.3	39.0 ± 3.2	39.7 ± 2.8	38.6 ± 3.1[c]
MAP (mmHg)	81.7 ± 8.1	82.1 ± 7.9	82.7 ± 7.8	81.6 ± 7.9
BMI (kg/m^2)	21.9 ± 2.0	22.7 ± 2.0	24.4 ± 1.9	22.3 ± 2.2[b]
Macular CT (μm)	194.5 ± 50.3	201.9 ± 51.5	214.3 ± 52.3	192.7 ± 51.9[c]

AL axial length, D diopters, IOP intraocular pressure, MOPP mean ocular perfusion pressure, MAP mean arterial pressure, BMI body mass index, CT choroidal thickness
[a]$p < 0.05$ compared with the first, and second trimesters by t-test; [b]$p < 0.01$ compared with the third trimester by t-test; [c]$p < 0.05$ compared with the third trimester by t-test

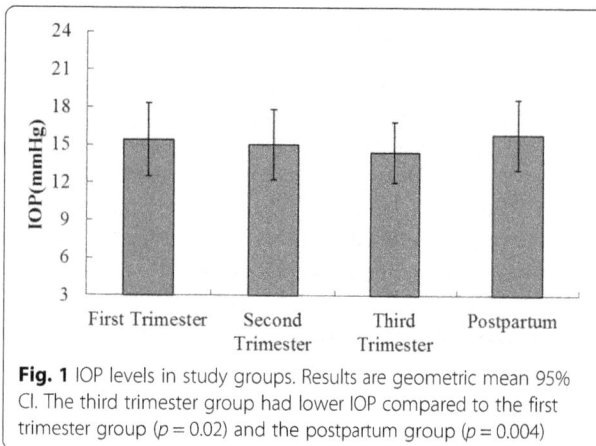

Fig. 1 IOP levels in study groups. Results are geometric mean 95% CI. The third trimester group had lower IOP compared to the first trimester group ($p = 0.02$) and the postpartum group ($p = 0.004$)

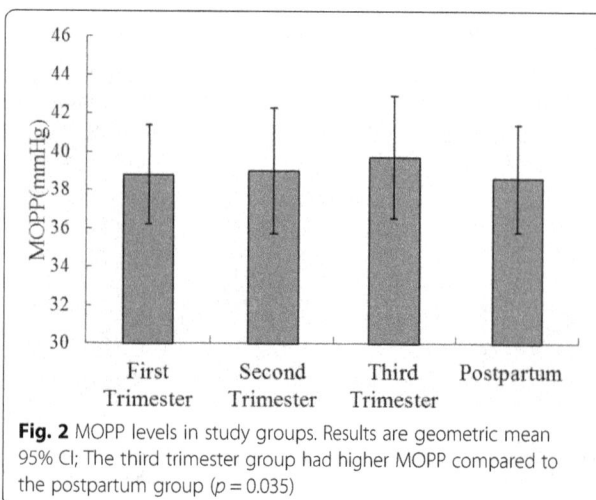

Fig. 3 Macular CT levels in study groups. Results are geometric mean 95% CI; The third trimester group had thicker CT compared to the postpartum group ($p = 0.014$)

maximum values (214.3 ± 52.3 μm), which were significantly greater compared to the postpartum group (192.7 ± 51.9 μm; $p = 0.014$). However, there were no differences compared with the first and second trimester ($p > 0.05$) groups, indicating that CTs didn't change significantly throughout pregnancy (Fig. 3). Such a finding is consistent with those of Kara et al. for normal pregnant women [4]. However, Takahashi et al. found that CTs did not differ significantly between pregnant and non-pregnant women [5]. The increases in CT may be due to an increased release of vasodilatory signaling molecules, e.g., nitric oxide, prostacyclin, and prostaglandins, all of which are key elements in the physiological systemic vasodilatation of pregnancy [17]. Our study provides the first in vivo demonstration of increased CT in HM pregnancy, including longitudinal data.

We found no significant differences in refractive errors in any of the trimester or postpartum groups ($p > 0.05$). Refractive changes during pregnancy are somewhat controversial. Mehdizadehkashi K et al. followed 107 pregnant women throughout the course of their pregnancies and 3 months postpartum, and reported no significant changes in refractive errors [9], findings identical to ours. Imafidon reported a ~ 1.25D myopic shift, attributing it to lens hydration [10]. Pizzarello reported that 15% of the women who complained of visual changes had experienced a myopic shift from pre-pregnancy levels [18]. We found a significant correlation between macular CT and refractive error during pregnancy ($p < 0.05$), indicating that choroidal thinning is prominent in highly myopic eyes, a finding consistent with another study of our group in non-pregnant highly myopic patients [15].

IOP can become lower throughout pregnancy [19]. We not only found IOP to be decreased during pregnancy, but also significantly so in the third trimester compared with first trimester, and postpartum groups (Fig. 1). The reasons for this are attributed to reduced episcleral venous pressure, greater aqueous outflow, and the effects of progesterone [20]. Similar investigations of pregnant women have shown a significant decrease in IOP compared with non-pregnant women [21]. Akar et al. also found that decreases in IOPs were greater during the third trimester [22]. In our study, we found no correlation between macular CT and IOP during pregnancy ($p > 0.05$).

Although the primary regulatory role of the choroid is well known, the in vivo clinical association of CT with MOPP has yet to be determined in HM pregnancy. Previous studies have reported that ocular blood flow increases throughout gestation [23]. In our study, we found that MOPP increased during the third trimester compared with postpartum groups ($p < 0.05$) (Fig. 2). However, no significant associations between CT and MOPP during pregnancy ($p > 0.05$) (Table 2) were found. These findings are in accordance with those of Kim et al., who found no significant correlation between subfoveal CT and MOPP ($p > 0.05$) in healthy subjects [24]. In contrast, Sayin et al. found subfoveal CT to be positively correlated with MOPP in pregnant women with no pre-eclampsia, while no correlation existed in pregnant women with pre-eclampsia [25]. The reasons for there

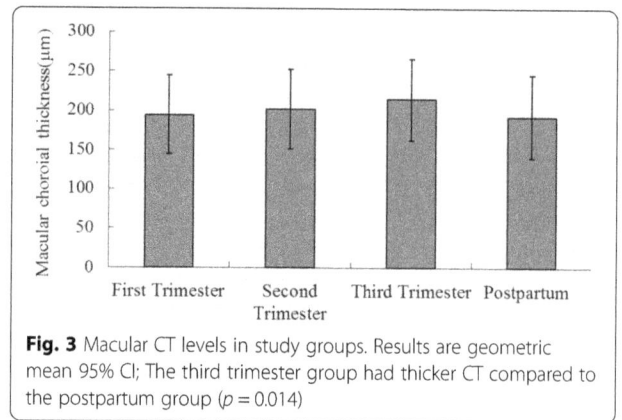

Fig. 2 MOPP levels in study groups. Results are geometric mean 95% CI; The third trimester group had higher MOPP compared to the postpartum group ($p = 0.035$)

Table 2 Correlations between macular CT and clinical and demographic factors

Factors	First trimester		Second trimester		Third trimester	
	Coefficient	p value	Coefficient	p value	Coefficient	p value
Age	−0.116	0.982	−1.297	0.791	−0.827	0.866
AL	−8.621	0.01	−8.268	0.013	−8.932	0.008
Refractive error	12.484	0.038	13.822	0.024	16.335	0.010
IOP	−2.398	0.597	−4.821	0.332	−4.181	0.422
MOPP	−7.430	0.060	−7.225	0.063	−7.676	0.058
MAP	−0.561	0.814	−1.579	0.712	−1.237	0.769
BMI	−6.614	0.205	−5.442	0.314	−5.623	0.315

CT choroidal thickness, *AL* axial length, *IOP* intraocular pressure, *MOPP* mean ocular perfusion pressure, *MAP* mean arterial pressure, *BMI* body mass index

being no significant correlation between macular CT and MOPP in our study may be the following. First, autoregulation of choroidal blood flow causes only slight changes in CT within normal ranges of IOP and ocular perfusion pressure (OPP) in healthy pregnant subjects. Second, the increase in CT may be secondary to the increase and accumulation of intrachoroidal or intrachoroidal cellular fluid substances.

Macular CT showed a negative correlation with AL ($p < 0.05$) throughout pregnancy (Table 2). These results are similar to those of Nishida et al. in their study of HM myopic eyes [26]. Meanwhile we found no significant association between macular CT and pregnancy-related factors, e.g. gestational age, BMI, or MAP (all $p > 0.05$) (Table 2).

Potential limitations to our study are as follows. First, the overall number of enrolled patients was relatively small. Large-scale studies are recommended in the future. Second, we were not able to measure all parameters before pregnancy in all patients to obtain longitudinal data for the whole study population. Third, there was some selection bias, as pregnant women were recruited from only one site. However, such a bias is not expected to be differential in nature. Fourth, CT measurements were performed manually, as there exist no precise automated software which only can reduce time and labor cost for measuring CT [27]. In the present study, two masked observers performed measurements, with adjudication if there was a difference of > 5% in agreement of measurements.

Conclusions

Our study demonstrates the presence of a significantly thicker choroid during the third trimester of pregnancy of HM women compared to 6-months after delivery. Macular CT positively correlated with refractive error and negatively correlated with AL during pregnancy, but did not correlate with gestational age, MOPP, IOP, MAP, or BMI. Improved in vivo visualization of the choroid and measurement of CT using EDI-OCT will go far to

improve our understanding of the morphologic changes occurring in the choroid in HM pregnancies.

Abbreviations
AL: Axial length; BMI: Body mass index; BP: Blood pressure; CI: Confidence interval; CT: Choroidal thickness; EDI-OCT: Enhanced-depth imaging (EDI)-optical coherence tomography; HM: High myopia; IOP: Intraocular pressure; MAP: Mean arterial pressure; MOPP: Mean ocular perfusion pressure; OPP: Ocular perfusion pressure; PP: Perfusion pressure; RPE: Retinal pigment epithelium; SD: Standard deviation; SE: Spherical equivalents; VA: Visual acuity

Acknowledgements
The authors wish to acknowledge the support of Bei Liu MD, Quan hong Han MD, Yan hua Chu MD, at the Clinical College of ophthalmology, Tianjin Medical University.

Funding
This research was funded by Tianjin Municipal Health Bureau Youth Fund-no.2012KY37 and no 2012KG124.

Authors' contributions
YZ: Design of the study; WC, LL, HYZ: Conduct of the study; LL: Statistical expertise; WC, HYZ, LL, YL, XC: Data collection; WC: Writing the article; YZ, XC: Critical revision of the article and final approval; WC, LL, HYZ, XC: Provision of materials, patients, or resources. All authors read and approved the final manuscript.

Competing interests
The authors declare that they have no competing interests.

Author details
[1]Clinical College of Ophthalmology, Tianjin Medical University, No.4, Gansu Road, Tianjin City, People's Republic of China. [2]Tianjin Central Hospital of Gynecology and Obstetrics, Tianjin, China.

References
1. Kim EC, Morgan IG, Kakizaki H, Kang S, Jee D. Prevalence and risk factors for refractive errors: Korean National Health and nutrition examination survey 2008-2011. PLoS One. 2013;8:e80361.

2. You QS, Peng XY, Xu L, Chen CX, Wang YX, Jonas JB. Myopic maculopathy imaged by optical coherence tomography: the bei jing eye study. Ophthalmology. 2014;121:220–4.
3. Dhoot DS, Huo S, Yuan A, et al. Evaluation of choroidal thickness in retinitis pigmentosa using enhanced depth imaging optical coherence tomography. Br J Ophthalmol. 2013;97:66–9.
4. Kara N, Sayin N, Pirhan D, et al. Evaluation of subfoveal choroidal thickness in pregnant women using enhanced depth imaging optical coherence tomography. Curr Eye Res. 2014;39:642–7.
5. Takahashi J, Kado M, Mizumoto K, Igarashi S, Kojo T. Choroidal thickness in pregnant women measured by enhanced depth imaging optical coherence tomography. Jpn J Ophthalmol. 2013;57:435–9.
6. Fujiwara T, Imamura Y, Margolis R, Slakter JS, Spaide RF. Enhanced depth imaging optical coherence tomography of the choroid in highly myopic eyes. Am J Ophthalmol. 2009;148:445–50.
7. Melchiorre K, Sharma R, Thilaganathan B. Cardiac structure and function in normal pregnancy. Curr Opin Obstet Gynecol. 2012;24:413–21.
8. Schmidl D, Garhofer G, Schmetterer L. The complex interaction between ocular perfusion pressure and ocular blood flow-relevance for glaucoma. Exp Eye Res. 2011;93:141–55.
9. Mehdizadehkashi K, Chaichian S, Mehdizadehkashi A, et al. Visual acuity changes during pregnancy and postpartum: a cross-sectional study in Iran. J Pregnancy. 2014;2014:675792.
10. Imafidon CO, Imafidon JE. Contact lenses in pregnancy. Br J Obstet Gynecol. 1992;99:865–7.
11. Chen W, Guan Y, He G, et al. Aqueous Levels of Pigment Epithelium-Derived Factor and Macular Choroidal Thickness in High Myopia. J Ophthalmol. 2015; 2015:731461.
12. Vera-Cala LM, Orostegui M, Valencia-Angel LI, López N, Bautista LE. Accuracy of the Omron HEM-705 CP for blood pressure measurement in large epidemiologic studies. Arq Bras Cardiol. 2011;96:393–8.
13. Rishi P, Rishi E, Mathur G, Raval V. Ocular perfusion pressure and choroidal thickness in eyes with polypoidal choroidal vasculopathy, wet-age-related macular degeneration, and normals. Eye (Lond). 2013;27:1038–43.
14. Skråstad RB, Hov GG, Blaas HG, Romundstad PR, Salvesen KÅ. A prospective study of screening for hypertensive disorders of pregnancy at 11 to 13 weeks in a Scandinavian population. Acta Obstet Gynecol Scand. 2014;93: 1238–47.
15. Chen W, Song H, Xie S, Han Q, Tang X, Chu Y. Correlation of macular choroidal thickness with concentrations of aqueous vascular endothelial growth factor in high myopia. Curr Eye Res. 2015;40:307–13.
16. Wang NK, Lai CC, Chu HY, et al. Classification of early dry-type myopic maculo- pathy with macular choroidal thickness. Am J Ophthalmol. 2012; 153:669–77. 677. e1–2
17. Clapp JF 3rd, Capeless E. Cardiovascular function before, during, and after the first and subsequent pregnancies. Am J Cardiol. 1997;80:1469–73.
18. Pizzarello LD. Refractive changes in pregnancy. Graefes Arch Clin Exp Ophthalmol. 2003;241:484–8.
19. Efe YK, Ugurbas SC, Alpay A, Ugurbas SH. The course of corneal and intraocular pressure changes during pregnancy. Can J Ophthalmol. 2012;47:150–4.
20. Grant AD, Chung SM. The eye in pregnancy: ophthalmologic and neuro-ophthalmologic changes. Clin Obstet Gynecol. 2013;56:397–412.
21. Ebeigbe JA, Ebeigbe PN, Ighoroje AD. Intraocular pressure in pregnant and non-pregnant Nigerian women. Afr J Reprod Health. 2011;15:20–3.
22. Akar Y, Yucel I, Akar ME, Zorlu G, Ari ES. Effect of pregnancy on intraobserver and intertechnique agreement in intraocular pressure measurements. Ophthalmologica. 2005;219:36–42.
23. Centofanti M, Migliardi R, Bonini S, Manni G, Bucci MG, Pesavento CB, et al. Pulsatile ocular blood flow during pregnancy. *Eur J Ophthalmol.* 2002;12: 276–80.
24. Kim M, Kim SS, Kwon HJ, Koh HJ, Lee SC. Association between choroidal thickness and ocular perfusion pressure in young, healthy subjects: enhanced depth imaging optical coherence tomography study. Invest Ophthalmol Vis Sci. 2012;27(53):7710–7.
25. Sayin N, Kara N, Pirhan D, Vural A, Araz Ersan HB, Tekirdag AI, et al. Subfoveal choroidal thickness in preeclampsia: comparison with normal pregnant and nonpregnant women. Semin Ophthalmol. 2014;29:11–7.
26. Nishida Y, Fujiwara T, Imamura Y, Lima LH, Kurosaka D, Spaide RF. Choroidal thickness and visual acuity in highly myopic eyes. Retina. 2012;32:1229–36.
27. Lee S, Fallah N, Forooghian F, Ko A, Pakzad-Vaezi K, Merkur AB, et al. Comparative analysis of repeatability of manual and automated choroidal thickness measurements in nonneovascular age-related macular degeneration. Invest Ophthalmol Vis Sci. 2013;54:2864–71.

12

"If we're here, it's only because we have no money…" discrimination and violence in Mexican maternity wards

Rosario Valdez Santiago, Luz Arenas Monreal, Anabel Rojas Carmona and Mario Sánchez Domínguez[*] ⓘ

Abstract

Background: Structural and gender violence in Mexico take on various forms, obstetric violence among them. The objective of our study consisted in analyzing experiences of structural and gender discrimination against women during childbirth care at two public hospitals in Mexico.

Methods: We conducted a cross-sectional mixed methods study including a survey of closed questions administered to all women **who received health care** for vaginal or cesarean childbirth at two public hospitals from May 7 to June 7, 2012 ($N = 512$). Those who reported some form of abuse on the part of health-care professionals were then invited to complete a semi-structured interview (20 women agreed to participate). In addition, three focus groups were organized with health-care professionals from both institutions (31 participants): two were composed of nurses and one of obstetrician-gynecologists (OB-GYNs). This work deals with the qualitative component of the study.

Results: The narratives of the health-care professionals interviewed contained expressions of health discrimination relating to certain characteristics of their clients, namely poverty, ignorance, failure to understand instructions and being women. The women, on the other hand, perceived themselves as belonging to a low social class and, as a result, behaved passively with staff throughout their hospital stay. They reported both physical and psychological abuse during care. The first included having their legs manipulated roughly, being strapped to the bed, and being subjected to multiple and careless pelvic examinations. Psychological abuse included reprimands, insults, disrespectful remarks, neglect and scowling gestures when requesting assistance.

Conclusions: The results of our study bear implications for the doctor-client relationship and for the health system in general. They suggest a need to dismantle medical practice – particularly with regard to obstetrics and gynecology - as it has been historically learned and internalized in Mexico. It is imperative to design public policies and strategies based on targeted interventions for dismantling the multiple forms of structural and gender violence replicated daily by actors in the health system.

Keywords: Obstetric violence, Discrimination, Mexico

* Correspondence: mario.sanchez@insp.mx
Center for Health Systems Research, The National Institute of Public Health in Mexico, Av. Universidad 655, Col. Santa María Ahuacatitlán, 62100 Cuernavaca, Morelos, Mexico

Background

The concept of structural violence includes various forms of social vulnerability [1] to discriminatory actions based on differences in social class, physical appearance, ethnicity and gender, among other characteristics. These actions, which normally pass unnoticed, are mirrored in the contrasting treatment of people exhibiting these differences [2].

According to Krieger [3], discrimination is a socially structured and sanctioned phenomenon identifiable by the preeminence of a dominant social group. Justified by the ideology of the dominant actors, discrimination translates into individual and institutional interactions that ensure the privileges of the dominant group. The forms and types of discrimination vary depending on who exerts or endures it. Krieger affirms that comparing the health outcomes of subordinate versus dominant social actors provides only an indirect perspective on the consequences of discrimination.

The study of violence in specific vulnerable groups (e.g., women, minors, refugees and older adults) has traditionally revolved around individual determinants rather than using an explicatory model where the association between structural and other forms of violence can be clearly traced. With regard to women, some forms of violence (e.g., intimate partner violence) have been spotlighted by studies and public policies while others (e.g., femicide) have occurred away from the public eye [4]. A salient example of the latter, obstetric violence [5] has been described as abuse and disrespect during the provision of health-care services [4]. This form of violence is perpetrated by health-care professionals (predominantly by the medical and nursing staff) against pregnant, laboring and postpartum women.

A consensus has not been reached on how to define or measure obstetric violence, with the result that prevalence rates in the literature vary considerably; for Latin America, for instance, reported rates range between 5.4 and 29.1% [6–9].

In recent years, abuse and violence against women during the provision of childbirth services have been classified under typologies including neglect, discrimination, and physical, sexual and verbal violence [5, 10, 11].

However, obstetric violence needs to be viewed as part of a wider picture, not only as a care quality issue. In addition to human rights violations, women victims of obstetric violence [12] experience numerous consequences from these acts. Physically, they undergo practices that range from painful procedures without prior informed consent or anesthesia to injuries and complications resulting from negligence or from excessive medicalization [11, 13]. Psychological consequences have also been reported involving a sense of loss of autonomy, denial of care, and discrimination [12]. These can lead to reduced acceptability and accessibility of obstetric services [14].

Thus far, the study of obstetric violence has centered on the doctor- woman relationship, without considering that this interaction does not occur in a social vacuum, but is intimately linked to expressions of structural and institutional violence which have been legitimized and normalized in the health sector, in public policy and in interpersonal relations overall: expressions which are rooted in the organization of the health system itself and in the education of health-care professionals [15].

Evidence of this can be seen in the configuration of what Good [16] has defined as the medical culture, where different disciplines intertwine (medicine-nursing). Abusive relationships not only exist within the various medical strata, but are learned and internalized from the very onset of a health professional's education [8, 10, 17].

Castro [18] suggests that a structural link exists between the overall education received by medical students and the authoritarian traits they eventually exhibit in their professional practice. These traits find their most favorable vehicle in the medical habitus [9].

In light of the foregoing, it is clear that the approach to the problem of obstetric violence needs to extend beyond the dominant-subordinate relationship (health-care professionals versus clients). It is important to bear in mind that the power mechanisms underlying the doctor-client relationship have been internalized and legitimized by institutionalized medical practice. They are no longer questioned by the actors (health-care personnel, authorities, or the women themselves in their role as patients). The qualitative approach used in our study enriched our analysis with the voices of health-service users and providers describing the ways in which structural factors shape the manifestations of obstetric violence.

The objective of our study involved analyzing experiences of structural and gender discrimination against women during childbirth care at two public hospitals in Mexico.

Methods

Our study adopted a cross-sectional mixed methods design featuring a survey of closed questions directed at all the women who received health care for either vaginal or cesarean childbirth at two public hospitals in Mexico, from May 7 to June 7, 2012. Methodological triangulation allowed for embodying prevalence data which, although important, proves insufficient to determine the magnitude of obstetric violence.

As a first step, we administered a questionnaire composed of 34 items on (a) socio-demographic characteristics (10 items); (b) prior obstetric experience (9 items);

(c) exposure to violence during the obstetric-care process (11 items); (d) information and consent to medical procedures (31 items); and (e) exposure to intimate partner violence during pregnancy (8 items). The results of the quantitative component have been published elsewhere (Valdez et al., abstract, [8]).

Women who reported some form of abuse on the part of health-care professionals were invited to complete a semi-structured interview. Three focus groups were organized with health-care professionals (two with nursing staff; the other with medical staff, specifically with obstetrician-gynecologists-OB-GYNs) from the same institutions where the women had received health care in a medical setting. This work presents only the qualitative data derived from the interviews with the women and from the focus groups with health-care professionals. Our research protocol was approved by the Research and Ethics Committees of the National Institute of Public Health in Mexico (*INSP* by its Spanish initials). The women and health-care professionals interviewed signed a letter of informed consent prior to participating in the study.

Population
Health-care users (20 women) and personnel (physicians and nurses from the obstetrics and gynecology department) at two public hospitals in Mexico (31 health-care professionals).

Instruments
(A) A semi-structured interview guide for exploring how women were cared for in a medical setting during their delivery and postpartum processes; (B) a guide for interviewing nursing personnel; and (C) a guide for interviewing OB-GYNs.

Procedure
We conducted and audio-recorded semi-structured interviews with the women, whose authorization was obtained prior to the recordings. The interviews were held within 6 to 24 h of delivery in the participating hospital facilities. We also organized three focus groups with physicians and nurses from the obstetrics and gynecology department at the hospitals where the women had been attended to.

Two focus groups were organized with nursing staff, each composed of six individuals. Mostly women, participants were aged 25–52 years, held a bachelor degree in nursing, and had 2–24 years' work experience.

The focus group with medical staff gathered OB-GYN specialists responsible for attending births in the two hospitals. They included seven women and two men aged 30–38 years and with 1–10 years' work experience.

All the groups, coordinated by two members of the research team, were held in the participating hospital facilities.

Data analysis
Information from the interviews and focus groups was transcribed and analyzed using Atlas ti V 7 software. Analysis was broken down into five phases: (1) reading of interview and focus group transcriptions to identify codes; (2) discussion and agreements among research team members to define codes; (3) re-reading of transcriptions to establish coding; (4) analysis by code to find regularities and differentials; and (5) elaboration of data concentration tables and matrices based on findings.

Analysis included the processes of open coding, axial coding and construction of a conditional matrix representing the characteristics, consequences and actions pertaining to the phenomenon under study. Having reached the point of theoretical saturation, the team found a conceptual scheme for identifying the central category, or phenomenon around which the other categories were built. The central category was abuse perpetrated by health-care professionals against women, and the related sub-categories were non-consensual care; non-confidential care; undignified medical care; abandonment of care; and health discrimination.

For the purposes of this study, the central category was defined as any action or omission that results in abuse (physical or emotional) or disrespect against women on the part of health-care personnel during childbirth care.

This manuscript discusses the central and the health discrimination categories, both of which clearly reflect the discrimination to which women were submitted by health services during childbirth care.

Results
Participants
Sociodemographic correlates of abuse
The sample was composed of 512 women: the majority were young adults (aged 13–44 years) dedicated to housework and affiliated with the *Seguro Popular*. They had middle-school education (nine years of schooling), had a partner, and identified themselves as Catholics. Table 1 presents their socio-demographic characteristics by reported abuse.

Abuse during childbirth care
Prevalence of abuse reached 29% ($n = 149$), with no differences observed between hospitals ($p = 0.815$). We were only able to interview 20 of the abused women (16 from hospital 1 and 4 from Hospital 2) (Table 2).

Table 1 Socio-demographic characteristics of abused women (by abuse)

Characteristics	Abuse		Total	p value*
	Yes	No		
	(n = 138)	(n = 374)	(n = 512)	
Age (years)				0.610
13–19	26	74	30	
20–24	27	73	34	
25–29	23	77	18	
30–34	38	62	9	
35–39	26	74	7	
40–44	30	70	2	
Education				0.050
None/elementary school	21	79	24	
Middle school	25	75	43	
High school	35	65	28	
University	32	68	5	
Religion				0.503
Catholic	26	74	77	
Other	30	70	18	
None	35	65	5	
Indigenous language				0.081
Yes	47	53	3	
No	26	74	97	
Marital status				0.321
Currently with partner	26	74	87	
Currently without partner	32	68	13	
Labor status				0.177
Works	30	70	7	
Studies	55	45	2	
Housewife	26	74	85	
Disability	0	100	1	
Does not work	36	64	5	
Insurance				0.477
Seguro Popular	27	73	96	
Other	0	100	1	
None	21	79	3	
Number of pregnancies				0.321
1	29	71	45	
2	27	73	26	
3	26	74	17	
4	28	72	7	
5 or more	8	92	5	

Table 1 Socio-demographic characteristics of abused women (by abuse) *(Continued)*

Characteristics	Abuse		Total	p value*
	Yes	No		
	(n = 138)	(n = 374)	(n = 512)	
Type of childbirth				0.060
Vaginal	32	68	43	
Cesarean	24	76	50	
Scheduled cesarean	18	82	7	

Source: authors elaboration *p value chi square test

Table 2 Socio-demographic characteristics of abused women

Caracterísics	Proportion (n = 20)
Age (years)	
13–19	39
20–24	39
25–29	11
30–34	6
35–39	5
Education	
None/elementary school	17
Middle school	55
High school	28
Religion	
Catholic	72
Other	28
Indigenous language	
Yes	6
No	94
Marital status	
Currently with partner	72
Currently without partner	28
Labor status	
Student	11
Housewife	89
Insurance	
Seguro Popular	100
Number of pregnancies	
1	50
2	33
3	11
4	6
Type of childbirth	
Vaginal	22
Cesarean	78

Source: authors elaboration

The health-care personnel who exerted abuse consisted of nurses (40%), female doctors (30%) and male doctors (30%).

Health discrimination

Expressions denoting stigmatization and discrimination against women on the part of health-care professionals were identified in the narratives of both women and professionals with regard to the following characteristics: (a) physical appearance, (b) poverty and (c) status as women. Furthermore, the self-perception of belonging to a disadvantaged social class was identified in the narratives of the women as a decisive factor in their submissive behavior towards health-care professionals during delivery care.

Because they are poor: The voices of health-care professionals

Health-care professionals stigmatized the behavior of poor women (e.g., eating with the food tray on the bed rather than on the table and piling up dirty diapers from their babies on the table) and reported that these actions "drove them crazy." They also mentioned repeatedly that, because these women were poor, they should make health decisions related to (a) exclusive breastfeeding and (b) contraceptive use. While both proposals are in themselves highly recommended for preserving the health of the mother and newborn, citing poverty as the primary reason for adopting them reflects a discriminatory attitude. Coupled with these comments, the health-care professionals continuously disparaged women for their limited understanding of medical instructions, recommendations and decisions. The following dialogue between a nurse and a woman is an example of this:

According to the nurse, "The mothers here, the majority, are very, what's the word? Strange. They're very reluctant to accept the information we give them."

"On breastfeeding or in general?" inquired the interviewer.

"In general." replied the nurse. "Here, we place a lot of emphasis on breastfeeding because they always ask for formula milk, but when we give them information, they act very reluctantly." She was referring to exclusive breastfeeding (Nurses FG).

Health-care professionals argued that the women had difficulty understanding their instructions and requests and that, as a result, their communication was ineffective. They held that the women understood the information at the beginning but quickly forgot it. This was an underlying belief among staff, who described this behavior as annoying and exasperating. They used the phrase "demanding and rude" in their descriptions of these women and attributed their behavior to their "low cultural level" (an expression they commonly used in reference to the women's low academic level).

They also employed the term "crazy" in reference to their limited schooling (desertion), early gestation (some were adolescent mothers), numerous births, and lack of knowledge about pregnancy and childbirth.

"I think that, here, what this implies, the heart of the matter, is the education of the patients." (OB-GYNs FG).

"You can explain things to them a lot, but they end up coming back to the same…" (Nurses FG).

"Maybe they understand, but you know, no matter how many times you show them slides, [use] the whiteboard and present [the information], some people are simply blocked. That's happened to me and it's exasperating." (OB-GYNs FG.)

In addition, the health-care professionals repeatedly expressed their annoyance with the demanding attitudes of the women by virtue of their being affiliated with the *Seguro Popular*.[1] What underlay this complaint, however, was not the affiliation in itself: these women believed that, being poor, they had no right to receive "free" medical care nor to demand that services be of high quality and offer a reasonable level of comfort - as if being poor implied having no rights at all. Once again, stigmatization and discrimination derived from structural social elements such as socioeconomic class were identified and translated into inequalities in care. Furthermore, aspects of the interpersonal relationships between health-care professionals and users marked by entrenched institutional hierarchies and high levels of vulnerability on the part of the users resulted in abuses of power by the former. The following testimony illustrates the points above:

"An angry woman comes up to me and says, 'Well, you know what? Thanks to me you have work.' And, although I usually don't respond, I tell her, 'Well, thanks to me you have *Seguro Popular*, because I pay my taxes,[2] and I didn't give her the bedpan.[3] I told her she had already gotten up to bathe, I mean, why did she want a comfortable bedpan when she had already, I mean, when a patient stays in bed it makes things more complicated, so I grabbed it and didn't give it to her." (Nurses FG; underlining is the authors').

In their narratives, the health-care professionals referred explicitly to what was permitted in public hospitals (e.g., multiple pelvic examinations), being teaching hospitals, as opposed to private hospitals, where it is understood that women who pay for services will not be examined as many times as "teaching" requires. The following testimony illustrates this contrasting perspective between what in fact *can* be done with women receiving health care at public (poor women) versus private hospitals (women with the means to pay for services). It demonstrates the unequal care provided to women with the same health-care needs but different means and conditions with which to confront them:

"Yes, there are resident doctors (in private medical facilities), yes, but fewer. Why? Because as a private patient, you [the OB-GYN] can't allow the 15 residents who are still in school to be tampering with her. So the physician in charge of the private patient assigns one [to the case]: 'Look, man [referring to the resident in training], you're going to examine her only when necessary. Otherwise, talk to me and I'll decide what to do, because I get paid 30 thousand pesos'.[4]" (OB-GYNs FG).

Social-class discrimination: The voices of women
Self-perception of social class

Testimonies reflected the self-perception of the women regarding poverty and explained their behavior: in identifying themselves as poor, they did not believe they could protect themselves from the insults of attending personnel. The majority of women interviewed did not see themselves as citizens with rights. Because they had no money to pay for other services, most were affiliated with the *Seguro Popular*. They felt, therefore, that they had no choice but to tolerate the treatment they were given; this, in addition to experiencing a constant fear that something would happen to their babies. Whether from shame or fear of being treated even worse, they did not respond to reprimands from the staff for not being knowledgeable about the physiological processes of infant care, or to their comments concerning their economic situation. Furthermore, the women reported that, having received an education, the professional staff believed they were superior to them and felt they had the right to accentuate that the reason they were giving birth in a public hospital was for lack of money. The following testimony illustrates how one of the interviewees assumed that she had to remain silent and put up with abuse:

"'So be quiet, because you're not the only one; there are many of you here.' [commentary of one physician to a woman]. So I had to be quiet. I couldn't do anything. We had no money to pay for private services. We had to be there no matter what, right?" (18-year-old first-time mother).

Abuse of women by health-care professionals

The testimonies of the women revealed basically two forms of abuse: physical and psychological. The health-care professionals reported the same information but did not accept the fact that they were perpetrating violence: they justified their rudeness as necessary for making the women understand instructions and, at times, for saving their lives.

Physical abuse

The physical abuse reported by the women was characterized by the following actions: having their legs manipulated roughly, being slapped, pinched and strapped to the bed. The following testimony justifies the violent actions exerted against women by health-care professionals:

"Well I tied her to the gurney, grabbed some bandages and put them on her hands and legs. I put them there like that, and that was the only way I could remove the placenta and stop the bleeding. So, to what extent can this be considered an aggression if I'm saving her life? Because I had no other choice but to tie her up so that I could get the baby out, because she wasn't listening, she wasn't paying attention to me even though I explained it to her and everything. What do you do [in these cases]?" (OB-GYNs FG).

Physical abuse also translated into poorly practiced routine clinical procedures, for example, sticking women numerous times in the attempt to administer anesthesia or intravenous (IV) serum, performing medical procedures, such as an episiotomy, without anesthesia, and repeating pelvic examinations carelessly and without providing an explanation. Painful in themselves, these are aggravated when conducted without the proper technique. The following testimony details how these procedures were carried out:

The interviewer asked one of the women in the study sample, "Did you know what they were injecting you with?".

"Well, no," replied the woman, "it was like...when I asked [they said], 'it was to speed it up [the delivery],' but I felt something burning on my back. They had to bend me over and they kept touching my back. The nurse kept on doing it wrong. It would have been better if the doctor did it, right? And again she did it wrong and kept on asking. I mean, they gave me the injection [epidural] three times." (15-year-old first-time mother).

Psychological abuse

This form of abuse was characterized by screaming, verbal humiliation, offensive jokes, reprimands for expressing pain or requesting service, scowling gestures and disapproving faces.

Screaming and humiliation were described as a routine form of communication: "You're not at home;" "You're not alone, so be quiet!" Ill-treatment extended to the newborns as well: "Do you do this by kilos?" [referring to a large baby], and "This product is for men" [referring to a female baby]. These are vivid examples of the objectification of the female body - even that of female babies.

According to the women's self-reports, gestures and expressions of disapproval were expressed by OB-GYNs and nurses at various moments during care, particularly when the women requested assistance in climbing onto the gurney, going to the lavatory, and bathing the day after giving birth.

Scowls of disapproval were as severe as stigmatizing of bad mothers, particularly for the unfamiliarity of the women with the physiological processes of pregnancy and childbirth, a lack of knowledge which was exacerbated in the case of adolescent or first-time mothers: "Are you stupid? You don't know what pregnancy is?"

In addition to the above, it was common practice for health-care professionals to hold the women accountable for any possible adverse results in the health of their newborns. In the delivery room,[5] allusions to eroticism in the women's lives were generalized, referring to the sexual enjoyment exclusively of the women, and presuming the moral authority to punish. And there were always those to remind them: "Don't cry. Deal with it. Remember how you did it. You liked it then and now you're screaming. So deal with it." (21-year-old multiparous woman).

The women interviewed reported being repeatedly neglected by staff during their care. Neglect took different forms: from not permitting visits from their families or children, ignoring requests from their relatives, and failing to provide assistance with activities which would have allowed them to move, to not/authorizing the entrance of family members to the women's rooms at their sole discretion.

The interviewer inquired, "And why are some women allowed to bring a family member with them and you aren't?".

"Because she came up yesterday night, the one over there, on that side," responded the woman, "and she brought a family member to stay with her. But me, no, they brought me up yesterday morning, and yesterday morning they wouldn't let my mother stay" (21-year-old first-time mother).

In addition to the actions outlined above, neglect acquired particular importance after delivery, when mothers awaited information about their newborns. A number of reports indicated that health-care professionals did not show the babies to the mothers at that time, nor offered information to their family members. Below is one of the most relevant testimonies:

The interviewer inquired, "Did they show you your baby when it was born?".

"They didn't show him to me," responded the woman. "They were checking him. I turned around and looked. They kept on checking him and took him away." (17-year-old first-time mother).

Discussion

We identified abusive practices – physical, verbal and discriminatory actions - against women during delivery care at the sampled hospitals. Relating mostly to the social vulnerability of the women, these practices reflect open discrimination against the majority of Mexican women. Our results are consistent with the national, regional and international literature on the topic [7, 11, 19, 20].

Our findings indicate that being poor and holding Seguro Popular (SP) insurance are grounds for discrimination. This bears far-reaching implications, given that the SP is the most important public policy ever implemented by the Mexican government to protect the health of the most vulnerable populations. Moreover, the SP was designed as a means for reversing segregation in the Mexican health system [21, 22]. According to Link, this form of discrimination in health institutions falls within the category of structural discrimination, as it involves professional health practices undertaken against women within institutional spaces [23].

Our findings provide evidence of violations of individuals' sexual and reproductive rights, specifically of the right to non-discrimination on social status [24]. The abusive practices observed are opposed to international and national regulations. Internationally, the UN Committee on Economic, Social and Cultural Rights (CESCR) defines health as a "fundamental human right indispensable for the exercise of other human rights" [25].

At the national level, in conformity with Article 4 of the Mexican Constitution, the regulation in force provides that "...every person has the right to health protection" [26]. Furthermore, the Supreme Court of Justice of the Nation established the right to health as a subjective public right, and determined that "the right to health protection pursues, inter alia, the enjoyment of health and social wellbeing services that meet the needs of the population" [27].

Another aspect that warrants particular attention concerns the annoyance expressed by health professionals at the women's inability to understand the instructions and processes relative to pregnancy and childbirth. They attribute this deficit to ignorance on the part of poor women, without bearing in mind that maternal health literacy involves "cognitive and social skills that determine the motivation and ability of women to gain access to, understand, and use information in a way that promotes and maintains their health and that of their children" [28]. They overlook the fact that maternal health literacy should be the outcome of quality prenatal care; in other words, that it is not a matter of personal ignorance, but rather a vacuum fostered by inadequate primary-care services.

This chasm between health-care professionals and the population should be deemed is sufficient grounds for reassessing the medical and nursing academic curricula. Established programs should encompass the ethical aspects of health care [10], the interculturality of service [29], and the notion of citizenship in health-care users [30]. The curricula should also provide sensitivity training in the human, sexual and reproductive rights of women [31].

Our findings indicate that health-care professionals are not aware that they engage in practices of violence and discrimination against women. They interpret their behavior as actions that "save lives" and are therefore justified as necessary [11]. Our results in Mexico resemble those obtained in other countries [29] regarding women with specific characteristics including single-mother maternity and ethnicity [32, 33].

Over two million births are attended annually in Mexico [34], the majority in public health institutions, which are the only option accessible to the poorest women. As documented in the present study, approaching these institutions involves having contact with a health system that violates their sexual and reproductive rights, among others.

Subsequent to studies conducted in Mexico [8, 10, 18, 20], decision-makers from the Ministry of Health have implemented a number of strategies to reverse this problem (e.g., the Strategy for the promotion of proper treatment during pregnancy, childbirth and the postpartum period) [35]. However, no evidence is available thus far for identifying the scope and impact of these interventions. Given the complexity of the problem, efforts in this area should be continuous and long-term.

Limitations

The principal limitation to our study is the fact that our quantitative sample was selected under convenience sampling.

Conclusions

Our findings support the argument that obstetric violence research must follow an integral approach. Account should be taken of the macro social context, rather than confining analysis to individuals [health-care professionals vs. women demanding obstetric care] who converge in a specific space at a specific time (public hospital-childbirth care).

The encounter between health-care professionals and their clients is conditioned by the characteristics of the health-care system itself. Additionally, it occurs in a social context where not only human relations but also health organizations are permeated by violence [15]. In particular, the naturalization of gender violence against women sustains its reproduction in different contexts; health-care spaces are not an exception. Notwithstanding progress made in information services and the national legal framework, Mexico continues to yield devastating indicators on violence against women including violations of their rights.

In Mexico, as in other countries, health institutions engage in structural discrimination against women. It is expressed in the delivery rooms and by health-care professionals.

Endnotes

[1] A government insurance scheme featuring a service catalog for affiliates (*CAUSES* by its Spanish initials). *CAUSES* is based on agreements with a variety of public and private health-care providers in all the states of Mexico (http://www.seguropopular.org/) last consulted on February 3, 2016).

[2] The underlying message in this comment was that, owing to their poverty, poor individuals did not pay taxes. This is technically erroneous, as all consumers pay taxes when they acquire consumer goods.

[3] A shallow receptacle for the urine and feces of persons confined to bed, particularly in a hospital.

[4] In 2012 equivalent to $ 2308 USD [36].

[5] An area in the labor and delivery unit of a hospital where women are assisted during the second stage of labor.

Abbreviations

CESCR: Committee on Economic, Social and Cultural Rights (United Nations); INSP: National Institute of Public Health in Mexico (by its Spanish initials); OB-GYNs: obstetrician-gynecologists; SP: Seguro Popular (by its Spanish initials)

Acknowledgements

We would first like to thank the women who agreed to participate in the study and replied to our questions at such a highly sensitive time in their lives. We are also grateful to the local and national authorities who facilitated our work despite resistance from the medical community to address the problem under consideration. Finally, special thanks go to Dr. Luis Villanueva Egan, at the time of our study Associate Director of the National Center for Gender Equity and Reproductive Health, the organization that funded our project.

Funding

We received funding from the National Center for Gender Equity and Reproductive Health (Ministry of Health and Health Services of the State of Morelos).

Authors' contributions

RVS was involved in the original study design; she also analyzed and interpreted the data. LAM analyzed and interpreted the data, and participated in the drafting of the manuscript. ARC collected and interpreted the data. She also participated in the drafting of the manuscript. MSD interpreted the data and participated in the drafting of the manuscript. All authors read and approved the final manuscript.

Competing interests

The authors declare that they have no competing interests.

References

1. François Delor MH. Revisiting the concept of "vulnerability". Soc Sci Med. 2000;50:1557–70. https://doi.org/10.1016/S0277-9536(99)00465-7.
2. Estigma GE. La identidad deteriorada. Buenos Aires; 1970. https://sociologiaycultura.files.wordpress.com/2014/02/goffman-estigma.pdf. Accessed 22 Nov 2017.
3. Krieger N. Discrimination and health. Soc Epidemiol. 2000;1:36–75.
4. Ramos Lira L, Saucedo González I, Saltijeral Méndez MT. Crimen organizado y violencia contra las mujeres: discurso oficial y percepción ciudadana. Rev Mex Sociol. 2016;78:655–84. http://www.scielo.org.mx/scielo.php?script=sci_arttext&pid=S0188-25032016000400655. Accessed 22 Nov 2017
5. Terán P, Castellanos C, González Blanco M, Ramos D. Violencia obstétrica: percepción de las usuarias. Rev Obstet Ginecol Venez. 2013;73:171–80.
6. Narchi NZ, Diniz CSG, Azenha C de AV, Schenck CA. Women's satisfaction with childbirth' experience in different models of care: a descriptive study. Online Brazilian J Nurs. 2010;9. https://doi.org/10.5935/1676-4285.20103102.
7. Arandy L, Romero Quiroz M de los A, Córdoba Avila MA, Campos Castolo M. Percepción del trato digno por la mujer embarazada en la atención obstétrica de enfermería. Rev CONAMED. 1997;16:5–5s11. http://biblat.unam.mx/pt/revista/revista-conamed/articulo/percepcion-del-trato-digno-por-la-mujer-embarazada-en-la-atencion-obstetrica-de-enfermeria. Accessed 22 Nov 2017.
8. Santiago RV, Solórzano EH, Iñiguez MM, Monreal LMA. Nueva evidencia a un viejo problema: el abuso de las mujeres en las salas de parto. Rev CONAMED. 2015;18 http://www.dgdi-conamed.salud.gob.mx/ojs-conamed/index.php/revconamed/article/view/96. Accessed 22 Nov 2017
9. Venturi G, Godinho T. Mulheres brasileiras e gênero nos espaços público e privado: uma década de mudanças na opinião pública. Perseu Abramo; 2013.
10. Villanueva Egan LA. El maltrato en las salas de parto: reflexiones de un gineco-obstetra. Rev CONAMED. 2010;15 http://www.dgdi-conamed.salud.gob.mx/ojs-conamed/index.php/revconamed/article/view/282. Accessed 22 Nov 2017
11. Bohren MA, Vogel JP, Hunter EC, Lutsiv O, Makh SK, Souza JP, et al. The mistreatment of women during childbirth in health facilities globally: a mixed-methods systematic review. PLoS Med. 2015;12:e1001847. https://doi.org/10.1371/journal.pmed.1001847.
12. Vacaflor CH. Obstetric violence: a new framework for identifying challenges to maternal healthcare in Argentina. Reprod Health Matters. 2016;24:65–73. https://doi.org/10.1016/j.rhm.2016.05.001
13. Oliveira VJ, Penna CM de M, Oliveira VJ, Penna CM de M. Discussing obstetric violence through the voices of women and health professionals. Texto Context - Enferm. 2017;26 https://doi.org/10.1590/0104-07072017006500015.
14. Ishola F, Owolabi O, Filippi V. Disrespect and abuse of women during childbirth in Nigeria: a systematic review. PLoS One. 2017;12:e0174084. https://doi.org/10.1371/journal.pone.0174084.
15. Villanueva Egan LA. Reflexiones sobre la violencia organizacional en los servicios de salud: del trabajo enajenado a la violencia obstétrica. Salud Probl. 2017;11 http://saludproblema.xoc.uam.mx/tabla_contenido.php?id=784. Accessed 22 Nov 2017
16. Salud OM de la . Prevención y erradicación de la falta de respeto y el maltrato durante la atención del parto en centros de salud. 2014.
17. Brüggemann AJ, Wijma B, Swahnberg K. Abuse in health care: a concept analysis. Scand J Caring Sci. 2012;26:123–32. https://doi.org/10.1111/j.1471-6712.2011.00918.x.
18. Castro R. Génesis y práctica del habitus médico autoritario en México. Rev Mex Sociol. 2014;76:167–97.
19. Cecilia M, dos RAP. Re-significando a dor e superando a solidão& 58; experiências do parto entre adolescentes de classes populares atendidas em uma maternidade pública de Salvador, Bahia, Brasil. https://www.ncbi.nlm.nih.gov/pubmed/27578340. Accessed 22 Nov 2017.
20. Víctimas CCE de A a. Diagnóstico sobre victimización a causa de violencia obstétrica en México ÍNDICE. http://www.scielo.br/scielo.php?script=sci_arttext&pid=S0104-07072017000200331. Accessed 22 Nov 2017.
21. Daniel C, Gómez-Dantés O, Knaul F, Atun R, Barreto IC HC, Cetrángolo O, et al. La lucha contra la segregación social en la atención de salud en América Latina. In: MEDICC; 1999. http://new.medigraphic.com/cgi-bin/resumen.cgi?IDARTICULO=64561. Accessed 22 Nov 2017.
22. Frenk J. La salud en transición. Nexos. 1988;22:25–30.
23. Link BG, Phelan JC. Conceptualizing stigma. Annu Rev Sociol. 2001;27:363–85. https://doi.org/10.1146/annurev.soc.27.1.363.
24. Cook RJ, Dickens BM, Fathalla MF. Reproductive health and human rights: integrating medicine, ethics, and law: Clarendon Press; 2003.
25. Rights O of the UNHC for H. The right to health. Geneva; 2008. http://www.ohchr.org/Documents/Publications/Factsheet31.pdf. Accessed 22 Nov 2017.
26. De Diputados C, De DHC. Unión L. In: Constitución Política De Los Estados Unidos Mexicanos; 2017. http://www.diputados.gob.mx/LeyesBiblio/pdf/1_150917.pdf. Accessed 23 Nov 2017.
27. Nación SSC de J de la. Tesis P. XIX / 2000, Seminario Judicial de la Federación y su Gaceta, Noveno Período, Volumen XI, marzo de 2000. México; 2000. https://apublica.org/wp-content/uploads/2013/03/JanainaMAguiar.pdf.
28. Renkert S, Nutbeam D. Opportunities to improve maternal health literacy through antenatal education: an exploratory study. Health Promot Int. 2001;16:381–8. https://doi.org/10.1093/heapro/16.4.381.
29. Aguiar JM de, d'Oliveira A. Violência institucional em maternidades públicas: hostilidade ao invés de acolhimento como uma questão de gênero. São Paulo Univ São Paulo 2010.
30. Herrera C. Invisible al ojo clínico : violencia de pareja y políticas de salud en México.

31. Consejo C. Viesca-Treviño C. Ética y relaciones de poder en la formación de médicos residentes e internos: Algunas reflexiones a la luz de Foucault y Bourdieu @BULLET Bol Mex His Fil Med. 2008;11:16–20. http://www.medigraphic.com/pdfs/bmhfm/hf-2008/hf081d.pdf. Accessed 22 Nov 2017

32. Amroussia N, Hernandez A, Vives-Cases C, Goicolea I. "Is the doctor god to punish me?!" an intersectional examination of disrespectful and abusive care during childbirth against single mothers in Tunisia. Reprod Health. 2017;14:32. https://doi.org/10.1186/s12978-017-0290-9.

33. Watson HL, Downe S. Discrimination against childbearing Romani women in maternity care in Europe: a mixed-methods systematic review. Reprod Health. 2017;14(1) https://doi.org/10.1186/s12978-016-0263-4.

34. INEGI. Natalidad y fecundidad. Censos y conteos. Población y Vivienda, Registros administrativos. Vitales. Natalidad. Matrimonios. 2017. http://www.beta.inegi.org.mx/temas/natalidad/. Accessed 22 Nov 2017.

35. García Ruíz G. Estrategia de capacitación para la promoción del buen trato durante la atención del embarazo, parto y puerperio en salas de obstetricia de los servicios de salud. México; 2014.

36. Secretaría de Hacienda y Crédito Público. Tipos de cambio de divisas extranjeras para el cierre contable al 31 de diciembre de 2012. Unidad de contabilidad gubernamental. 2013:1. http://www.hacienda.gob.mx/LASHCP/MarcoJuridico/ContabilidadGubernamental/SCG_2013/2013/tabla_de_tipo_de_cambio_cierre_2012.pdf. Accessed 6 Dec 2017.

13

Improving shared decision-making in a clinical obstetric ward by using the three questions intervention

S. W. E. Baijens[1], A. G. Huppelschoten[2], J. Van Dillen[3*] (iD) and J. W. M. Aarts[3]

Abstract

Background: Shared decision-making (SDM) is an important aspect of modern health care. Many studies evaluated different interventions to improve SDM, however, none in an inpatient clinical setting. A tool that has been proven effective in an outpatient department is the three questions intervention. These questions are created for patients to get optimal information from their medical team and to make an informed medical decision. In this study, we evaluated the feasibility and effectiveness of this simple intervention on SDM in the obstetric inpatient department of a university hospital in the Netherlands.

Method: This is a clinical pilot before and after study, using mixed methods with quantitative and qualitative data collection. The three questions were stated on a card; (i.e. 1) What are my options; 2) What are the possible benefits and harms of those options; 3) How likely are each of those benefits and harms to happen to me?). The study period lasted 6 weeks in which all patients admitted to the obstetric ward were asked to participate in the study. In the first 3 weeks patients did not receive the three questions intervention (pre-intervention group). In the final 3 weeks all patients included received the intervention (intervention group). The main quantitative outcome measure was the level of SDM measured using the SDM-Q9 questionnaire at discharge (range 0–100). In addition, interviews with four patients of the intervention group were conducted and qualitatively analyzed.

Results: Thirty-three patients were included in the pre-intervention group, 29 patients in the intervention group. The mean score of the SDM-Q9 in the pre-intervention group was 65.5 (SD 22.83) and in the intervention group 63.2 (SD 20.21), a not statistically significant difference. In the interviews, patients reported the three questions to be very useful. They used the questions mainly as a prompt and encouragement to ask more specific questions.

Discussion: No difference in SDM was found between the two groups, possibly because of a small sample size. Yet the intervention appeared to be feasible and simple to use in an inpatient department. Further studies are needed to evaluate the impact of implementation of these three questions on a larger scale.

Keywords: Shared decision making, Inpatient department, Three questions intervention, Obstetrics

Background

Shared decision making (SDM) is an important aspect of modern health care. Patients prefer to be involved in making their own medical decisions [1]. However, currently, patients reported not receiving enough information about options and corresponding advantages and disadvantages [2, 3]. In addition, patients' preferences are often not taken into account when making health decisions [4]. In other words, patients are not provided with optimal personalized information [5], while these aspects are crucial in the process of SDM. Aside from an ethical imperative, SDM can result in better outcomes, such as increased understanding of their health condition, lower anxiety and greater compliance to treatment plans [6]. Many interventions have been designed and evaluated to improve SDM. These interventions can be provider-directed (e.g. training) [7] or patient-directed, such as patient decisions aids [8].

* Correspondence: Jeroen.vanDillen1@radboudumc.nl
[3]Gynaecology and Obstetrics Department, Radboudumc, Geert Grooteplein Zuid, 10 6525 GA Nijmegen, the Netherlands
Full list of author information is available at the end of the article

Decision aids are developed to improve patients' knowledge about their medical condition and risk perception. Ultimately, it helps them in making an informed decision based on their personal preferences.

A simple patient-directed intervention to improve SDM was introduced by Shepherd and colleagues and showed promising results [9]. Patients visiting their general practitioner in an outpatient clinical setting were shown a 4-min video-clip, a pamphlet and a website and appeared to be successful in prompting participants to ask three questions in the consultation with their doctor. These questions were conducted from a consumer advocacy program 'Patient first program' in Western Australia and a health advise book 'Smart health choices' [10]. The goal of this program was to create three questions for patients stimulating healthcare providers to give patients the most optimal information and allow patients to make an informed medical decision. The three questions were:

1. What are my options/possibilities?
2. What are the benefits and harms of these options?
3. How likely are each of these benefits and harms to happen to me?

This study showed that 87% of the patients ($N = 197$) attending an outpatient family planning clinic and making a medical decision, asked all three questions. It provided patients with more suitable information about their options. It also improved patients' involvement in decision-making. This study also showed that patients preferred making the primary decision and wanting to get all the information possible from their care provider.

Studies on SDM in obstetrics [11–13] indicated that women prefer to be more involved in medical decisions. Moreover, in the Netherlands, a 2016 interdisciplinary protocol for integral pregnancy care [14] introduced SDM as an important point of attention. In this protocol the three questions are mentioned as a tool to improve SDM. However, to the best of our knowledge none of the SDM interventions have been tested in an inpatient clinical setting. This is remarkable as it is common knowledge that patients admitted to an inpatient department are usually very dependent of the medical staff and control is an important factor for the patients comfort [15]. Patients frequently get mixed messages from different doctors while hospitalized [16] and most patients do not feel involved in decision-making while in hospital [17]. Given the simple nature of the 'three questions' intervention, we aimed to evaluate the feasibility and effectiveness on SDM of this intervention in an inpatient department. Additionally, as this is a pilot study, testing the feasibility of conducting a larger scale study on this topic is also an aim.

Methods

Design

This is a clinical pilot study evaluating the feasibility and effectiveness of the three questions intervention on SDM in a clinical inpatient setting. We carried out a mix-method study, in which we combined a quantitative pre- and postintervention study including qualitative in-depth interviews with a selection of participants from the intervention group.

Setting and participants

All patients older than 18 years and admitted to the obstetrics inpatient unit of the Radboud university medical center in the Netherlands were asked to participate. These patients were hospitalized requiring tertiary care because of severe and complicated problems during their pregnancy or problems after childbirth. Non-Dutch speaking patients were excluded. Recruitment took place in June and July 2016. All patients admitted in the study period were informed and those willing to participate signed an informed consent form.

Total duration of the study was 6 weeks. In the first 3 weeks patients who participated did not receive the three questions intervention (pre-intervention group). In the last 3 weeks, all participating patients received the three questions intervention at admission (intervention group). The three questions were printed on a card, so patients could conveniently keep it with them.

Patients were encouraged to use these questions during ward rounds on the department. Typically, physicians (i.e. obstetricians and obstetrics trainees), did ward rounds on patients with pregnancy- related problems or complex postpartum. A hospital-based midwife did ward rounds on the majority of postpartum patients. An observer (SB) was present during ward rounds for the entire 6 weeks to measure the length of each consultation between physician or midwife and patient. To provide a complete and adequate description of the intervention we used the TIDieR checklist as a guideline, since this checklist has shown to be useful in adequate reporting of interventions [18].

Before commencing the study both an e-mail and presentation with information about the study and a presentation was provided to all medical staff (physicians, midwives, nurses). This included information about the study design, the 'three question' intervention, and the primary and secondary outcomes of the study. At admission all patients received an information pamphlet to inform them about the study. The three questions were not specifically mentioned in this pamphlet, as patients in the control group would be biased. One of the researchers (SB) then approached individual patients, and asked them to participate in this study. During the first 3 weeks patients in the pre-intervention group were asked to act as they normally would do and ask the questions they would normally ask during clinical ward rounds. During the last 3 weeks patients in the intervention group received the card with the three questions. One of the researchers (SB) gave information about the three questions and encouraged patients to use this card and its questions during daily ward rounds during their hospital stay. Medical staff was aware which patients received the intervention, because we had specific timeframes for the pre-intervention and intervention period (i.e. 3 weeks) and because of the visibility of the card. Physicians and midwives were instructed to perform their ward rounds as they would normally do.

Data collection

Our primary outcome was the patient's perceived level of SDM, as measured with the Shared Decision Making questionnaire (SDM-Q9). The SDM-Q9 contains nine items relevant to shared decision making, e.g. 'My doctor made clear that a decision needs to be made.' The items rate from 0 until 6 on a Likert scale (0 = completely disagree to 6 = completely agree) with a continuous scale and with a scoring range from 0 to 54. This questionnaire is widely used and translated in multiple languages [19–23]. A study of Rodenburg-Vandenbussche [21] showed a good acceptance, internal consistency and reliability of the Dutch version of the SDM-Q9. Patients of both the pre-intervention and intervention group were asked to complete the SDM-Q9 questionnaire at discharge. Patients, who were hospitalized for more than 1 week, filled out the questionnaire weekly. In addition, at inclusion patients were asked to complete a questionnaire with seven general background questions, such as age, educational level, ethnicity, reason for admission, number of pregnancies, duration of hospital stay and number of admissions to the ward during the current pregnancy. Also, they were asked about their preferences about their involvement in decision making and information provision, as was done in the study by Shepherd et al. [9].

Finally, we purposively selected four patients from the intervention group for an interview, to substantiate the interpretation of our results and to establish future recommendations for the three questions intervention. These interviews had an open and semi-structured character using an interview guide (see Additional file 1). Questions that were included were for example: 'What did you think when you saw the questions for the first time?' and 'What do you think we want to accomplish with these questions?'. The interviews were performed during the last week of the intervention period

Analysis

As we performed a pilot study to evaluate the feasibility of the use of the three questions in a clinical inpatient setting, we aimed at including 25 to 50 patients per group.

The participants' demographics and background characteristics were analyzed using descriptive statistics. Using the Chi-squared test we calculated the statistically significant differences between the demographics of the patients and reason for admission were tested between the pre- intervention and intervention group. Differences in duration of hospital stay were calculated with an independent sample T-test, because of the numerical, continuous outcome. Because the SDM-Q9 questionnaire has an unfamiliar range (0-54), we rescaled these scores to a more practical range of 0-100 [20]. To study the difference between the two study groups on the SDM-Q9 questionnaire and the length of consultations during ward rounds we used an independent sample T-test for numerical, continuous outcomes. In case of statistically significant differences in baseline characteristics between the two study groups, we performed multivariate regression analyses to account for this difference. Statistically significance for all analyses was set at $P<0.05$. All analyses were done using Statistical Package for the Social Sciences (SPSS), version 22.

Results

A total of 104 patients were eligible to participate in the study: 62 patients in the pre-intervention group and 42 patients in the intervention group (Fig. 1). Of the 62 eligible patients of the pre- intervention group, 13 patients did not speak the Dutch language adequately, 10 patients did not want to participate and four patients were not able to participate, due to the severity of their illness. Eventually, 35 patients were included. In the intervention group, six patients did not have an adequate level of the Dutch language, two patients did not want to participate and three patients were not able to participate, due to the severity of their illness. The intervention group finally contained of 31 participants. In both groups, two participants were excluded, because they had not completed the SDM-Q9 questionnaire at discharge. This resulted in 33 patients for the pre- intervention group and 29 patients for the intervention group.

Mean age of participating patients was 31 years old in the pre-intervention group and 32 years old in the intervention group (P=0.092) (Table 1). The majority of patients was Dutch (95.2%), had a high educational level (61.3%), and was admitted for the first time during the current pregnancy (79.0%) being pregnant of their first child (56.5%). Background characteristics were comparable between the two groups and did not differ

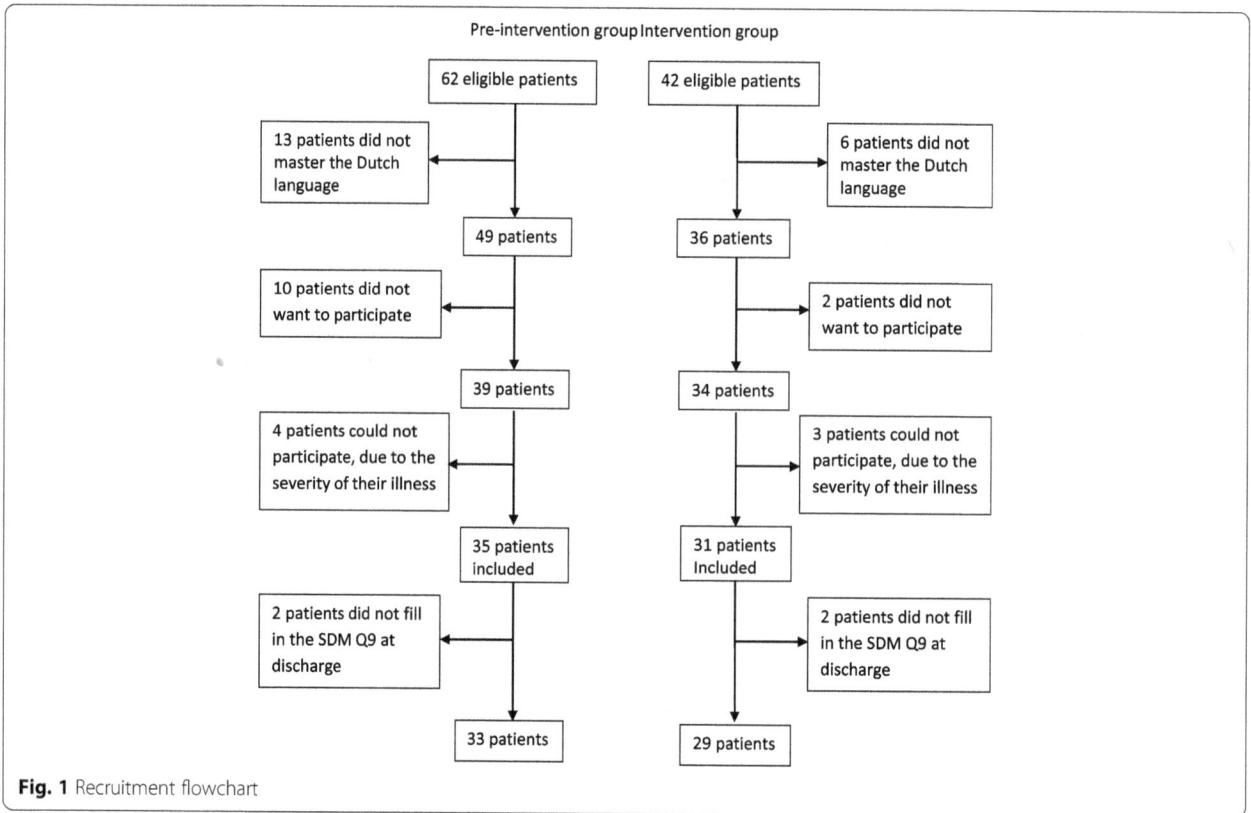

Fig. 1 Recruitment flowchart

statistically significant. The reason for admission was the only variable to be statistically significant different (P=0.005) between the two groups. The main reason for admission in the pre-intervention group was a pregnancy-related problem (81.8%), whereas the main reason in the intervention group was a postpartum medical problem (51.7%). These results are presented in Table 1.

The duration of hospitalization was statistically significant different (P=<0.001, 95% CI 0.72-7.56) between the two groups. The pre-intervention group had a mean hospitalization period of 8.2 days (SD 9.33) compared to 4.1 days (SD 2.41) in the intervention group. Two patients in the pre-intervention group had a long hospital stay, namely 43 and 30 days. When excluding these patients from the analysis the difference between the two groups was still statistically significant (P= <0.001, 95% CI 0.031-4.601). Patients in both groups had similar involvement and information preferences (Table 2). The majority of patients in both groups preferred the doctor to make the decision, but only after the doctor explicitly considered the patient's needs and priorities (pre-intervention 60.6% and intervention group 51.7%). For information preferences, 20 patients (60.6%) in the pre-intervention group and 11 patients (37.9%) in the intervention group preferred as many details as possible about the choice that needed to be make.

The mean score of the SDM-Q9 in the pre-intervention group was 65.5 (SD 22.86) and in the intervention group 63.2 (SD 20.21). This was not a statistically significant difference (P=0.64). Also when correcting for the reason of admission and duration of hospitalization, using multivariate analysis, no statistically significant difference (P=0.41) in SDM-Q9 scores between the two groups was found.

With respect to the secondary outcome, multivariate analysis showed a significant difference in duration of consultation between the two groups: 6min 33 sec in the pre-intervention group versus 7min 26 sec in the intervention group (P=0.03) (Table 3).

Six patients participating in the intervention group were approached for an interview and four of them agreed. All four patients believed that the questions were a method to gain more information from the physician. The three questions were primarily used as a prompt and reminder to ask more specific questions. Patients reported that the three questions were not always applicable. Before receiving the intervention, treatment plans were usually already known, most of the three questions were already answered and patients were often waiting to recover or to go into labor while hospitalized. However, if a new problem occurred while in the ward the questions were useful immediately. A selection of quotes can be seen in Table 4.

Table 1 Characteristics of study sample (pre-intervention group n = 33, intervention group n = 29)

	Pre-intervention group N %		Intervention group N %		P value
Age					
18–24	1	3.0	2	6.9	
25–30	13	39.4	8	27.6	
30–35	13	39.4	6	20.7	
> 35	6	18.2	13	44.8	0.092
Ethnicity					
Dutch	32	97.0	27	93.1	
Other	1	3.0	2	6.9	0.365
Education level					
Medium - Low	14	42.5	10	34.4	
High	19	57.5	19	65.6	0.522
Reason for admission					
Problem in pregnancy	27	81.8	14	48.3	
Postpartum	6	18.2	15	51.7	0.005
Hospitalizations in this pregnancy					
First	26	78.8	23	79.3	
Second	4	12.1	4	13.8	
Third	0	0	2	6.9	
Fourth	3	9.1	0	0	0.176
Total pregnancies					
First	17	51.5	18	62.1	
Second	11	33.3	9	31.0	
Third	4	12.1	1	3.5	
Fourth	1	3.0	1	3.5	0.620

Table 2 Involvement and information preference concerning SDM compared between pre-intervention group and intervention group

	Pre-intervention group N %		Intervention group N %		P value
Involvement preferences					
The doctor should make the decisions using all that's known about the treatments	2	6.1	2	6.9	
The doctor should make the decisions but strongly consider my needs and priorities	20	60.6	15	51.7	
The doctor and I should make the decisions together on an equal basis	4	12.1	5	17.2	
I should make the decisions, but strongly consider the doctor's opinion	6	18.2	7	24.1	
I should make the decisions using all I know or learn about the treatments	1	3.0	0	0	0.800
Information preferences					
Prefer as many as details as possible	20	60.6	11	37.9	
I want only information needed to care for myself properly	5	15.2	8	27.6	
I want additional information only if it is good news	0	0	0	0	
I want as much information as possible, good and bad	8	24.2	10	34.5	0.194

Table 3 Statistics of SDM-Q9 score and duration of consultation during ward rounds, compared between pre- intervention group and intervention group

	N	Mean (SD)	Mean difference	95% confidence interval
Score of SDM-Q9 (range 0–100)				
Pre-intervention group	54	65.47 (±22.86)		
Intervention group	31	63.20 (±20.21)	4.780	−7.272 – 11.801
Duration of consultation (seconds)				
Pre- intervention group	135	392.94 (±278.60)		
Intervention group	71	445.73 (±254.35)	38.550	− 128.947 – 23.364

Discussion

This study introduced the 'three questions' as an intervention to improve SDM in a clinical inpatient setting. This study showed no difference in SDM between patients in an inpatient clinical setting with and without using the three questions intervention. The duration of the consultations during ward rounds was statistically significant higher in the intervention group (53 seconds). From in-depth interviews we learned that patients thought that the questions were very convenient to gain more information from care providers. The 'three questions' intervention prompted patients to ask more, but also more specific questions. This suggests that the three questions stimulated the awareness of patients to ask questions to their medical team. The card with the three questions seems a simple and feasible method to improve SDM. The implementation of this intervention to daily care routines seemed easy and did not encounter any problems. Effortless implementation on a larger scale is therefore likely, if shortcomings of this study are taken into account.

To the best of our knowledge, this is the first study to evaluate a SDM intervention in an inpatient obstetric

Table 4 Comments from in-depth interviews with four patients concerning SDM

I think the questions are very good and handy. They are general questions, so applicable in different situations, as a reminder to ask more questions.

These questions are to accomplish better communication between doctor and patient, I think. So patients will get more information about the treatment options and so forth. I believe doctors should in any case give answers to these questions, but I understand that this is not always the case. Also you never know exactly what the patient wants to know, so these questions are very helpful for the patient to ask more specific questions.

I didn't use the three questions literally in the consultation with the doctor. I used the three questions to form more specific questions, which were more applicable to my situation.

These three questions are not so much applicable while you're admitted in the hospital and the whole plan is already known. While admitted the patient is usually waiting. There are very little changes [during the hospital stay]. Therefore you have few questions. If a new situation occurs, then I would definitely use the three questions to gain more information. I also think it is convenient that the patient has the questions in advance, so you can use them immediately, if necessary.

department. Strength of the study is the addition of in-depth interviews to the quantitative data. The qualitative data did provided some more insight into the quantitative results, although only four interviews were conducted because of the small sample size of this pilot study, in which saturation was reached.

However, some limitations of the study should be mentioned as well. First, this study had a small sample size, which might have resulted in the lack of significant findings on our main outcome measure. In general this is a common phenomenon in pilot and feasibility studies. This was also the reason for choosing a non-randomized design. Nevertheless, this limitation should be taken into account when interpreting the results. Second, different healthcare providers consulted patients that participated in this study. Physicians were lead care providers for patients admitted for pregnancy-related problems, whereas hospital-based midwives led the ward rounds for most patients with postpartum problems. Although physicians and hospital-based midwives in the Netherlands both get training in communication with patients, the approach, techniques and focus during conversations with patients could be different. Finally, both groups were not comparable because there was a significant difference in reason for admission between groups (i.e. problem in pregnancy vs. postpartum problem).

Furthermore, blinding of patients and care providers was not possible, because of the visibility of the card containing the three questions during clinical ward rounds. It was attempted to minimize bias by keeping patients in the pre-intervention group oblivious for the purpose of the study. Finally, care providers were aware of the aim of the study. This could have affected the conversation between them and the patient, which can result in a response bias.

Shepherd et al [9] developed and evaluated the 'three questions' intervention in an outpatient setting. Also, they did not specifically evaluate the impact of this intervention on the process of SDM. The qualitative part of our study showed that the three questions were primarily used as a reminder to ask more questions, and to form new questions better suitable for the patient's particular situation. The questions were not literally used during ward rounds. This in contrast to Shepherd's study [9]. This study was designed to encourage patients to literally use the questions in the consultation with their care provider. Also opposed to Shepherd et al. [9], we found a statistically significant increase of consultation duration when patients used the three questions. However, in our study patients had either a physicians or a midwife as the lead care provider during ward rounds, which might explain this difference. Also, the number of consultations per patient might affect the length of consultations. We did not collect that information in this study.

During the interviews, we found that the three questions were not always suitable for a clinical inpatient setting. For example, in this hospital patients are often first evaluated in an outpatient assessment unit before admitted to the ward. We noticed that some of the care providers already provided patients with a lot of information at admission about the reason for admission and treatment plan, in which also patients' view on these things are discussed. It could be argued that the three questions intervention needs to be implemented immediately at admission in the outpatient assessment unit, where most of the information about the reason for admission and the management plan is provided and deliberated. This is similar to the results of other studies reporting that SDM was not or less possible because of the specific clinical setting [1, 24].

Because this study is conducted in an obstetrics inpatient unit, all participants included were women. Studies of LaCousiere [25] and Nussbaum [26] showed that women have a say in over 80% of the health-care decisions they make and are usually the primary decision maker. On the contrary, men are more likely to prefer a paternalistic approach of physicians compared to women. The same accounts for older and less educated patients [1]. In our study, we found that most patients wanted to make the primary decision about their medical situation. Therefore, our patient group seems to be a representative group of women.

We have chosen to exclude patients who do not speak Dutch adequately. However, this might be a group of patients that could particularly benefit from this intervention. Patients having a language barrier are more prone of being miss- or under informed while hospitalized, especially in patient-physician communication about diagnosis, risks and emergency situations [27]. A recent meta-analysis [13] showed that SDM decision aids have a greater positive effect on disadvantaged groups, compared to a normal population. Especially their knowledge, participation, decisional conflict and self-efficacy increases when using decision aids. With respect to the three questions intervention, this intervention could be translated into different languages and accompanied with visual sign to increase SDM in patients with a language barrier.

Conclusion

This pilot study was a brief evaluation of the three questions intervention on SDM in an inpatient clinical setting. We recommend that more attention should be given to studies that focus on the improvement of SDM in an inpatient clinical setting, as this is lacking in current literature. The 'three questions' intervention seems simple and feasible. It might be at least helpful in prompting patients to be more actively involved in decision-making and ask more questions to medical staff. Further research is needed to study the impact of this intervention on SDM on a larger scale and in different settings.

Abbreviations
SD: Standard deviation; SDM: Shared decision making; SDM-Q9: Shared decision making questionnaire 9 SPSS = statistical package for the social sciences; TIDieR: Template for intervention description and replication

Acknowledgements
We thank the participating doctors and nurses, clinic staff and patients who enabled completion of this study.

Funding
No funding was needed and used for this research.

Authors' contributions
AH and JA conceived the study. SWEB, AGH, JD and JWMA designed the study. SWEB coordinated the running of the study, the data collection and carried out the initial statistical analysis. SWEB wrote the first draft of the manuscript. SWEB, AGH, JD and JWMA assisted with further analysis and contributed to the interpretation of the analysis and the writing of the manuscript. All authors read and approved the final manuscript.

Competing interests
The authors declare that they have no competing interests. JvD is associate editor of BMC Pregnancy and Childbirth.

Author details
[1]Gynaecology and Obstetrics Department, Meander Medical Hospital, Maatweg 3, 3813 TZ Amersfoort, the Netherlands. [2]Gynaecology and Obstetrics Department, Jeroen Bosch Hospital, Henri Dunantstraat 1, 5223 GZ 's-Hertogenbosch, the Netherlands. [3]Gynaecology and Obstetrics Department, Radboudumc, Geert Grooteplein Zuid, 10 6525 GA Nijmegen, the Netherlands.

References

1. Benbassat J, Pilpel D, Tidhar M. Patients' preferences for participation in clinical decision making: a review of published surveys. Behav Med. 1998; 24(2):81–8.
2. Boberg EW, Gustafson DH, Hawkins RP, Offord KP, Koch C, Wen KY, et al. Assessing the unmet information, support and care delivery needs of men with prostate cancer. Patient Educ Couns. 2003;49(3):233–42.
3. Jenkins V, Fallowfield L, Saul J. Information needs of patients with cancer: results from a large study in UK cancer centres. Br J Cancer. 2001;84(1):48.
4. van Haastert C, Lekkerkerk T. Meldactie 'Samen beslissen'. Nederlandse Patienten Consumenten Federatie; 2014.
5. McNair AG, MacKichan F, Donovan J, Brookes S, Avery K, Griffin S, et al. What surgeons tell patients and what patients want to know before major cancer surgery: a qualitative study. BMC Cancer. 2016;16(1):1.
6. Stacey D, Legare F, Col NF, Bennett CL, Barry MJ, Eden KB, Holmes-Rovner M, Llewellyn-Thomas H, Lyddiatt A, Thomson R, Trevena L, Wu JHC. Decision aids for people facing health treatment or screening decisions. Cochrane Database Syst. Rev. 2014;(1):Cd001431. https://doi.org/10.1002/14651858.CD001431.pub4.
7. Dwamena F, Holmes-Rovner M, Gaulden CM, Jorgenson S, Sadigh G, Sikorskii A, Lewin S, Smith RC, Coffey J, Olomu A, Beasley M. Interventions for providers to promote a patient-centred approach in clinical consultations. Cochrane Database Syst Rev. 2012;12. Art. No.: CD003267. https://doi.org/10.1002/14651858.CD003267.pub2.
8. Kinnersley P, Edwards A, Hood K, Cadbury N, Ryan R, Prout H, Owen D, MacBeth F, Butow P, Butler C. Interventions before consultations for helping patients address their information needs. Cochrane Database Syst Rev. 2007; 3. Art. No.: CD004565. https://doi.org/10.1002/14651858.CD004565.pub2.
9. Shepherd HL, Barratt A, Jones A, Bateson D, Carey K, Trevena LJ, et al. Can consumers learn to ask three questions to improve shared decision making? A feasibility study of the ASK (AskShareKnow) patient–clinician communication model® intervention in a primary health-care setting. Health Expect. 2015;2016;(5):1160–8.
10. Irwig L, Irwig J, Trevena L, Sweet M. Smart health choices: making sense of health advice. London: Hammersmith Press. Professor Les Irwig, Judy Irwig, Dr Lyndal Trevena, Melissa Sweet; 2008.
11. Vlemmix F, Warendorf JK, Rosman AN, Kok M, Mol BW, Morris JM, et al. Decision aids to improve informed decision-making in pregnancy care: a systematic review. BJOG. 2013;120(3):257–66.
12. Horey D, Kealy M, Davey MA, Small R, Crowther CA. Interventions for supporting pregnant women's decision-making about mode of birth after a caesarean. Cochrane Database Syst Rev 2013(7):Cd010041. https://doi.org/10.1002/14651858.CD010041.pub2.
13. Durand MA, Carpenter L, Dolan H, Bravo P, Mann M, Bunn F, et al. Do interventions designed to support shared decision-making reduce health inequalities? A systematic review and meta- analysis. PLoS One. 2014;9(4): e94670.
14. Geboortezorg EZI. Zorgstandaard Integrale geboortezorg. 2016 28–06-2016.
15. Williams AM, Irurita VF. Enhancing the therapeutic potential of hospital environments by increasing the personal control and emotional comfort of hospitalized patients. Appl Nurs Res. 2005;18(1):22–8.
16. Smith S, Nicol K, Devereux J, Cornbleet M. Encounters with doctors: quantity and quality. Palliat Med. 1999;13(3):217–23.
17. Marshall A, Kitson A, Zeitz K. Patients' views of patient-centred care: a phenomenological case study in one surgical unit. J Adv Nurs. 2012;68(12): 2664–73.
18. Hoffmann TC, Glasziou PP, Boutron I, Milne R, Perera R, Moher D, et al. Better reporting of interventions: template for intervention description and replication (TIDieR) checklist and guide. BMJ. 2014;348:g1687.
19. Scholl I, Kriston L, Dirmaier J, Buchholz A, Harter M. Development and psychometric properties of the shared decision making questionnaire–physician version (SDM-Q-doc). Patient Educ Couns. 2012;88(2):284–90.
20. Kriston L, Scholl I, Holzel L, Simon D, Loh A, Harter M. The 9-item shared decision making questionnaire (SDM-Q-9). Development and psychometric properties in a primary care sample. Patient Educ Couns. 2010;80(1):94–9.
21. Rodenburg-Vandenbussche S, Pieterse AH, Kroonenberg PM, Scholl I, van der Weijden T, Luyten GP, et al. Dutch translation and psychometric testing of the 9-item shared decision making questionnaire (SDM-Q-9) and shared decision making questionnaire-physician version (SDM-Q-doc) in primary and secondary care. PLoS One. 2015;10(7):e0132158.
22. Glass KE, Wills CE, Holloman C, Olson J, Hechmer C, Miller CK, et al. Shared decision making and other variables as correlates of satisfaction with health care decisions in a United States national survey. Patient Educ Couns. 2012; 88(1):100–5.
23. De las Cuevas C, Perestelo-Perez L, Rivero-Santana A, Cebolla-Marti A, Scholl I, Harter M. Validation of the Spanish version of the 9-item shared decision-making questionnaire. Health Expect. 2015;18(6):2143–53.
24. Rodriguez-Osorio CA, Dominguez-Cherit G. Medical decision making: paternalism versus patient-centered (autonomous) care. Curr Opin Crit Care. 2008;14(6):708–13.
25. LaCoursiere SP. A theory of online social support. Adv Nurs Sci. 2001;24(1): 60–77.
26. Nussbaum R. Studies of women's health care: selected results. Perm J. 2000; 4(3):62–7.
27. van Rosse F, de Bruijne M, Suurmond J, Essink-Bot ML, Wagner C. Language barriers and patient safety risks in hospital care. A mixed methods study. Int J Nurs Stud. 2016;54:45–53.

14

The effect of advanced maternal age on perinatal outcomes in nulliparous singleton pregnancies

Bekir Kahveci[1], Rauf Melekoglu[2]* (iD), Ismail Cuneyt Evruke[3] and Cihan Cetin[3]

Abstract

Background: Pregnancy at advanced maternal age has become more common in both developed and developing countries over the last decades. The association between adverse perinatal outcomes and advanced maternal age has been a matter of controversy in several studies. The objective of this study is to investigate the impact of advanced maternal age on perinatal and neonatal outcomes of nulliparous singleton pregnancies.

Methods: Records of patients admitted to the Department of Obstetrics and Gynecology, University of Cukurova School of Medicine, between January 2011 and July 2015 for routine mid-trimester fetal ultrasonography were retrospectively reviewed. The control (age: 18–34 years), advanced maternal age (35–39 years), and very advanced maternal age (> 40 years) groups included 471, 399, and 87 women, respectively.

Results: Gestational diabetes, gestational hypertension, and cesarean delivery rates were more common in the very advanced maternal age group, with compared with the advanced maternal age and the younger age group. There were no significant differences in regarding rates of spontaneous preterm delivery before 34 weeks of gestation, prolonged rupture of membranes, large for gestational age infants, and operative vaginal delivery rates between the groups. Also, there were no significant differences regarding in APGAR scores, the rate of low birth weight infants, and neonatal morbidity rates between the groups. However, admission to the neonatal intensive care unit requirement was more common in the two advanced maternal age groups compared with the control group.

Conclusion: Advanced maternal age is a risk factor for gestational diabetes mellitus, gestational hypertension, preeclampsia, small for gestational age infants, spontaneous late preterm delivery, and cesarean section, with significant potential clinical implications.

Keywords: Maternal age, Nulliparity, Preeclampsia, Pregnancy outcomes, Small for gestational age

Background

Pregnancy at advanced maternal age has become more common in both developed and developing countries over the last decades [1]. Advanced maternal age is commonly considered to be 35 years or older, whereas very advanced maternal age is defined as older than 40 or 45 years [2, 3]. Widespread use of family planning measures, postponing pregnancy because of career goals, and advances in assisted reproductive techniques contribute to this increment [4]. Accordingly, concerns about adverse effects of advanced maternal age on perinatal outcomes have also increased steadily over the past years. The association between adverse perinatal outcomes and advanced maternal age has been a matter of controversy in several studies. While some researchers have noted an increased rate of adverse pregnancy outcomes in women older than 35 years, others have failed to find any association between advanced maternal age and adverse perinatal outcomes [5, 6]. This discordance in conclusions could be attributed to the heterogeneity of study populations, differences in the definition of pregnancy outcomes, and failure to adjust for potential confounders. Therefore, we aimed to investigate the impact of advanced maternal age

* Correspondence: rmelekoglu@gmail.com
The institute where the work was conducted: Cukurova University School of Medicine Department of Obstetrics and Gynecology
[2]Faculty of Medicine, Department of Obstetrics and Gynecology, The University of Inonu, 44280 Malatya, Turkey
Full list of author information is available at the end of the article

on perinatal and neonatal outcomes of nulliparous single-ton pregnancies in this study. We hypothesized that gesta-tional diabetes mellitus (GDM), gestational hypertension and increased cesarean delivery rate would be associated with advanced maternal age.

Methods

The study was approved by the ethics committee of Cukur-ova University Faculty of Medicine. Written consent was obtained from all participants for the use of their clinical data in analysis and reporting before mid-trimester fetal ultrasonography scan. The retrospective analyses of the prospectively collected database of patients admitted to the Department of Obstetrics and Gynecology, University of Cukurova School of Medicine, between January 1, 2011, and July 1, 2015, for routine mid-trimester fetal ultrasonog-raphy was performed. Patients who met the following cri-teria were enrolled: 1) maternal age of 18–45 years, 2) viable singleton pregnancy, 3) nulliparity, 4) admission at 18–23 weeks of gestation for mid-trimester fetal ultrason-ography, and 5) unremarkable obstetric history. The exclu-sion criteria were 1) any concomitant chronic disease (diabetes, hypertension, chronic renal disease), 2) body mass index > 35 kg/m^2, 3) a history of intrauterine insemin-ation and in vitro fertilization/intracytoplasmic sperm injection 4) a history of uterine surgery, 5) any known Mullerian anomaly, 6) presence of any uterine and adnexal mass, 5) multiple pregnancies, 6) smoking and alcohol use, 7) and any fatal congenital anomalies or chromosomal ab-normalities. Main outcome variables included, gestational hypertension, preeclampsia, ablatio placenta, placenta pre-via, spontaneous preterm delivery before 34 weeks of gesta-tion, spontaneous preterm delivery between 34 and 37 weeks of gestation, prolonged rupture of membranes, delivery of a (SGA) or (LGA) fetus, post-term pregnancy, operative vaginal delivery and Cesarean delivery.

GDM was diagnosed based on a positive 75-g oral glu-cose tolerance test result, according to the one-step diag-nostic approach between 24 and 28 weeks of gestation. The diagnosis of GDM was defined based on a single glu-cose concentration that met or exceeded the threshold value (fasting value, 92 mg/dl; 1-h value, 180 mg/dl; and 2-h value, 153 mg/dl). Gestational hypertension was defined as systolic blood pressure ≥ 140 mmHg and/or diastolic blood pressure ≥ 90 mmHg on at least two occasions 4 h apart, developing after 20 weeks' gestation in a previously normotensive woman in the absence of significant proteinuria and end-organ dysfunction (thrombocytopenia, renal insufficiency, impaired liver function, pulmonary edema and cerebral or visual symp-toms). fined as gestational hypertension with proteinuria of ≥300 mg in 24 h, or the new-onset end-organ dysfunc-tion. Placental abruption was defined as the premature separation of the placenta and placenta previa was described as the insertion of the placenta close to the in-ternal cervical os. Spontaneous preterm delivery included those with spontaneous onset of labor before 37 com-pleted weeks of pregnancy. Prolonged rupture of mem-branes was defined rupture of membranes occurring at least 18 h before the onset of labor. SGA and LGA were defined as those with estimated fetal weight below the 10th percentile or above the 90th percentile for gestation, respectively. Post-term pregnancy was defined as pregnan-cies at or beyond 42 0/7 weeks of gestation. Operative vaginal delivery was described as the accomplishment of delivery by applying direct traction on the fetal skull with forceps or by applying traction to the fetal scalp using a vacuum extractor. Cesarean delivery was defined as a surgical procedure to use the delivery of a fetus by abdom-inal route. The neonatal intensive care unit (NICU) admission criteria were defined as follow; low birthweight (< 2500 g), prematurity (36 weeks gestation or less), respiratory problems (apnea or cyanotic episodes, any respiratory distress causing concern), suspicion of infec-tion with clinical concern, gastrointestinal problems (feed-ing problems, bile stained vomiting, or other clinical signs suggesting bowel obstruction), metabolic problems, cen-tral nervous system problems (convulsion, neonatal encephalopathy), cardiovascular problems requiring moni-toring or intervention and any baby that is causing con-cern to the attending doctor that the baby requires observation or treatment in NICU.

A total of 957 women met the study criteria, of which 471 were assigned to the control group (aged 18–34 years) whereas 399 and 87, respectively, formed the advanced maternal age (35–39 years) and very advanced maternal age (40 years or more) groups. Antenatal care and delivery for patients included in this study took place at our clinic, according to the standard protocols. Maternal characteris-tics, perinatal and neonatal outcomes were obtained from medical records.

The statistical software package IBM SPSS, version 22.0 (SPSS IBM, Armonk, NY, USA), was used for all data analyses. Thus, adjusted odds ratios and 95% confi-dence intervals were calculated for maternal age and potential confounding factors in relation to pregnancy outcome. Differences were considered significant when p-values were < 0.05.

Results

During the study period, 2617 singleton deliveries oc-curred at the University of Cukurova School of Medicine Department of Obstetrics and Gynecology. Of these, 957 met the study criteria. The demographic characteristics of the study population are summarized in Table 1. There were no significant differences between the groups regard-ing age, gravidity, the degree of consanguinity with the spouse, and educational status. In contrast, invasive

Table 1 Patient characteristics

Maternal characteristics	Maternal Age Groups			p		
	< 35 years (a) (n = 471)	35–39 years (b) (n = 399)	≥40 years (c) (n = 87)	a vs. b	a vs. c	b vs. c
Age (year)[a]	27.6 ± 4.2	36.6 ± 1.4	41.71 ± 2.0	< 0.001	< 0.001	0.035
Gravidity[b]	1.0 (1.0–2.0)	1.0 (1.0–3.0)	1.0 (0.0–3.0)	0.865	0.759	0.980
Body Mass Index (kg/m²)[a]	28.7 ± 4.1	29.9 ± 5.8	30.1 ± 4.6	0.450	0.375	0.681
Consanguinity between spouses (first or second degree)[c]	26 (5.5)	19 (4.7)	3 (3.4)	0.284	0.120	0.330
Underwent invasive prenatal diagnosis procedure[c]	24 (5.1)	26 (6.5)	23 (26.4)	0.530	< 0.001	< 0.001
Educational status[c]				0.101	0.085	0.253
Primary school	12 (2.5)	19 (4.7)	6 (6.9)			
High school	81 (17.2)	76 (19.1)	17 (19.5)			
Graduated or higher	378 (80.3)	304 (76.2)	77 (88.5)			

[a]Data are given as mean ± SD
[b]Data are given as median (minimum-maximum)
[c]Data are presented as n (%)
Values with the same superscript letter within a row do not differ significantly at the 0.05 level

prenatal diagnostic procedures were performed more often in patients aged 40 years or older.

Gestational hypertension, GDM, and cesarean delivery rates were higher in the very advanced maternal age group than in the advanced maternal age and control groups. While the frequencies of preeclampsia and SGA were similar in patients aged 35–39 years and 40 years or older, the risk of preeclampsia and SGA was significantly lower in women younger than 35 years. Post-term pregnancy was significantly more common in the < 35 years age group than in the other groups. There were no significant differences in spontaneous preterm delivery before 34 weeks of gestation, prolonged rupture of membranes, ablatio placentae, placenta previa, LGA, and operative vaginal delivery rates between the groups. The frequencies of complications according to maternal age group are described in Table 2.

The rates of low birth weight and first- and fifth-minute APGAR scores of neonates were similar between the groups. While admission to the neonatal intensive care unit was more frequent in the advanced and very advanced maternal age groups compared with the control group, the neonatal morbidity rates were similar among the groups. The neonatal outcomes are shown in Table 3.

According to the results of unadjusted logistic regression analysis, the rates of perinatal outcomes such as gestational diabetes, gestational hypertension, spontaneous preterm delivery before 34 weeks of gestation spontaneous late preterm delivery between 34 and 37 weeks of gestation, SGA, and cesarean delivery increased with maternal age, with the most substantial increases seen in gestational diabetes and cesarean delivery rates in the very advanced age group (OR 2.41, 95% CI 2.13–3.76; OR 2.67, 95% CI 1.90–3.82, respectively). However, there was little evidence of increased risk of ablatio placentae,

prolonged rupture of membranes, LGA, and operative vaginal delivery. Babies born to older women were at higher odds of neonatal intensive care unit admission (OR 1.54, CI 95% 1.13–2.12; OR 1.69, CI 95% 1.02–2.76 at 35–39 years old and ≥ 40 old, respectively). After adjusting for gravidity, educational status, consanguinity status, and cesarean delivery rates, all these adverse outcomes remained significantly higher in older primiparae. Crude and adjusted ORs for adverse perinatal and neonatal outcomes according to maternal age are shown in Table 4.

Discussion

Several studies investigating the impact of advanced age on pregnancy outcomes [7–9] produced conflicting results because of differences in study group homogeneity and inadequate control for variables like maternal diseases, assisted conception, obesity, multiple pregnancies, and parity. The results of this study, in which all of these variables were controlled for, demonstrate that advanced maternal age nulliparous women with no previous chronic diseases, including obesity, there is an increased odds of adverse perinatal and neonatal outcomes, including gestational diabetes, gestational hypertension, preeclampsia, SGA, spontaneous late preterm delivery between 34 and 37 weeks of gestation, and cesarean delivery, but not spontaneous preterm delivery before 34 weeks, ablatio placentae, prolonged rupture of membranes, placenta previa, LGA, and operative vaginal delivery. These evidence-based conclusions should be of interest to both advanced maternal age women and medical professionals. Consistently with the current results, Khalil et al. demonstrated that preeclampsia, SGA, GDM, and cesarean delivery were more common in advanced maternal age pregnancies. However, they

Table 2 Frequency of perinatal outcomes according to maternal age group

| Perinatal Outcomes | Total | Maternal Age Groups | | | p | | |
		< 35 years (a) (n = 471)	35–39 years (b) (n = 399)	≥40 years (c) (n = 87)	a vs.b	a vs. c	b vs. c
Gestational diabetes mellitus	101	27 (5.7)	57 (14.3)	15 (17.2)	< 0.001	< 0.001	0.041
Gestational hypertension	58	20 (4.2)	29 (7.2)	8 (9.2)	< 0.001	< 0.001	0.035
Pre-eclampsia	62	22 (4.6)	31 (7.7)	8 (9.2)	0.033	< 0.001	0.457
Ablatio placenta	7	2 (0.4)	4 (1.0)	1 (1.1)	0.073	0.051	0.865
Spontaneous preterm delivery before 34 weeks	83	39 (8.2)	36 (9.0)	7 (8.0)	0.469	0.754	0.601
Spontaneous late preterm delivery between 34 and 37 weeks of gestation	71	34 (7.2)	28 (7.0)	9 (10.3)	0.342	0.044	0.038
Prolonged rupture of membranes	41	21 (4.5)	16 (4.0)	4 (4.6)	0.780	0.913	0.612
Small for gestational age	80	21 (4.5)	48 (12.0)	11 (11.5)	< 0.001	< 0.001	0.560
Large for gestational age	21	7 (1.5)	12 (3.0)	2 (2.3)	0.072	0.134	0.411
Placenta previa	24	13 (2.8)	9 (2.2)	2 (2.3)	0.613	0.218	0.891
Post-term pregnancy	66	41 (8.7)	21 (5.3)	4 (4.6)	0.021	< 0.001	0.139
Operative vaginal delivery	16	9 (1.9)	6 (1.5)	1 (1.1)	0.451	0.112	0.207
Cesarean delivery	396	175 (37.1)	167 (41.8)	44 (50.5)	0.029	< 0.001	0.040

Data are presented as n (%)

found that gestational hypertension and spontaneous preterm delivery rates were similar after adjustment for maternal characteristics and obstetric history, and only an increased risk of iatrogenic early preterm delivery attributed to the increased rates of preeclampsia and SGA was observed in this age group [10]. In a retrospective cohort study of the impact of parity on adverse perinatal outcomes in advanced maternal age pregnancy conducted by Baser et al., preterm delivery rates were higher in the advanced maternal age group (OR 1.08, 95% CI 0.95–1.12) [11]. These contradictory results regarding the relationship between maternal age and the increased preterm delivery rate could be attributed to methodological differences, in particular, the definition of gestational age of preterm delivery, which ranged between 37, 34, and 32 weeks.

In this study, the risks of preeclampsia and gestational hypertension were significantly higher in pregnant women aged over 35 years compared with younger controls. In agreement, Duckitt et al. demonstrated that maternal age greater than 40 years doubles the risk of preeclampsia [12]. Furthermore, Saftlas et al. showed that the risk of preeclampsia increases by 30% per year after the age of 35 years old [13]. In contrast, Cleary-Goldman et al. did not find any association between hypertensive disorders of pregnancy and maternal age in The First and Second Trimester Evaluation of Risk trial. This was interpreted to be a consequence of controlling for covariates associated with gestational hypertension and preeclampsia, such as parity and assisted reproductive care [14].

The incidence of glucose intolerance increases with age owing to reduced insulin sensitivity and increased level of serum lipids. In this study, the risk of GDM increased with maternal age. However, we did not observe an age-related increase in the risk of LGA. Fulop et al. explained the reduction in insulin sensitivity with age by progressive deterioration of pancreatic β-cell function [15]. In a population-based study conducted by Carolan et al. to

Table 3 Frequency of neonatal outcomes according to maternal age group

| Neonatal Outcomes | Total | Maternal Age Groups | | | p | | |
		< 35 years (a) (n = 471)	35–39 years (b) (n = 399)	≥40 years (c) (n = 87)	a vs.b	a vs. c	b vs. c
Low birthweight < 2500 g	110	54 (11.4)	46 (11.5)	10 (11.4)	0.980	0.999	0.987
First minute APGAR score < 7	194	91 (19.3)	83 (20.8)	18 (20.7)	0.793	0.788	0.960
Fifth minute APGAR score < 7	42	22 (4.6)	17 (4.2)	3 (3.4)	0.810	0.209	0.311
Neonatal intensive care unit requirement	185	77 (16.3)	89 (22.3)	17 (19.5)	0.019	0.041	0.027
Neonatal morbidity	66	32 (6.8)	27 (6.7)	6 (6.8)	0.955	0.989	0.881

Data are presented as n (%)
Neonatal morbidity includes; sepsis, pneumonia, respiratory distress syndrome, bronchopulmonary dysplasia, intraventricular hemorrhage, necrotizing enterocolitis

Table 4 Crude and adjusted Odds ratios (95% confidence intervals) for maternal and neonatal outcomes at advanced and very advanced maternal age groups compared with < 35 years group

Perinatal Outcomes	Maternal Age Groups			
	35–39 years		≥40 years	
	Crude OR (95% CI)[b]	Adjusted OR[a] (95% CI)[b]	Crude OR (95% CI)[b]	Adjusted OR[a] (95% CI)[b]
Gestational diabetes	1.15 (1.01–1.27) p < 0.15	1.21 (0.82–1.27) p < 0.01	2.41 (2.13–3.76) p < 0.15	2.23 (0.25–3.96) p < 0.01
Gestational hypertension	1.57 (1.16–2.07) p < 0.15	1.55 (1.32–1.78) p < 0.01	1.70 (1.12–2.63) p < 0.15	1.68 (0.69–4.16) p < 0.01
Pre-eclampsia	1.26 (1.15–1.39) p < 0.15	1.34 (1.11–1.62) p < 0.01	1.44 (1.21–1.67) p < 0.15	1.37 (1.13–1.48) p < 0.01
Ablatio placenta	1.00 (0.63–1.57) p = 0.99	1.00 (0.42–1.68) p = 1.00	1.00 (0.39–2.64) p = 1.00	1.03 (0.91–1.12) p = 0.88
Spontaneous preterm delivery before 34 weeks	0.86 (0.68–0.98) p < 0.15	0.90 (0.75–1.16) p = 0.03	1.35 (0.95–1.91) p < 0.15	1.33 (1.21–1.49) p = 0.24
Spontaneous late preterm delivery between 34 and 37 weeks of gestation	0.61 (0.29–1.32) p = 0.20	0.82 (0.72–1.08) p = 0.35	1.22 (1.10–1.64) p < 0.15	1.41 (1.29–1.57) p < 0.01
Prolonged rupture of Membranes	0.87 (0.85–0.91) p = 0.78	0.91 (0.71–1.15) p = 0.81	0.83 (0.72–0.95) p = 0.94	1.05 (0.72–1.08) p = 0.98
SGA (<10th centile)[b]	1.71 (1.44–2.49) p < 0.15	1.65 (0.71–3.05) p < 0.01	1.63 (1.38–2.11) p < 0.15	1.55 (1.41–1.88) p < 0.01
LGA (>90th centile)[b]	1.10 (0.93–1.32) p = 0.27	1.12 (0.81–1.52) p = 0.35	0.68 (0.34–1.37) p = 0.27	0.54 (0.50–0.64) p = 0.11
Placenta previa	1.00 (0.84–1.23) p = 0.95	1.05 (0.81–1.15) p = 0.88	0.78 (0.66–0.98) p = 0.15	1.03 (0.76–1.34) p = 0.25
Post-term pregnancy	1.05 (0.75–1.54) p = 0.61	1.02 (0.74–1.67) p = 0.77	0.68 (0.45–1.03) p = 0.21	0.54 (0.41–0.67) p = 0.18
Operative vaginal delivery	0.72 (0.46–1.18) p = 0.19	0.68 (0.51–0.88) p = 0.34	0.81 (0.72–0.96) p = 0.15	0.73 (0.56–0.94) p = 0.33
Cesarean delivery	1.75 (1.61–1.95) p < 0.15	1.87 (1.44–2.25) p < 0.01	2.67 (1.90–3.82) p < 0.15	2.76 (1.70–4.65) p < 0.01
Low birth weight < 2500 g	1.23 (1.08–1.41) p < 0.15	1.27 (1.14–1.59) p < 0.01	1.20 (0.84–1.23) p < 0.15	1.19 (1.09–1.35) p < 0.01
First minute APGAR score < 7	1.14 (0.91–1.49) p < 0.15	1.10 (0.73–1.56) p = 0.08	1.27 (0.95–1.71) p < 0.15	1.26 (1.01–1.55) p = 0.04
Fifth minute APGAR score < 7	0.94 (0.71–1.30) p = 0.74	1.00 (0.99–1.05) p = 0.96	1.04 (0.95–1.15) p < 0.15	1.05 (1.00–1.08) p = 0.04
Neonatal intensive care unit requirement	1.69 (1.02–2.76) p < 0.15	1.68 (1.42–2.15) p < 0.01	1.54 (1.13–2.12) p < 0.15	1.52 (1.21–1.92) p < 0.01
Neonatal morbidity	0.93 (0.27–3.10) p = 0.93	0.86 (0.70–1.09) p = 0.25	1.12 (0.82–1.55) p = 0.48	1.09 (0.90–1.33) p = 0.23

[a] Adjusted for gravidity, educational status, consanguinity status and C/S rates
[b] CI confidence interval, LGA large-for-gestational age, OR odds ratio, SGA small-for-gestational age

determine maternal and perinatal outcomes of pregnancies in women aged 45 years or older, the odds of gestational diabetes (OR 2.05, 95% CI 1.3–3.3) were greater in this age group, with the GDM incidence of 9.7% [16].

In this study, the rate of cesarean section increased linearly with maternal age, which is consistent with previous studies. In a systematic review of twenty-one studies, Bayrampour et al. found an increased risk of cesarean birth among women of advanced maternal age compared with younger women for both nulliparas and multiparas [17]. This increasing rate of the CS could be explained by the age-related weakening of the myometrium, reduction in the number of oxytocin receptors, the lower clinical threshold for obstetric interventions, and increased rates of maternal systemic diseases and obstetric complications. The result of this study also indicated increased cesarean rate as high as 37.1% in nulliparous young age women that may be accepted as low-risk pregnancies by considering the exclusion and inclusion criteria of the study. Consistently, a recent observational study revealed an increasing CS rate in low-risk pregnancies, and it was demonstrated that this rising trend in CS rates is most prominent in nulliparous women with a term cephalic in spontaneous labor [18].

Despite the data from large-scale studies implying that optimal CS rates are between 15 and 19% [19], current CS rates both worldwide and even in Turkey considerably higher than these recommended optimal primary CS rates. Reasons for this high prevalence of CS rates are complex and appear to demographic, sociocultural, and institutional factors.

The relationship between SGA and maternal age is believed to be U-shaped, with an increased risk in women under the age of 30 and over the age of 40 years old. We demonstrated that advanced maternal age is associated with a risk of SGA. Previously, Odibo et al. identified a positive dose-response relationship between advanced maternal age and increased risk of intrauterine growth restriction (IUGR). They noted that advanced maternal age is an independent risk factor for IUGR and suggested that screening for IUGR should be conducted among women aged 35 years or older [20]. Although the exact mechanism of the association between advanced maternal age and SGA has not been demonstrated clearly, it has been suggested that poor oxygen exchange may be the underlying factor.

In this study, we also examined the impact of advanced maternal age on neonatal outcomes. Admission to a NICU was more likely in the advanced maternal age groups (OR 1.69, 95% CI 1.02–2.76; OR 1.54, 95% CI 1.13–2.12 in the 35–39 and > 40 years old groups, respectively), but there were no significant differences in APGAR scores, occurrence of low birth weight, and neonatal morbidity rates between the groups. Mutz-Dehbalaie et al. investigated the impact of advanced maternal age on the rate of perinatal mortality in 56,517 singleton hospital deliveries between 1999 and 2008 in Austria. They found that the rate of perinatal mortality was more than two-fold greater in women older than 40 years than in younger women. However, there was no significant correlation between neonatal mortality rate and maternal age [21]. Delbaere et al. found increased rates of low birth weight (adjusted OR 1.69, 95% CI 1.47–1.94), very low birth weight (adjusted OR 1.62, 95% CI 1.15–2.28), and extremely low birth weight (adjusted OR 2.14, 95% CI 1.29–3.56) in primiparas of advanced maternal age after controlling for confounding factors [22]. The observed inconsistencies in the occurrence of low birth weight could be explained by the inability to control for congenital malformations and maternal diseases in the study group.

The main limitation of this study was that the results of this study are applicable to a narrow population of patients for the large list of exclusion criteria. No inferences can be made to women with previous births, history of diabetes, obesity and the other excluded variables. This failure to examine the different population may be addressed in future studies. Other limitations include the single center population, small number of women in the sample with age > 40 years and the lack of data on race/ethnicity, subfertility issues and the reasons of women for delayed pregnancy.

Conclusions

This study showed a significant association between advanced maternal age and gestational diabetes, gestational hypertension, preeclampsia, increased cesarean section rates, SGA, and spontaneous late preterm delivery. These findings may have significant implications in clinical practice. Modification of follow-up protocols to account for these age-related risk factors could improve pregnancy outcomes in women of advanced maternal age.

Abbreviations

CI: Confidence interval; IUGR: Intrauterine growth restriction; LGA: Large for gestational age; NICU: Neonatal intensive care unit; OR: Odds ratio; SGA: Small for gestational age

Authors' contributions

BK contributed to the project development, data collection, data analysis, data interpretation and presentation, manuscript construction and presentation. RM, ICE, and CC contributed to the data collection, data interpretation and presentation, and manuscript construct and presentation. All authors read and approved the final manuscript.

Competing interests

The authors declare that they have no competing interests.

Author details
[1]Department of Obstetrics and Gynecology, Diyarbakır Gazi Yaşargil Training and Research Hospital, 21010 Diyarbakır, Turkey. [2]Faculty of Medicine, Department of Obstetrics and Gynecology, The University of Inonu, 44280 Malatya, Turkey. [3]Faculty of Medicine, Department of Obstetrics and Gynecology, The University of Cukurova, 01330 Adana, Turkey.

References

1. Montan S. Increased risk in the elderly parturient. Curr Opin Obstet Gynecol. 2007;19:110–2.
2. Traisrisilp K, Tongsong T. Pregnancy outcomes of mothers with very advanced maternal age (40 years or more). J Med Assoc Thail. 2015; 98(2):117–22.
3. Yogev Y, Melamed N, Bardin R, Tenenbaum-Gavish K, Ben-Shitrit G, Ben-Haroush A. Pregnancy outcome at extremely advanced maternal age. Am J Obstet Gynecol. 2010;203(6):558.e1–7.
4. Wennberg AL, Opdahl S, Bergh C, Aaris Henningsen AK, Gissler M, Romundstad LB, Pinborg A, Tiitinen A, Skjærven R, Wennerholm UB. Effect of maternal age on maternal and neonatal outcomes after assisted reproductive technology. Fertil Steril. 2016;106(5):1142–1149.e14.
5. Dulitzki M, Soriano D, Schiff E, Chetrit A, Mashiach S, Seidman DS. Effect of very advanced maternal age on pregnancy outcome and rate of cesarean delivery. Obstet Gynecol. 1998;92(6):935–9.
6. Balayla J, Azoulay L, Assayag J, Benjamin A, Abenhaim HA. Effect of maternal age on the risk of stillbirth: a population-based cohort study on 37 million births in the United States. Am J Perinatol. 2011;28:643–50.
7. Ludford I, Scheil W, Tucker G, Grivell R. Pregnancy outcomes for nulliparous women of advanced maternal age in South Australia, 1998–2008. Aust N Z J Obstet Gynaecol. 2012;52:235–41.
8. Favilli A, Pericoli S, Acanfora MM, Bini V, Di Renzo GC, Gerli S. Pregnancy outcome in women aged 40 years or more. J Matern Fetal Neonatal Med. 2012;25:1260–3.
9. Alshami HA, Kadasne AR, Khalfan M, Iqbal SZ, Mirghani HM. Pregnancy outcome in late maternal age in a high income developing country. Arch Gynecol Obstet. 2011;284:1113–6.
10. Khalil A, Syngelaki A, Maiz N, Zinevich Y, Nicolaides KH. Maternal age and adverse pregnancy outcome: a cohort study. Ultrasound Obstet Gynecol. 2013;42(6):634–43.
11. Başer E, Seçkin KD, Erkılınç S, Karslı MF, Yeral IM, Kaymak O, Cağlar T, Danışman N. The impact of parity on perinatal outcomes in pregnancies complicated by advanced maternal age. J Turk Ger Gynecol Assoc. 2013; 14(4):205–9.
12. Duckitt K, Harrington D. Risk factors for pre-eclampsia at antenatal booking: systematic review of controlled studies. BMJ. 2005;330:565.

13. Saftlas AF, Olson DR, Franks AL, Atrash HK, Pokras R. Epidemiology of preeclampsia and eclampsia in the United States, 1979–1986. Am J Obstet Gynecol. 1990;163:460–5.

14. Cleary-Goldman J, Malone FD, Vidaver J, Ball RH, Nyberg DA, Comstock CH, Saade GR, Eddleman KA, Klugman S, Dugoff L, Timor-Tritsch IE, Craigo SD, Carr SR, Wolfe HM, Bianchi DW, D'Alton M, FASTER Consortium. Impact of maternal age on obstetric outcome. Obstet Gynecol. 2005;105(5 Pt 1):983–90.

15. Fulop T, Larbi A, Douziech N. Insulin receptor and ageing. Pathol Biol (Paris). 2003;51:574–80.

16. Carolan MC, Davey MA, Biro M, Kealy M. Very advanced maternal age and morbidity in Victoria, Australia: a population based study. BMC Pregnancy Childbirth. 2013;13:80.

17. Bayrampour H, Heaman M. Advanced maternal age and the risk of cesarean birth: a systematic review. Birth. 2010;37:219–26.

18. Delbaere I, Cammu H, Martens E, Tency I, Martens G, Temmerman M. Limiting the caesarean section rate in low risk pregnancies is key to lowering the trend of increased abdominal deliveries: an observational study. BMC Pregnancy Childbirth. 2012;12:3.

19. Montoya-Williams D, Lemas DJ, Spiryda L, Patel K, Neu J, Carson TL. What are optimal cesarean section rates in the U.S. and how do we get there? A review of evidence-based recommendations and interventions. J Women's Health (Larchmt). 2017;26(12):1285–91.

20. Odibo AO, Nelson D, Stamilio DM, Sehdev HM, Macones GA. Advanced maternal age is an independent risk factor for intrauterine growth restriction. Am J Perinatol. 2006;23:325–8.

21. Mutz-Dehbalaie I, Scheier M, Jerabek-Klestil S, Brantner C, Windbichler GH, Leitner H, Egle D, Ramoni A, Oberaigner W. Perinatal mortality and advanced maternal age. Gynecol Obstet Investig. 2014;77(1):50–7.

22. Delbaere I, Verstraelen H, Goetgeluk S, Martens G, De Backer G, Temmerman M. Pregnancy outcome in primiparae of advanced maternal age. Eur J Obstet Gynecol Reprod Biol. 2007;135(1):41–6.

15

The effect of uterine artery ligation in patients with central placenta pevia

Ahmad Sameer Sanad*, Ahmad E. Mahran⊙, Mahmoud Elmorsi Aboulfotouh, Hany Hassan Kamel,
Hashem Fares Mohammed, Haitham A. Bahaa, Reham R. Elkateeb, Alaa Gamal Abdelazim,
Mohamed Ahmed Zeen El-Din and Hossam El-Din Shawki

Abstract

Background: Placenta previa is major obstetric surgical risk as it is associated with higher percentage of intraoperative and postpartum hemorrhage (PPH), increased requirement of blood transfusion and further surgical procedures. The current study aimed to evaluate uterine artery ligation prior to uterine incision as a procedure to minimize blood loss during cesarean section in patients with central placenta previa.

Methods: One hundred and four patients diagnosed with central placenta previa antenatally and planned to have elective caesarean section were recruited from the antenatal clinic at Minia Maternity University hospital. Patients were randomly allocated into either ligation group or control group.

Results: Both groups were similar regarding demographic features and preoperative risk factors for bleeding. The intraoperative blood loss was significantly lower in the ligation group as compared with the control group (569.3 ± 202.1 mL vs. 805.1 ± 224.5 mL respectively, $p = 0.002$). There was a significant increase in the requirement for blood transfusion in the control group as compared with the ligation group (786 ± 83 mL vs. 755 ± 56 mL respectively, $p = 0.03$) Three cases in the control group required further surgical interventions to control intraoperative bleeding, while no cases in the ligation required further surgical techniques and that was statistically significant ($p = 0.001$).

Conclusion: Uterine artery ligation prior to uterine incision may be a helpful procedure to minimize intraoperative and postpartum blood loss in cases with central placenta previa.

Trial registration: Retrospectively registered in ClinicalTrials.gov Identifier: NCT02002026- December 8, 2013.

Keywords: Central placenta previa, Uterine artery ligation, Cesarean section

Background

Placenta previa is a potentially serious obstetric complication where the placental tissue abnormally lies within the lower uterine segment [1, 2]. The exact pathophysiology of this serious condition is not exactly known. However uterine scaring is a potential risk factor. Other risk factors for placenta previa include advanced maternal age, high parity, history of placenta previa and congenital uterine malformations [3–6].

The prevalence of placenta previa is estimated to be 5.2 per 1000 pregnancies. However, there is evidence of regional variation [7]. In Minia maternity University hospital where the study was conducted, data from labor ward registry showed that 5% of caesarean deliveries were performed due to placenta previa and its variants. This rate is expected to rise in the coming years due to high rate of caesarean deliveries and subsequently more pregnancies with uterine scarring.

Placenta previa is associated with higher incidence of intraoperative bleeding and postpartum hemorrhage (PPH), need for blood transfusion and further surgical procedures like devascularization and emergency hysterectomy

* Correspondence: ahmed.sameer@mu.edu.eg
Obstetrics and Gynecology, Faculty of Medicine, Minia Maternity University Hospital, Minia University, PO Box 61111, Minia, Egypt

[8, 9]. In addition, women with placenta previa are at higher risk of delivering premature babies with lower Apgar scores and with higher rates of neonatal intensive care (NICU) admission, stillbirth and neonatal death [10, 11].

In 2014, the total number of deliveries in Minia Maternity University Hospital was 10,854. There were 332 cases with antepartum hemorrhage, 224 of them were diagnosed as placenta previa.

In this study, we introduced uterine artery ligation prior to uterine incision as a novel technique to reduce intraoperative blood loss in patients with central placenta previa. It is proposed that the procedure is associated with reduction of the blood flow to the lower uterine segment and consequently leads to reduction of blood loss during placental separation.

The aim of this study was to evaluate the effect of uterine artery ligation prior to uterine incision in patients with central placenta previa on blood loss during caesarean section.

Methods

Project no.: MUH201310127

The study protocol was approved by scientific ethical committee of the Department of Obstetrics and Gynecology, Faculty of Medicine, Minia University in September 2013. The study procedure was explained to all eligible patients. All patients signed informed consent that include their agreement to participate in the study.

This study is a randomized controlled study including 104 patients diagnosed with central placenta previa antenatally and were planned to have elective cesarean section. Patients were recruited from attendees of the antenatal clinic at Minia Maternity University Hospital in the period between January 2014 and December 2016.

Patients were randomly allocated into study or control group. The random allocation was based on computer-generated random numbers sealed in consecutively numbered opaque envelopes that were picked up by the patients outside the operating theatre. As major outcomes were not patient-dependent or patient-reported, the patients and the surgeons were not blind to group allocation.

We included patients diagnosed with central placenta previa diagnosed with two-dimensional ultrasound scan at 28 weeks' gestation and remained so till the time of planned cesarean delivery. Central placenta previa was defined as placental localization in the lower uterine segment either anteriorly or posteriorly. Laterally situated placenta was not considered "central". We excluded patients with; a) known bleeding disorder, b) patients with hypertensive disorders or developed preeclampsia (PET) during the study, c) patients who had antepartum hemorrhage (APH) and delivered by emergency caesarean section, and d) patients with anterior placenta previa that were diagnosed antenatally with color Doppler

ultrasound and MRI to have placenta accreta. These criteria were designed prior to initiation of the study.

Thorough assessment of the risk factors associated with each case was done. Patients were followed up with regular ultrasound scans every 2 weeks to ensure fetal wellbeing and placental localization till the time of planned delivery. Deliveries were planned to take place between 36 and 38 weeks according to each case situation. Preoperative hemoglobin (Hb) assessment was done and four to six blood units were cross matched for each case before planned cesarean section. Each cesarean section was performed by two consultant obstetricians with experience in operative management of placenta previa and placenta accreta. The two consultants were assisting each other in each case to ensure uniformity of the procedure in all patients. Postoperative hemoglobin level was checked 24 h after the CS (day 1) or after at least 6 h from the blood transfusion. We adhered to the CONSORT guidelines Fig. 1.

Sample size calculation

Sample size was calculated to prevent type II error. The average intraoperative blood loss in cases of central placenta previa at the hospital where the study was conducted was estimated to be 800 ml (figure obtained from the hospital audit report for the year preceding the trial). To be of clinical significance, it was assumed that uterine artery ligation prior to uterine incision should reduce intraoperative blood loss by 50%. Based on these data, we would need to study 27 patients in each arm to be able to reject the null hypothesis that the rates for study and control groups are equal in intraoperative blood loss at a probability of 80%. The type one error probability associated with this test for the null hypothesis is 0.05. To compensate for patients' withdrawal or cases in which the procedure cannot be performed, we recruited 35 patients in each arm.

Procedure

- Skin incision through Pfannenstiel approach and anterior abdominal wall layers were incised separately.
- The loose peritoneum covering the lower uterine segment is dissected to expose the lower uterine segment and mobilize the urinary bladder downwards.
- Uterine artery ligation was performed by grasping the broad ligament on each side with thumb anterior and the index finger posterior lifting the base below the site uterine incision; the uterine artery was singly ligated with No. 1 vicryl suture. Uterine vessels were ligated and not damaged through inclusion of myometrium. The procedure was then repeated on the other side.
- A curvilinear transverse lower uterine segment incision was performed as usual. Higher incisions

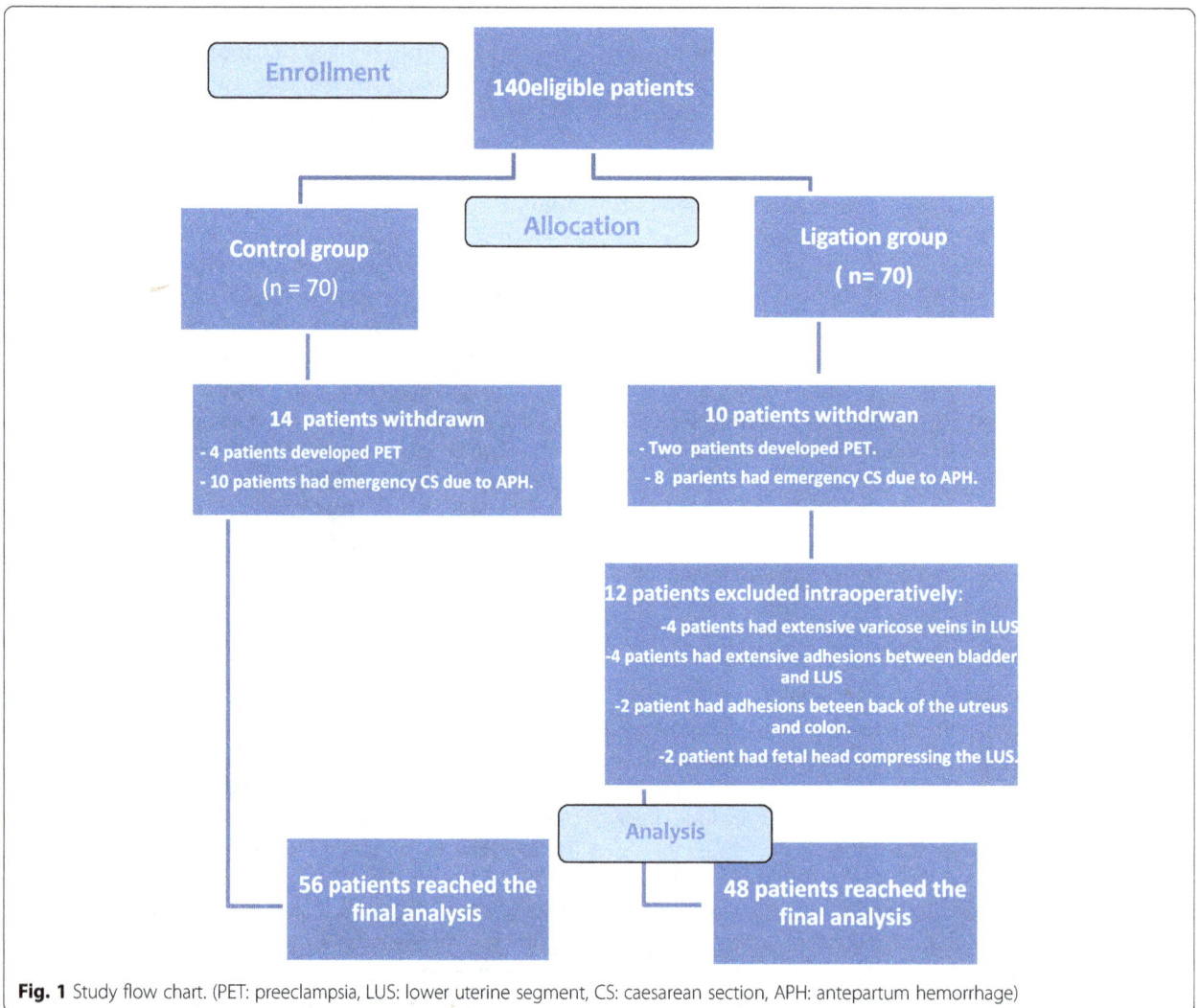

Fig. 1 Study flow chart. (PET: preeclampsia, LUS: lower uterine segment, CS: caesarean section, APH: antepartum hemorrhage)

were performed in cases where the traditional incision was expected to be directly through the placenta.
- Delivery of the baby and placenta.
- Closure of the uterine incision in 2 layers with no. 1 vicryl suture.
- Closure of the anterior abdominal wall in layers.

In the control group, lower segment caesarean section was performed in the classic way.

Assessment of intraoperative blood loss
The intraoperative blood loss was measured using the alkaline hematin method [12]. All the blood-stained swabs, diapers and pads and the contents in the drainage bottles were collected, put in a plastic bag and blended with 5% NaOH solution. The plastic bag was then transferred to the Stomacher Lab Blender (Model 3500, Seward Laboratories, London, UK) and processed for few minutes to extract hemoglobin. A portion of the fluid was collected

and diluted with 5% NaOH solution. The concentration of alkaline hematin was obtained by assay in a spectrophotometer at 546 nm with the appropriate NaOH as a blank. The intra-assay coefficient for analyzing the concentration is 1%. The blood loss was then calculated using the patient's preoperative hemoglobin as a reference.

Outcome measures
The primary outcome measures of the study were:

- The amount of intra-operative blood loss.
- The change in pre and post-partum hemoglobin.

The secondary outcome measures were:

- The need for blood transfusion.
- The need for further surgical intervention to control intraoperative bleeding.
- The operative time.

Statistical methodology

Statistical analysis was performed using the Statistical Package for Social Science (SPSS Inc., NY) version 21 for Microsoft Windows. Data was described in terms of mean ± SD (standard deviation) for continuous variables and frequencies (number of cases) and percentages for categorical data. Independent Student's t-test was used to compare quantitative variables and Chi square test was used to compare categorical data. A p value < 0.05% was considered significant.

Results

We initially recruited 140 patients in this study. In the study group, 10 cases were withdrawn from the study (8 developed APH and had emergency CS and 2 developed PET). In the control group, 14 cases were withdrawn (10 cases developed APH and had emergency CS and 4 cases developed PET).

Difficulties during the procedure

In the study group, 12 cases were excluded intra-operatively due to difficulty in performing the procedure as:

1. Extensive varicosities over the lower uterine segment (LUS) in 6 cases
2. Extensive adhesions between the urinary bladder and LUS in cases with repeat cesarean sections in 3 cases,
3. Adhesions between the colon and the back of the uterus or the broad ligament in 2 cases,
4. Fetal head compressing over the lower uterine segment making fetal head injury possible during the procedure in one case,

In these cases, the procedure was not done, and patients were excluded from the final analysis. However, these cases were analyzed initially within the ligation group. Results remained significant by comparing 56 patients in the control group versus 60 patients in the ligation group (Additional file 1: Table S1, Additional file 2: Table S2, Additional file 3: Table S3 and Additional file 4: Table S4).

At the end, 104 patients reached the final analysis; 48 patients in the study (ligation) group and 56 patients in the control group. Study flow chart is shown in Fig. 1.

There was no statistically significant difference between the study and control groups regarding the demographic features and risk factors associated with placenta previa as shown in Table 1. The ultrasonographic features of the placentae in the study population are summarized in Table 2.

Patients in the ligation group had higher postoperative hemoglobin, which was statistically significant ($p <$ 0.0001), shorter operative time that was not significant ($p = 0.2$). The intraoperative blood loss and requirements for blood transfusion were significantly lower in the ligation group compared with the control group

Table 1 Characteristics and risk factors in the study population

	ligation group ($n = 48$)	control group ($n = 56$)	p value
· Maternal age (years)	33.5 ± 4.8	34.1 ± 4.7	0.8
· BMI (kg/m2)	28.9.2 ± 4.7	29.2 ± 5.1	0.7
· Occupation:			
➢ housewife	28	38	0.6
➢ nonprofessional	14	12	
➢ professional	6	6	
· Residence:			
➢ Rural	34	42	0.6
➢ Urban	14	14	
· Smoking	1	0	0.5
· Parity	4.1 ± .0.9	4.3 ± 1.1	0.7
· Previous uterine surgery:			
➢ Caesarean section	20	23	0.6
➢ Dilatation and curettage	8	7	
➢ Myomectomy	2	1	
➢ Resection of septum	0	1	
➢ Resection of intrauterine adhesions	0	2	
➢ Repair of uterine rupture	2	2	
➢ B-lynch suture	0	1	
Previous placenta previa:			
➢ Minor	6	7	0.5
➢ Major	4	5	
· Manual removal of placenta	2	1	0.6
· Placenta previa and previous uterine surgery	8	12	0.7
· Pregnancy with assisted conception	2	4	0.5

Data are presented as mean ± SD or frequency and percentages

(569.3 ± 202.1 mL vs. 805.1 ± 224.5 mL, $p < 0.0001$ and 755 ± 56 mL vs. 786 ± 83 mL, $p = 0.03$ respectively) Three cases in the control group required further surgical interventions to control intraoperative bleeding; two cases of internal iliac artery (IIA) ligation and one case of supravaginal hysterectomy. In spite that patients with anterior placenta previa that were diagnosed antenatally with color Doppler and MRI to have placenta accrete were excluded from the study, one patient in the control group was discovered intra-operatively to have placenta accrete and that was the case in whom supravaginal hysterectomy was performed. No cases needed further surgical interventions in the study group. Two cases developed PPH in the control group compared to no cases in the ligation group (3.8% vs. 0%, $p = 0.02$). There were three cases of bladder injuries; one in the ligation group and two in the control group. Bleeding from varicosities over the bladder

Table 3 Outcome measures in the ligation and control groups

	Ligation group (n = 48)	Control group (n = 56)	p value
• Preoperative Hb (g/dL)	11.1 ± 0.61	11.2 ± 0.6	0.6
• Postoperative Hb (g/dL)	10.2 ± 0.34	9.3 ± 0.56	0.0001*
• Intraoperative blood loss (mL)	569.3 ± 202.1	805.1 ± 224.5	0.0001*
• Operative time (min)	54.2 ± 11.2	57 ± 10.9	0.2
• Amount of blood transfusion (mL)	755 ± 56	786 ± 83	0.03*
• Further surgical interventions:	0	3 (5.4%)	
➢ IIA ligation	0	2 (3.6%)	0.001*
➢ Supravaginal hysterectomy	0	1 (1.8%)	
• Urinary bladder injury	1 (2.1%)	2 (3.6%)	0.2
• Bleeding from varicosities over bladder surface	2 (4.2%)	3 (5.4%)	0.6
• Postpartum hemorrhage (n)	0	2 (3.6%)	0.02*

12 cases were excluded from ligation group in the final analysis due failure of the procedure. Results remained significant by comparing 56 patients in the control group versus 60 patients in the ligation group
Data is presented as mean ± SD or frequency and percentages
HB hemoglobin, IIA Internal iliac artery
*p < 0.05

surface was encountered in five cases; two in the ligation group and three cases in the control group. These differences were insignificant. Outcome measures in both groups are summarized in Table 3.

Table 2 The ultra-sonographic criteria of the placenta in the study population

	Ligation group (n = 48)	Control group (n = 56)	p value
• Location:			
➢ Placenta previa anterior.	20(41.7%)	26(46.4%)	0.6
➢ Placenta previa posterior	28(58.3%)	30(53.6%)	0.8
Distance from internal os:			
➢ Incomplete Centralis	38(79.2%)	46(82.2%)	0.5
➢ Centralis	10(20.8%)	10(17.8%)	0.6
Color Doppler:			
➢ Normal	34(70.8%)	40(71.4%)	0.8
➢ Retro-placental hypervascularity	14(29.2%)	16(28.6%)	0.7
Clear zone:			
➢ Present	32(66.7%)	38(67.9%)	0.9
➢ Absent	16(33.3%)	18(32.1%)	0.7
Lacunae:			
➢ Present	8(16.7%)	10(17.9%)	0.8
➢ Absent	40(83.3%)	46(82.1%)	0.9

Data is presented as frequency and percentages

Regional anesthesia was used in all cases at the beginning. In the control group, six cases were converted to general anesthesia (GA) as spinal anesthesia worked off and additional surgical procedures were required and consumed longer time (two cases of internal iliac artery "IIA" ligation and one case of supravaginal hysterectomy). In these three cases, placenta was anterior. No cases in the study group required conversion to GA (0% vs. 23.1%, p = 0.001). There was no significant difference in the experience of anesthetist between the two groups. Anesthetic details are summarized in Table 4.

The mean gestational age at time of CS was 36.2 ± 1.1 weeks in the study group and 36.3 ± 0.9 weeks in the control group (p = 0.7). There was no significant difference between the two groups regarding the perinatal outcome difference as shown in Table 4.

Discussion

To our knowledge, it is the first study to assess the technique of uterine artery ligation in patients with central placenta previa. We recruited patients diagnosed with central placenta previa at 28 weeks' gestation by 2D ultrasound. We used the alkaline hematin test to allow objective assessment of the intraoperative blood loss.

The new procedure evaluated in this study was found to minimize the intraoperative blood loss and shorten the operative time. Patients in the study group had

Table 4 Anesthetic details of CS and Perinatal outcome in the study population

	Ligation group (n = 48)	Control group (n = 56)	p value
• Type of anesthesia:			
➢ Spinal	38 (79.1%)	43 (76.8%)	
➢ Epidural	10 (20.9%)	13 (23.2%)	
➢ GA↑↑	0 (0%)	3 (5.3%)	
• Gestational age at time of CS (weeks)	36.2 ± 1.1	36.3 ± 0.9	0.7
• Birth weight (gram)	2875.6 ± 253.5	2976.5 ± 265.2	0.5
• Apgar score at 5 min:			
➢ 1–2	2(4.2%)	2(3.6%)	0.7
➢ 3–6	12(25%)	16(28.6%)	0.6
➢ ≥7	34(70.8%)	38(67.8%)	0.8
• Neonatal outcome:			
➢ Early neonatal death	1(2.1%)	1(1.8%)	0.88
➢ NICU admission	4(8.4%)	4(7.2%)	0.9
➢ Hospital discharge	44(91.6%)	51(91%)	0.91

Data is presented as frequency and percentages or mean ± SD
GA general anesthesia
↑↑: Conversion from spinal to general anesthesia as spinal worked off (2 cases of IIA ligation and 1 case of supravaginal hysterectomy)

higher postoperative hemoglobin and lower require-ment for blood transfusion. In addition, none of the pa-tients underwent the procedure needed further surgical interventions to control intraoperative bleeding, while three patients in the control group needed another sur-gical intervention; two IIA ligation and one case needed supravaginal hysterectomy.

The procedure was not easy in all cases and was not possible in some patients as those with extensive adhe-sions between the LUS and the urinary bladder, exten-sive varicose veins in the LUS. In these cases, the procedure was not done as we believed there would be a great risk of urinary bladder injury or severe bleeding from varicose veins. In some occasions, the fetal head was compressing LUS, and the ligation was not done.

Ligation of Internal iliac artery, used to be performed to overcome massive pelvic hemorrhage, is not the technique of choice for control of atonic PPH due to placenta previa. Apart from its efficacy it requires more time for dissection and effort for training [13]. In a comprehensive research for 30 years, O'Leary had sug-gested the procedure of uterine artery ligation as an ef-ficient and alternate procedure to internal iliac artery ligation although in his trial, 10 out of 265 cases failed to respond [14]. In another excellent study concerning massive PPH due to uterine atony. The authors con-cluded that arterial embolization as effective as uterine artery ligation with success rate approaching 100%. Embolization can be performed after vaginal delivery in stable patients but it needs expertise and facilities [15].

The strengths of this study are the nature of the study (RCT) and reporting a novel technique in management of a serious obstetric condition as central placenta pre-via with potential for implication in clinical practice. The limitation of the study is the relatively small num-ber of patients included.

Conclusion

Uterine artery ligation prior to uterine incision could be an effective method to reduce the intraoperative blood loss in patients with central placenta previa undergoing elective CS. Larger studies are required to reach a firm conclusion about the procedure.

Additional files

Additional file 1: Table S1. Characteristics and risk factors in the study population before exclusion. This table shows the socio-demographic and clinical data of all patients before exclusion. (DOCX 18 kb)

Additional file 2: Table S2. The ultra-sonographic criteria of the placenta in the study population before exclusion. This table shows the ultrasound findings of all patients before enrollment. (DOCX 17 kb)

Additional file 3: Table S3. Outcome measures in the ligation and control groups before exclusion. This tables shows postoperative outcome of all patients. (DOCX 18 kb)

Acknowledgements
The authors are grateful to the entire medical, nursing and laboratory staff at Minia Maternity University Hospital for their help and cooperation throughout the research work.

Authors' contributions
ASS: Design the study methodology, diagnosis of cases, operative management, data collection, results preparation, and manuscript writing. AEM: Design the study methodology, diagnosis of cases, operative management, data collection, results preparation, and manuscript writing. MEA: Design the study methodology data analysis, results preparation, and manuscript writing. HHK: Design the study methodology, operative management, diagnosis of clinical cases program, and data collection. HAB: Design the study methodology, operative management, diagnosis of cases. HFM: Design the study methodology, diagnosis of clinical cases program, and data collection. RRE: Design the study methodology, diagnosis of clinical cases program, and data collection. AGA: Design the study methodology, operative management, data collection, results preparation and manuscript writing. MAZ: Design the study methodology, diagnosis of cases, operative management, data collection, results preparation and manuscript writing. HES: Assist us in ethical consideration, help in reviewing the work, was involved in revising the manuscript and provide final approval of the version to be published. All authors read and approved the final manuscript.

Competing interests
The authors declare that they have no competing interests.

References
1. Getahun D, Oyelese Y, Salihu HM, Ananth CV. Previous cesarean delivery and risks of placenta previa and placental abruption. Obstet Gynecol. 2006;107(4):771–8.
2. Brace V, Kernaghan D, Penney G. Learning from adverse clinical outcomes: major obstetric haemorrhage in Scotland, 2003-05. BJOG. 2007;114(11):1388–96.
3. Olive EC, Roberts CL, Algert CS, Morris JM. Placenta praevia: maternal morbidity and place of birth. Aust N Z J Obstet Gynaecol. 2005;45(6):499–504.
4. Oyelese Y, Smulian JC. Placenta previa, placenta accreta, and vasa previa. Obstet Gynecol. 2006;107(4):927–41.
5. Gurol-Urganci I, Cromwell DA, Edozien LC, Smith GC, Onwere C, Mahmood TA, et al. Risk of placenta previa in second birth after first birth cesarean section: a population-based study and meta-analysis. BMC Pregnancy Childbirth. 2011;11:95.
6. Arlier S, Seyfettinoglu S, Yilmaz E, Nazik H, Adiguzel C, Eskimez E, et al. Incidence of adhesions and maternal and neonatal morbidity after repeat cesarean section. Arch Gynecol Obstet. 2017;295(2):303–11.
7. Cresswell JA, Ronsmans C, Calvert C, Filippi V. Prevalence of placenta praevia by world region: a systematic review and meta-analysis. Tropical Med Int Health. 2013;18(6):712–24.
8. Tuzovic L. Complete versus incomplete placenta previa and obstetric outcome. Int J Gynaecol Obstet. 2006;93(2):110–7.
9. Onwere C, Gurol-Urganci I, Cromwell DA, Mahmood TA, Templeton A, van der Meulen JH. Maternal morbidity associated with placenta praevia among women who had elective cesarean section. Eur J Obstet Gynecol Reprod Biol. 2011;159(1):62–6.
10. Rosenberg T, Pariente G, Sergienko R, Wiznitzer A, Sheiner E. Critical analysis of risk factors and outcome of placenta previa. Arch Gynecol Obstet. 2011;284(1):47–51.
11. Schneiderman M, Balayla J. A comparative study of neonatal outcomes in placenta previa versus cesarean for other indication at term. J Matern Fetal Neonatal Med. 2013;26(11):1121–7.
12. Fraser IS, Warner P, Marantos PA. Estimating menstrual blood loss in women with normal and excessive menstrual fluid volume. Obstet Gynecol. 2001; 98(5 Pt 1):806–14.
13. Evans S, McShane P. The efficacy of internal iliac artery ligation in obstetric hemorrhage. Surg Gynecol Obstet. 1985;160(3):250–3.
14. O'Leary JA. Uterine artery ligation in the control of postcesarean hemorrhage. J Reprod Med. 1995;40(3):189–93.
15. Sergent F, Resch B, Verspyck E, Rachet B, Clavier E, Marpeau L. Intractable postpartum haemorrhages: where is the place of vascular ligations, emergency peripartum hysterectomy or arterial embolization? Gynecol Obstet Fertil. 2004;32(4):320–9.

'If I do 10–15 normal deliveries in a month I hardly ever sleep at home.' A qualitative study of health providers' reasons for high rates of caesarean deliveries in private sector maternity care in Delhi, India

Alison Peel[1], Abhishek Bhartia[2], Neil Spicer[3] and Meenakshi Gautham[3]*

Abstract

Background: Although the overall rate of caesarean deliveries in India remains low, rates are higher in private than in public facilities. In a household survey in Delhi, for instance, more than half of women delivering in private facilities reported a caesarean section. Evidence suggests that not all caesarean sections are clinically necessary and may even increase morbidity. We present providers' perspectives of the reasons behind the high rates of caesarean births in private facilities, and possible solutions to counter the trend.

Methods: Fourteen in-depth interviews were conducted with high-end private sector obstetricians and other allied providers in Delhi and its neighbouring cities, Gurgaon and Ghaziabad.

Results: Respondents were of the common view that private sector caesarean rates were unreasonably high and perceived time and doctors' convenience as the foremost reasons. Financial incentives had an indirect effect on decision-making. Obstetricians felt that they must maintain high patient loads to be commercially successful. Many alluded to their busy working lives, which made it challenging for them to monitor every delivery individually. Besides fearing for patient safety in these situations, they were fearful of legal action if anything went wrong. A lack of context specific guidelines and inadequate support from junior staff and nurses exacerbated these problems. Maternal demand also played a role, as the consumer-provider relationship in private healthcare incentivised obstetricians to fulfil patient demands for caesarean section. Suggested solutions included more support, from either well-trained midwives and junior staff or using a 'shared practice' model; guidelines introduced by an Indian body; increased regulation within the sector and public disclosure of providers' caesarean rates.

Conclusions: Commercial interests contribute indirectly to high caesarean rates, as solo obstetricians juggle the need to maintain high patient loads with inadequate support staff. Perceptions amongst providers and consumers of caesarean section as the 'safe' option have re-defined caesareans as the new 'normal', even for low-risk deliveries. At the policy level, guidelines and public disclosures, strong initiatives to develop professional midwifery, and increasing public awareness, could bring about a sustainable reduction in the present high rates.

Keywords: Caesarean section rates, Private sector, Qualitative interviews, Delhi, India

* Correspondence: Meenakshi.gautham@lshtm.ac.uk
[3]Department of Global Health and Development, Faculty of Public Health and Policy, London School of Hygiene and Tropical Medicine, London, UK
Full list of author information is available at the end of the article

Background

Caesarean section can be a life-saving intervention during deliveries where the mother or baby is at significant risk of adverse outcome. Many high maternal mortality regions struggle to provide safe and timely caesarean sections in such circumstances [1], yet women worldwide are increasingly undergoing procedures for which there is little clinical justification [2]. These 'unnecessary' caesarean sections have been associated with increased maternal risk of severe morbidity and even mortality [3, 4]. High rates of caesarean sections also have economic repercussions on patients and their families, as financial costs for the procedure are higher than for vaginal birth and a longer period of hospitalization is necessary. This is especially true in low- and middle-income countries where medical care is often purchased 'out-of-pocket' [5]. It is widely accepted, including by the World Health Organization (WHO), that caesarean deliveries should only be undertaken where medically necessary [3, 4, 6, 7].

Caesarean section rates vary widely across the globe, ranging from as low as 1% in parts of Sub-Saharan Africa to 30% in the USA and 45% in Brazil [5]. Following debate over the most appropriate rates of caesarean sections at national and regional levels, the WHO issued a statement in 2015 recommending that every effort should be made to provide caesarean sections to women *in need*, rather than striving to achieve specific population-level rates [6]. At the facility-level, it is recommended the 'Robson classification' system be used as it allows for comparison of caesarean rates within and across different risk groups of women [6, 8].

A wide variety of explanations have been proposed for rising caesarean rates, ranging from medical and demographic factors to changing patient expectations and provider practices. Repeat caesareans are an important contributor to high rates, as previous caesarean delivery pre-empts need for the procedure in successive deliveries. The risk of morbidity increases with each procedure [9].

Studies in multiple settings have found high rates of caesarean sections associated with non-medical factors. Higher caesarean rates are consistently associated with delivery by private providers, and thus have often been linked to financial incentives [10–19]. Research in private facilities has also shown that both planned and unplanned caesarean sections, including some emergency ones, are more likely to occur on weekdays or during daylight hours [20–22]. It is possible that elective procedures account for many of these daytime caesareans, and that some emergency caesareans may be held over until day staff come on duty, rested and alert, to ensure better outcomes. However, these studies [20–22] also suggest that physician factors, including convenient timing of deliveries and desire for increased leisure time, are significant predictors of caesarean sections. Obstetricians' fears of complaints and

legal action have also been indicated as determinants of caesarean delivery [23–27], and it has been suggested that providers perceive fewer risks, both legal and medical, associated with caesarean versus vaginal deliveries [4, 26]. Another concept frequently cited in literature is the influence of patient-related factors, such as maternal request for caesarean section. Maternal demand could be motivated by a number of non-medical factors including fear of vaginal birth, need for control, and cultural acceptability of the procedure [28]. One study in the UK suggested that doctors perceived maternal request as the most important factor driving caesarean rates, although few actually reported receiving a large number of requests or performing caesareans on request themselves [26].

The Indian context

India has made significant progress in improving maternal health, with the current maternal mortality ratio almost half of what it was in 2000 [29]. As mortality rates fall and increasing numbers of women gain access to formally trained maternity care providers, improving quality of care is becoming a priority for policy-makers. Indeed, some data suggest that quality of care is generally poor, though variable, in both the public and private healthcare sectors [30]. The private sector currently accounts for more than 70% of primary healthcare in India following rapid growth in recent decades [31]. This expansion has been accompanied by very little regulation or quality assurance, and insufficient standardisation of treatments, protocols and pricing. Private medical insurance is becoming increasingly common, although a large proportion of people still pay for care 'out-of-pocket' and are vulnerable to financial impoverishment if they require expensive surgeries or medication [32].

Private providers play a significant role in maternity care in India, accounting for 48% of institutional childbirths in urban areas and 24% in rural areas [31]. In Delhi, as in many other large cities in India, the vast majority of deliveries in the private sector are undertaken by obstetricians, who typically operate fee-for-service solo practices. There is very little practice of midwifery in urban hospitals and obstetricians often assume the role of the primary carer during deliveries, with limited support from other healthcare staff, especially midwives [33]. The size and structure of private sector facilities varies widely, from small nursing homes to large hospitals that are part of multi-national corporate chains [14].

Although the overall rate of caesarean deliveries in India is around 17%, rates have risen rapidly over the last ten years from 8.5% in 2005–06 to 17.2% in 2015–16 [34], driven particularly by increases in the private sector and in urban areas. Data collected over 2 years in the city of Chennai in south India indicated a caesarean rate of 47% in private healthcare [18]. Other studies have reported that women in the states of Kerala, Goa, Andhra Pradesh, Bihar, Gujarat, Karnataka, Punjab, Uttar Pradesh, Delhi, Maharashtra, and Tamil Nadu are far more likely to deliver by caesarean if they receive private care [11, 13, 15]. A community-based household survey indicated that 54% of women delivering in the private sector in Delhi underwent caesarean section, compared with a 24% rate in the public sector [14]. Although rates were not classified according to women's risk-status, this figure appears to indicate overuse of the procedure.

A small number of studies have presented data that begin to explain *why* caesarean section rates in the Indian private sector are higher than in the public sector. An analysis of supplier-induced demand in Madhya Pradesh and Gujarat [35] found that direct economic incentives led to increases in caesarean rates whilst financial disincentives led to decreasing rates. This suggests that private obstetricians induce maternal demand for caesarean section due to profit-making motives. Other studies have identified a positive correlation between maternal educational level and likelihood of caesarean delivery in private facilities, suggesting that maternal demand also plays a role, particularly amongst women with a higher level of education [15, 17]. Despite these findings, one of the studies [15] suggests that rising rates of caesarean delivery are more a result of supply factors (relating to the obstetrician) than maternal demand.

A number of studies reporting high rates of caesarean sections in the private healthcare sector in India have hypothesized that these reflect financial incentives, time pressures, the custom of solo practice, fear of litigation, maternal request, and use of intensive foetal monitoring [13, 14, 18]. However, it was not within the remit of the studies to test these hypotheses, and so the evidence remains lacking. No studies have explored providers' perspectives of the reasons for high caesarean rates in their private practices in India. The small quantity of data generated in other settings, especially high-income countries, may not be applicable to the Indian private sector. Our study sought to explore the perspectives of private healthcare professionals involved in maternity care in Delhi on reasons for high caesarean section rates, and solutions to reverse the trend of high rates in private maternity care in Delhi. The study is among the first to explore provider-side perspectives on this issue in the Indian setting.

Methods
Study setting
The study was located in Delhi and its neighbouring suburbs of Gurgaon and Ghaziabad, all in the National Capital Region (NCR) of India. Maternity care is delivered by a wide range of private and public facilities that vary greatly in size, structure, and staffing arrangements in these three settings. There are more than 560 private hospitals and nursing homes in Delhi alone [36]. Women of high socio-economic status are more likely to pay for private maternity care, with more than 80% attending private facilities. A substantial proportion of middle and low socio-economic status women (40 and 16%, respectively) also opt for private maternity care. Caesarean sections are more common in private facilities, where the rate is 54% compared with 24% in the public sector [14]. Our study focused on private maternity care providers in this setting. We collaborated with a private medical hospital and research institute based in South Delhi.

Study design
Fourteen in-depth qualitative interviews were conducted during July and August 2015. We approached key informants who could offer insights from the perspective of a private sector maternity care provider. To get an all-round providers' perspective, we purposively selected practicing obstetricians and a small number of other healthcare professionals with involvement in maternity care - two paediatricians, the manager of a private maternity hospital and a 'doula' or birth companion, who is professionally trained to provide physical, emotional and educational support to the mother. This gave us the opportunity to compare and contrast the perspectives of obstetricians with those of other professionals with good knowledge of the sector.

The majority of study participants worked in South Delhi, with an additional participant working in East Delhi and two in other cities in the NCR, Gurgaon and Ghaziabad. As the sector is highly diverse, we selected providers from secondary and tertiary facilities of different sizes, with capacity for performing caesarean sections: small hospitals or nursing homes (< 50 beds), medium-sized hospitals (50–150 beds), and a large corporate hospital (> 150 beds). These included a mix of multi-specialty and super specialty private hospitals where a normal delivery can cost upwards of INR 40,000 (US$ 615), and a caesarean section in a super luxury room can be priced as high as INR 12,00,000 (US$ 18,461). These were amongst the more high-end private hospitals in the NCR, serving the wealthiest socio-economic sections of the population, who would typically seek only private sector maternity care.

With the help of our collaborating research institute, we drew up an initial list of 19 potential respondents and contacted them for interviews. Ten agreed to an interview during the period that the primary researcher was available, and with the help of these respondents, we identified and interviewed an additional four who agreed.

The interviews were conducted using an interview guide that explored participants' professional status and background, perceptions of current caesarean section rates in the private sector, awareness of guidelines regarding rates, reasons they attributed to high rates, and their suggested solutions for reducing rates.

Confidentiality was maintained by conducting the interviews in private rooms at participants' workplaces or homes. Interviews were audio-recorded where permission was given. In the case of three participants where permission was not given, detailed hand-written notes were taken. All interviews were carried out in English by a single interviewer.

Analysis

All audio-recorded interviews were transcribed. Transcripts and interview notes were coded manually using a coding frame developed both from concepts that emerged in the data and those found in the existing literature, for example financial incentives. Data were organised into matrices for each major topic to help systematize analysis, identify patterns in the data, and compare participants. A final list of key themes and sub-themes emerging from interviews was identified.

Results

Perceptions of caesarean rates in Delhi private sector

Most respondents were of the view that caesarean section rates in the private maternity homes they visited were unjustifiably high and that a substantial proportion of procedures were performed without clear medical need. Two obstetricians believed that rates could be as high as 90% in the different hospitals where they practiced. Others cited rates of 15–50% in their facilities. Most respondents acknowledged that, as high caesarean section rates were rarely discussed within the healthcare community, practitioners were unlikely to know precise facility-level or even personal rates and little self-auditing occurred in private hospitals.

> "It's not part of the Indian medical environment right now to really critically analyse their outcomes and compare it to standards." (Hospital chief executive)

Reasons for high rates of caesarean sections

Three groups of themes emerged in our analysis of participants' explanations for high caesarean rates in the Delhi and NCR private sector: provider-related, system-related, and patient-related factors. These are presented in the following sections.

Provider-related factors

Personal convenience The majority of respondents said that providers' convenience, in terms of time spent and timing of deliveries, was the most important consideration for doctors. Vaginal deliveries could involve more than 12 h of labour and occur at inconvenient times, particularly during the night. Caesareans allowed doctors to exercise control over the duration and timing of delivery so that they had more time for personal and professional activities.

> "One normal delivery costs me at least a night, sometimes 2 nights. If I do 10-15 normal deliveries in a month I hardly ever sleep at home. If I do 15 caesareans I'm not home late for coffee." (Private sector obstetrician)

Concerns about decision-making Many respondents spoke about the pressure of an obstetrician's demanding workload, which meant that doctors were unable to commit their full attention to every delivery because they were pre-occupied by other concerns or a lack of sleep. This could affect decision-making regarding deliveries.

> "Supposing one is awake the whole night for 2 days, the third night one will have a tendency to take weak decisions." (Private sector obstetrician)

Another common theme was the pressure of having sole responsibility for a delivery (due to the norm of working alone), and having to make difficult, subjective decisions about the safest option for a patient.

> "Decision-making is very tough. For caesarean anybody can make decision, but how long you have to wait for a normal delivery is very difficult to assess". (Private sector obstetrician)

Some spoke about fearing for the safety of patients and their babies during deliveries. This fear could lead them to decide in favour of a caesarean section earlier than necessary.

> "Whatever I was trained in just goes away...suddenly I think I have to give her a live baby" (Private sector obstetrician)

Fear of legal action by patients emerged as another important challenge to doctors' decision-making. Respondents explained that, according to the existing laws, if anything goes wrong the sole legal responsibility lies with the obstetrician. Therefore, they considered caesarean as the safer option for avoiding litigation, as one described it, a caesarean was *"a more comfortable and assured path..." (Private sector obstetrician).*

Some respondents suggested that use of technologies such as 'cardiotocography' machines for continuous foetal heart rate monitoring could also be increasing the frequency of decisions for caesarean deliveries. They described doctors panicking or becoming *"hyper"* when they saw decelerations in foetal heartrate, leading them to perform a caesarean section even though the labour may have progressed normally.

Training and continuing medical education Some interviewees explained that waiting for normal labour to progress might seem counterintuitive to doctors because of the training they have received. They argued that doctors are trained for pathological events and therefore they are predisposed to intervene, even during a physiologically normal birth.

"Doctors are not trained for sitting and watching and waiting, they are trained to intervene…they are people who need to jump in when something is going wrong" (Private sector paediatrician)

Aside from this, the providers interviewed thought that the initial training for obstetrics was adequate, although some expressed concern about obstetricians not updating themselves on current knowledge later in their careers. Although interviewees stated that continuing medical education was available for obstetricians, they indicated that many would not attend due to heavy workloads, or a perceived lack of need for additional training.

"Most of us don't do trainings, we just run our own clinics and the basic idea is the financial situation is fine, and if you're sensible enough, then you don't do any harm to your patients" (Private sector obstetrician)

Respondents believed that, due to a lack of continuing medical education, some obstetricians were unaware of current evidence-based guidelines and performed unnecessary caesareans as a result.

Non-compliance with guidelines was also an issue. Many obstetricians reported working in hospitals where a set of standard guidelines were available. However, one protested that there is little compulsion for visiting consultants to follow guidelines.

"You cannot enforce the guidelines on them… if we force them they will not bring the patient to the hospital, so hospital will lose those number of clients." (Private sector obstetrician)

As we report further on, respondents also expressed concerns over a lack of guidelines that were appropriate to the setting.

In addition, it emerged that many obstetricians associated little risk with caesarean deliveries. Respondents spoke about caesareans having become routine procedures, with doctors thinking of them as *"no big deal"*. Nevertheless, they also described adverse consequences associated with medically unindicated caesarean sections and believed that all obstetricians would be aware of these from their training. One respondent attempted to explain the disparity between these viewpoints:

"We all know what we're doing, but of course the mind is between knowing and using that knowledge" (Professor of obstetrics).

Some respondents reasoned that a vaginal delivery may appear more risky to obstetricians as there were more 'unknowns' compared with a caesarean section.

Commercial interests A few respondents mentioned financial incentives as a reason for high caesarean section rates in the private sector. However, they placed less weight on this than the other reasons. This could be because they felt uncomfortable admitting to monetary incentives in interviews, or because the financial benefits of caesarean deliveries affected them only indirectly.

Many respondents referred to hospitals, rather than individual doctors, being financially motivated. Several described how, in their experience, corporate hospitals were often run in a way where doctors were encouraged to take on as many patients as possible in order to generate revenue.

"[Hospitals] see the business that you are doing. They will not see how many caesareans or normal deliveries you're doing…the doctor is under pressure to have more patients because that's her power, her importance in the institution is what she brings to the hospital." (Private sector obstetrician)

It was also reported that patients paid more for caesarean than vaginal delivery, due to additional charges for operating theatre rent, anaesthetists, and other necessary arrangements. Some suggested that these dis-incentivised facilities to decrease caesarean rates.

"Hospitals earn about 30-50% more revenue as the result of a caesarean delivery compared to a normal delivery. And almost all of the additional revenue is additional margin. So, hospitals have a clear financial incentive to not mind a high caesarean section rate." (Hospital chief executive)

In contrast, some other interviewees were insistent that commercial incentives played no part in doctors' decisions to perform caesarean sections.

"No no no no no! ...the charges [fees charged by doctors] for caesarean and normal delivery are almost at one. So that is never a reason." (Private sector obstetrician)

This assertion that doctors' fee for both modes of delivery were the same or very similar was reiterated by several respondents. Many emphasised that obstetricians *"don't do it for money but to save time"*.

"An obstetrician would rather do a caesarean and go and save time, maximise the benefit of the time spent to do more deliveries, see more OPD patients." (Private sector paediatrician)

Even those who believed that financial incentives played a role stated that time was a more important factor. However, this was put into perspective by one obstetrician who pointed out that by attending to more patients in less time doctors could take on more clients and thus generate more revenue.

Furthermore, a number of other respondents indicated that the commercial nature of the private health sector's commercial nature prevents providers from lowering their caesarean rates. Doctors and hospital executives are compelled to maximise the number of patients they receive as it directly determines their income.

"If you want to do always what is right for the patient but you reward clinicians on volumes there's a misalignment." (Hospital chief executive)

As obstetricians were unlikely to turn patients away even if their workload was high, there was always great pressure on their time. This was especially likely for doctors visiting multiple hospitals, as one respondent described of an obstetrician she knew:

"She did clinics and had women waiting in labour at all of the hospitals. She was getting calls continuously. It's that sort of life, very hectic. That will increase caesarean rates." (Private sector paediatrician)

The norm of solo practice in the sector exacerbated this problem, as obstetricians could not rely on other doctors to assist them when they were short of time, unlike in a 'shared' practice.

System-related factors
Some interviewees believed that the structure of the private sector could be partially to blame for high caesarean rates. They emphasised lack of regulation as an important systemic factor. There were no government requirements for reporting on maternity care in the private sector, and some believed that this could be a reason for high rates.

"If I'm an obstetrician with a 70% caesarean rate I can go on that way for the next 30 years. Nobody will find out." (Hospital chief executive)

Many respondents believed that obstetricians would be less likely to perform unnecessary caesareans if they knew their practice was being monitored.

Some respondents also pointed to the lack of clinical guidelines for making decisions about caesarean sections issued by an Indian body. Indeed, several obstetricians reported using guidelines from other countries and some expressed concern about their use in an Indian setting. Others mentioned that the Federation of Obstetric and Gynaecological Societies of India issues a limited number of guidelines relating to caesarean sections, but these were not comprehensive and awareness of them was low amongst obstetricians.

Poor support systems were also cited as a cause of high caesarean rates. Respondents said that the standards of support from junior and nursing staff in the private sector varied greatly.

"The nurses are not trained in midwifery, they are not taking part in the antenatal period...I think they are underutilised, which is a big problem" (Private sector obstetrician)

One obstetrician explained that "...*as a result* [of poor support], *all of the decision-making responsibility flows straight up to the consultant" (private sector obstetrician)*, highlighting the additional pressure on doctors caused by these inadequate support systems.

Patient-related factors
Respondents reported that caesareans frequently occur because of patient demand, sometimes scheduled beforehand, but often requested during the process of labour. Many expressed that caesarean sections were perceived as the 'normal' mode of delivery amongst women.

"Caesarean has become the new normal. Chances are my friends, my mum, more people that I know have had caesarean deliveries rather than normal deliveries." (Hospital chief executive)

Respondents perceived that women viewed caesarean as an *"easy way out"* of the pain of labour, and spoke about women hearing accounts of traumatic experiences, through either word of mouth or the media, which led them to request caesarean deliveries. A couple of respondents also observed a link between fear of labour and women's bodies, saying that this led to the body not responding well to natural birth, so that a caesarean was necessary. Other patient-related factors included the convenience of a *"short-cut"* delivery and desire to schedule deliveries on auspicious dates.

Some respondents expressed concern about the sources from which patients obtained their information on deliveries, which they perceived to be primarily peer groups and family. Several stated that women did not fully understand the risks of a caesarean delivery, or that women perceived caesarean to be a safer choice than normal delivery. Many thought that counselling of patients by doctors, where the relative risks and benefits of delivery methods were explained, was often insufficient or entirely lacking.

Obstetricians often agreed to patients' demands and performed caesareans even though they were not medically necessary. This was attributed to the time and effort required to change a patient's mind.

> "The easiest approach is that I do what the patient is saying...the more I try to explain the more time is used...I might as well give her a date for caesarean in 5 minutes" (Private sector obstetrician)

Others spoke about patients who insisted on a caesarean delivery in spite of counselling, and felt that they could not *"force"* a woman to have a natural delivery. Some respondents said that patients' families put pressure on doctors to intervene during labour. Consumer-provider type relationships in the private sector implied that obstetricians were willing to satisfy patients' demands for caesarean sections. If they refused to perform a procedure the patient could easily go to a doctor who was more willing, and this would result in loss of patients. *"It's a demand and supply kind of thing"* said one private sector obstetrician, emphasising that private sector clients have more power to make demands than in the public sector because they are paying customers.

In addition to ideas about patient's expectations and choices, interviewees spoke about lifestyle changes, such as women having babies later in life or being more sedentary and overweight, which were related to the higher socio-economic status of patients using the private sector. Previous caesareans were another reason, as women were likely to require a caesarean section if they had had one previously, due to the increased risks of complications. One interviewee stated that vaginal birth after caesarean was *"almost zero"* in the private sector in Delhi.

Possible solutions to high caesarean rates

The most frequently mentioned solution was improved counselling by doctors, in order to reduce patient demand for caesareans.

> "Shaping women's attitudes and behaviour is a very important aspect of this challenge if we actually want to solve the caesarean problem." (Hospital chief executive)

Many respondents called for better education of pregnant women about the vaginal delivery process, the risks associated with caesarean sections, and maximising the chances of a natural delivery. This would help women cope with labour pains and could be imparted during existing sessions, such as antenatal workshops.

Acknowledging the present lack of guidelines, several respondents suggested that standardised evidence-based guidelines, issued by an Indian body and tailored to the Indian setting, would be effective in reducing caesarean rates. They expressed that guidelines should be introduced at the institutional level at the least, and that doctors should be encouraged to follow them. One obstetrician, who managed the mother and child unit of a hospital, stated that introducing standard guidelines had been the most effective method for lowering numbers of caesarean deliveries in their facility.

A number of respondents believed that regulation would be important for enforcing these guidelines. Some suggested the possibility of a higher-level regulatory body auditing caesarean rates and imposing penalties where unnecessary procedures were being performed. Others thought that promoting transparency could begin to tackle the problem.

> "If, as part of a professional code of conduct, I was required to disclose it [my caesarean rate], now suddenly women would know...there would be an incentive for everyone in the system to start rectifying the situation." (Hospital chief executive)

Another solution was to improve support for obstetricians from other medical staff. Respondents emphasised that nurses should receive training to provide more 'hands-on' support during labour. Some respondents suggested an expanded role for midwives as the primary carers in low-risk deliveries. A counter argument was that patients in private hospitals might not feel comfortable if they were attended by a midwife rather than a doctor. Therefore, an additional suggestion for improving support was the idea of 'shared practice', where obstetricians could rely on each other for help with decision-making and performing deliveries.

Discussion

The present study identifies a number of important factors that may be driving high rates of caesarean sections in the private healthcare sector in Delhi and its neighbourhood. The rates reported by some respondents for facilities where they practiced varied from 15 to 50%, and a small number reported rates as high as 90%. As self- or facility-level auditing of caesarean sections was not commonly practiced in these facilities, these rates may be considered as estimates rather than precise figures. Even so, the figure of 50% is comparable to rates reported by two household surveys in Delhi: the National Family Health Survey-4 [34] that reported 43% caesarean births in the private sector and another household survey conducted at a similar time [14] that found 54% caesarean section births in the private sector. The higher rate of 90% reported by a small number of our respondents could be more facility specific and indicative of the substantial variation likely to exist across facilities. Similar variation can be seen in reported rates ranging from 50 to 99% in a study of private health facilities providing delivery care in the state of Uttar Pradesh, which borders Delhi [37].

The respondents we interviewed were generally of the opinion that unnecessary use of caesarean sections was an important issue in this sector. Key contributors were identified as: obstetrician convenience and time pressures, particularly owing to the high prevalence of solo obstetric practice; a perception of caesarean deliveries as the 'safe' option, both in terms of maternal health and protection from litigation; and financial pressures associated with running a successful clinic, or working for a commercial hospital. Other important reasons for high rates of caesarean deliveries included system-related factors, especially the lack of comprehensive guidelines tailored to the Indian setting, and lack of well-trained support staff such as midwives, as well as patient-related factors such as maternal and family related fears and demands. Interestingly, none of our respondents mentioned emergency referrals from smaller, more poorly-equipped private facilities or from government facilities as an important reason for the high caesarean rates. In a recent study in Uttar Pradesh [37], emergency referrals for caesarean sections were commonly reported by secondary and tertiary private facilities located on the outskirts of big cities and in smaller urban centres. Our study sample was quite different from these types of peri-urban facilities. Our respondents were all located within a metropolis, where most delivery facilities, private as well as public, have the capacity for performing caesarean sections and do not need to refer frequently. Moreover, the clientele at these facilities belonged to the wealthiest socio-economic groups who could afford pregnancy and delivery care at the best equipped private facilities from the very beginning.

Although respondents gave a variety of reasons for high caesarean rates, many of these can be retraced to the commercial nature of private sector practice that incentivises growing practices even to the point that time pressures interfere with the ability to provide quality care. Obstetricians must maintain their patient loads in order to run commercially viable practices, leading to immense pressures on their time. They must protect their patients from any adverse outcomes, and themselves from litigation. It is not possible to monitor every delivery to its normal conclusion, and so obstetricians may opt for caesarean deliveries in order to ensure patient safety and sufficient time to attend to all of their patients. As a result, caesarean section has come to be considered as the 'safe' option, in spite of the associated risks. A culture amongst obstetricians of performing caesarean sections, where 'caesarean is seen as the new normal', reinforces this perception and may prevent providers from recognising high caesarean rates as abnormal or harmful. Furthermore, inadequate support systems, including very limited practice of midwifery in India, increase time pressures on obstetricians and the difficulty of decision-making regarding deliveries.

Maternal and family requests for caesarean section were also identified as a driver of caesarean rates. Providers perceived a culture where caesarean sections are considered an 'easy' option among women using private sector facilities. The apparent frequency with which obstetricians fulfil patients' requests for caesarean section reflects the provider-consumer type exchange between doctors and patients due to the commercial nature of their relationship. Doctors may feel obliged to fulfil patients' demands or refrain from taking a hard line during patient counselling in order to avoid losing that patient. Our data suggest that some women who request caesarean deliveries receive insufficient counselling regarding the associated risks, likely due to the pressures on obstetricians' time. Respondents did, however, identify physical factors, such as women postponing pregnancy until later in life or being overweight because they were leading more sedentary lifestyles, as a cause of rising caesarean rates, particularly amongst the high socio-economic status women who use private healthcare.

A lack of guidelines and regulation regarding caesarean sections amplify the effects of rising caesarean section rates, as obstetricians and institutions are not held accountable for their rates. The Indian government's most recent guidelines for dealing with obstetric complications were issued in 2005. These detail the complications for which a caesarean section may be necessary, but no thresholds for caesarean section are given and few associated risks are mentioned [38].

The solutions that respondents offered for reducing caesarean section rates reinforce these explanations. They suggested that the level of support from junior and nursing/midwifery staff be improved, by either expanding the roles of support staff or encouraging small groups of obstetricians to work in 'shared practice', providing professional support to one another where necessary. Expanding the role of midwives to be the primary carers during normal deliveries, with support from obstetricians only when complications occur, could significantly reduce the time pressures on doctors and thus help avoid unnecessary caesareans. Unfortunately, midwifery remains an under-developed and under-recognised profession in India [33], with neither legislative support nor training standards for independent midwifery. The currently available training in midwifery, which is limited to a few months and combined with more general nursing training, has been found inadequate for preparing confident and competent midwives [39]. Greater policy support is required to promote midwifery in India, although this is likely to be met with initial resistance from providers and patients who are accustomed to doctors being present throughout the delivery. Other suggestions were that comprehensive caesarean section guidelines be made available from an Indian medical body, and that individual and institutional caesarean section rates undergo auditing and regulation. Some form of peer review within the sector, or regulation by an external body, could help to improve obstetricians' awareness of their own rates and incentivise them to only perform procedures in cases where they are truly necessary.

The present study adds depth to the current understanding of high caesarean rates in the Indian private sector. Our findings support results from previous studies both in Indian and non-Indian settings, which emphasise obstetrician time and convenience factors [20–22], fear of litigation [23–27], financial incentives [10–19], perceptions of low risk [4, 26], and maternal demand [26, 28] as important reasons for high caesarean section rates. In addition, the present study identifies some previously undocumented factors that may contribute to high caesarean rates in the Indian setting: a lack of appropriate guidelines on caesarean sections, and the culture of private sector obstetricians working in solo practice, often with insufficient support systems, particularly well-trained midwives. Furthermore, our analysis highlights the 'missing' link between caesarean sections and obstetricians' high practice volumes as a result of financial incentives in the private sector.

Limitations

The small sample size of this study, due to resource constraints and the difficulties in accessing busy obstetricians and other maternity healthcare providers, limits its generalisability. Our sample was also mostly limited to the higher end obstetricians and multi-speciality/super-specialty private hospitals that cater to wealthier, urban clients that can afford to pay a high fee for institutional deliveries in big city hospitals. The situation in smaller, less expensive private hospitals in peri urban and rural areas is likely to be quite different and needs to be explored through other studies. Another limitation was that we could not access any documented data on caesarean rates from the facilities and, therefore, the rates we present here are reported estimates. However, it is unlikely that this information would have been available in many cases, as the respondents themselves reported that little self-auditing occurred amongst providers. We have also shown that the estimates are comparable to rates reported in the published literature. Finally, we did not interview any patients in this study, as our focus was on providers' perceptions. Patients' perceptions could be very different, and especially useful for understanding the extent to which maternal requests play a role in this setting. Nonetheless, the providers' perceptions reported in this article are a valuable addition to the literature. We have reached out to an important and challenging group of providers and gathered rich and in-depth insights on a sensitive topic that will be useful for exploring caesarean reduction strategies, and designing further research around this important topic.

Conclusions

A complex relationship exists between high caesarean rates and the commercial nature of the private sector. Although there may be no direct link between providers' decisions for a caesarean section and financial gain, obstetric practice in the private sector is dependent on maintaining high patient loads. This can lead to doctors taking on more patients than they can feasibly manage, and opting for caesarean deliveries in order to ensure patient safety, as well as protection from litigation.

Reducing high rates of caesarean deliveries in the Delhi private sector will depend on the introduction of comprehensive caesarean section guidelines, including indications and thresholds for which the procedure should be performed, and public disclosure of the caesarean rate for individual obstetricians and hospitals. However, regulations and guidelines may be insufficient without a parallel strengthening of professional midwifery support for obstetricians, before, during and after childbirth, and improved patient counselling and awareness. As India's most prominent obstetric body, the Federation of Obstetrics and Gynaecological Societies of India could play an important role in steering a comprehensive and sustainable caesarean reduction strategy in the higher end private sector in India.

Abbreviations
NCR: National Capital Region; UK: United Kingdom; USA: United States of America; WHO: World Health Organization

Acknowledgements
We are grateful to all the healthcare providers who participated in the study and to Sitaram Bhartia for facilitating the study.

Funding
AP received student funding for travel and fieldwork from the London School of Hygiene and Tropical Medicine. MG was AP's student supervisor, and India

Country Coordinator of LSHTM's IDEAS project. This work was supported by IDEAS-Informed Decisions for Actions to improve maternal and newborn health (https://ideas.lshtm.ac.uk/) which is funded through a grant from the Bill and Melinda Gates Foundation to the London School of Hygiene and Tropical Medicine (Gates Global Health Grant Number: OPP1017031).

Authors' contributions

The study design was developed by AP and MG. AP conducted data collection and initial analysis, with support from MG and AB. AP, MG, NS and AB all had input into the interpretation and presentation of results. AP drafted the initial manuscript with critical inputs from MG. All authors critically reviewed the drafts, offered revisions and approved the final manuscript.

Competing interests

The authors declare that they have no competing interests.

Author details

[1]London School of Hygiene and Tropical Medicine, London, UK. [2]Sitaram Bhartia Institute of Science and Research, New Delhi, India. [3]Department of Global Health and Development, Faculty of Public Health and Policy, London School of Hygiene and Tropical Medicine, London, UK.

References

1. Ronsmans C, Holtz S, Stanton C. Socioeconomic differentials in caesarean rates in developing countries: a retrospective analysis. Lancet. 2006; 368(9546):1516–23.
2. Lavender T, Hofmeyr GJ, Neilson JP, Kingdon C, Gyte GM. Caesarean section for non-medical reasons at term. Cochrane Database Syst Rev. 2012;3(3): CD004660. https://doi.org/10.1002/14651858.CD004660.pub3.
3. Lumbiganon P, Laopaiboon M, Gulmezoglu AM, Souza JP, Taneepanichskul S, Ruyan P, et al. Method of delivery and pregnancy outcomes in Asia: the WHO global survey on maternal and perinatal health 2007-08. Lancet. 2010; 375(9713):490–9.
4. Souza JP, Gulmezoglu A, Lumbiganon P, Laopaiboon M, Carroli G, Fawole B, et al. Caesarean section without medical indications is associated with an increased risk of adverse short-term maternal outcomes: the 2004-2008 WHO global survey on maternal and perinatal health. BMC Med. 2010;8:71.
5. Gibbons LBJ, Lauer JA, Betran AP, Merialdi M, Althabe F. The Global Numbers and Costs of Additionally Needed and Unnecessary Caesarean Sections Performed per Year: Overuse as a Barrier to Universal Coverage. World Health Report Background Paper 30. Geneva: World Health Organization; 2010.
6. World Health Organisation. WHO statement on caesarean section rates. Geneva: WHO; 2015.
7. Vogel JP, Betran AP, Vindevoghel N, Souza JP, Torloni MR, Zhang J, et al. Use of the Robson classification to assess caesarean section trends in 21 countries: a secondary analysis of two WHO multicountry surveys. Lancet Glob Health. 2015;3(5):e260–70.
8. Betrán AP, Vindevoghel N, Souza JP, Gülmezoglu AM, Torloni MR. A systematic review of the Robson classification for caesarean section: what works, Doesn't work and how to improve it. PLoS One. 2014;9(6):e97769.
9. Marshall NE, Fu R, Guise JM. Impact of multiple cesarean deliveries on maternal morbidity: a systematic review. Am J Obstet Gynecol. 2011;205(3):262.e1–8.
10. Gomes UA, Silva AA, Bettiol H, Barbieri MA. Risk factors for the increasing caesarean section rate in Southeast Brazil: a comparison of two birth cohorts, 1978-1979 and 1994. Int J Epidemiol. 1999;28(4):687–94.
11. Padmadas SS, Kumar S, Nair SB, Kumari A. Caesarean section delivery in Kerala, India: evidence from a National Family Health Survey. Soc Sci Med. 2000;51(4):511–21.
12. Phadungkiatwattana P, Tongsakul N. Analyzing the impact of private service on the cesarean section rate in public hospital Thailand. Arch Gynecol Obstet. 2011;284(6):1375–9.
13. Mishra US, Ramanathan M. Delivery-related complications and determinants of caesarean section rates in India. Health Policy Plan. 2002;17(1):90–8.
14. Nagpal J, Sachdeva A, Sengupta Dhar R, Bhargava VL, Bhartia A. Widespread non-adherence to evidence-based maternity care guidelines: a population-based cluster randomised household survey. BJOG. 2015;122(2):238–47.
15. Leone T. Demand and supply factors affecting the rising overmedicalization of birth in India. Int J Gynaecol Obstet. 2014;127:157–62.
16. Roberts CL, Tracy S, Peat B. Rates for obstetric intervention among private and public patients in Australia: population based descriptive study. BMJ. 2000;321(7254):137–41.
17. Neuman M, Alcock G, Azad K, Kuddus A, Osrin D, More NS, et al. Prevalence and determinants of caesarean section in private and public health facilities in underserved south Asian communities: cross-sectional analysis of data from Bangladesh. India and Nepal BMJ Open. 2014;4(12):e005982.
18. Sreevidya S, Sathiyasekaran BW. High caesarean rates in Madras (India): a population-based cross sectional study. BJOG. 2003;110(2):106–11.
19. Lutomski JE, Murphy M, Devane D, Meaney S, Greene RA. Private health care coverage and increased risk of obstetric intervention. BMC pregnancy and childbirth. 2014;14:13.
20. Brown HS 3rd. Physician demand for leisure: implications for cesarean section rates. J Health Econ. 1996;15(2):233–42.
21. Burns LR, Geller SE, Wholey DR. The effect of physician factors on the cesarean section decision. Med Care. 1995;33(4):365–82.
22. Mossialos E, Allin S, Karras K, Davaki K. An investigation of caesarean sections in three Greek hospitals: the impact of financial incentives and convenience. Eur J Pub Health. 2005;15(3):288–95.
23. Fuglenes D, Oian P, Kristiansen IS. Obstetricians' choice of cesarean delivery in ambiguous cases: is it influenced by risk attitude or fear of complaints and litigation? Am J Obstet Gynecol. 2009;200(1):48.e1–8.
24. Belizan JM, Quaranta P, Paquez E, Villar J. Caesarean section and fear of litigation. Lancet. 1991;338(8780):1462.
25. Minkoff H. Fear of litigation and cesarean section rates. Semin Perinatol. 2012;36(5):390–4.
26. Weaver JJ, Statham H, Richards M. Are there "unnecessary" cesarean sections? Perceptions of women and obstetricians about cesarean sections for nonclinical indications. Birth. 2007;34(1):32–41.
27. Chaillet N, Dube E, Dugas M, Francoeur D, Dube J, Gagnon S, et al. Identifying barriers and facilitators towards implementing guidelines to reduce caesarean section rates in Quebec. Bull World Health Organ. 2007;85(10):791–7.
28. Fuglenes D, Aas E, Botten G, Oian P, Kristiansen IS. Why do some pregnant women prefer cesarean? The influence of parity, delivery experiences, and fear. Am J Obstet Gynecol. 2011;205(1):45.e1–9.
29. WHO, UNFPA, World Bank. Trends in maternal mortality: 1990 to 2013. Geneva: World Health Organisation; 2014.
30. Sharma G, Powell-Jackson T, Haldar K, Bradley J, Filippi V. Quality of routine essential care during childbirth: clinical observations of uncomplicated births in Uttar Pradesh, India. Bull World Health Organ. 2017;95:419–29.
31. National Sample Survey Organization. Government of India. NSSO 71st round (Jan-Jun 2014). Report no. 574. Ministry of Statistics and Programme Implementation, Government of India: New Delhi; 2016.
32. National Commission on Macroeconomics and Health. Report of the national commission on macroeconomics and health. New Delhi: New Delhi: Ministry of Health and Family Welfare, Government of India; 2005.

33. Kumbhar K. Shunned for years, can trained midwives fix India's maternity mess? Quartz India. 2016. https://qz.com/629132/shunned-for-years-can-trained-midwives-fix-indias-maternity-mess. Accessed 23 March 2018.

34. IIPS. National Family Health Survey-4 (NFHS-4) 2015–16. India Factsheet. Government of India, 2015–16.

35. Bogg L, Diwan V, Vora KS, DeCosta A. Impact of alternative maternal demand-side financial support programs in India on the caesarean section rates: indications of supplier-induced demand. Maternal Child Health J. 2016;20(1):11–5.

36. Government of NCT of Delhi. Delhi Human Development Report 2006. New York, NY: Oxford University Press; 2006.

37. Goodman C, Gautham M, Iles R, Bruxvoort K, Subharwal M, Gupta S, Jain M. The nature of competition faced by private providers of maternal health services in Uttar Pradesh, India. A Report (unpublished). UK: London School of Hygiene and Tropical Medicine; 2017.

38. Guidelines for Pregnancy Care and Management of Common Obstetric Complications by Medical Officers. Maternal Health Division, DoFW, Minsitry of Health and Family Welfare, Government of India, New Delhi; 2005.

39. Sharma B, Hildingsson I, Johansson E, Prakasamma M, Ramani KV, Christensson K. Do the pre-service education programmes for midwives in India prepare confident 'registered midwives'? A survey from India. Glob Health Action. 2015;8(1):29553.

17

Risk factors for hypertensive disorders of pregnancy among mothers in Tigray region, Ethiopia: matched case-control study

Hailemariam Berhe Kahsay[1*], Fikre Enquselassie Gashe[2] and Wubegzier Mekonnen Ayele[2]

Abstract

Background: Hypertensive disorders of pregnancy are a global public health concern both in developed and developing countries. However, evidences regarding the risk factors of hypertensive disorders of pregnancy are limited particularly in Ethiopia. The aim of the study was to assess risk factors associated with hypertensive disorders of pregnancy among mothers in public hospitals of Tigray.

Methods: The study was conducted in seven public hospitals of Tigray region, Ethiopia from June 2017 to November 2017. A facility based matched case-control study was employed to select 110 cases and 220 controls who were pregnant women. Cases and controls were matched by parity status. A case was a mother diagnosed to have hypertensive disorders of pregnancy by an obstetrician in the antenatal period while a control was a mother who did not have a diagnosis of hypertensive disorders of pregnancy. Data were collected by face to face interview technique using a pretested questionnaire and a checklist. Conditional logistic regression analysis was used to identify the independent predictor variables. Adjusted matched odds ratio with its corresponding 95% confidence interval was used and significance was claimed at P-value less than 0.05. Overall findings were presented in texts and tables.

Results: Rural residents were at greater odds of suffering from hypertensive disorders (OR = 3.7, 95% CI; 1.9, 7.1). Similarly, mothers who consume less amount of fruits in their diet had 5 times higher odds of developing hypertensive disorders than those who consume fruits regularly (OR = 5.1, 95% CI; 2.4, 11.15). Overweight (BMI > 25 Kg/m2) mothers were also at risk of developing hypertensive disorders of pregnancy as compared with the normal and underweight mothers (AOR = 5.5 95% CI; 1.12, 27.6). The risk of developing hypertensive disorders of pregnancy was 5.4 times higher among diabetic mothers.

Conclusion: Rural residence, less fruit consumption, multiple pregnancy, presence of gestational diabetes mellitus and pre-pregnancy overweight were identified as independent risk factors in this study. It is recommended that health care givers may use these factors as a screening tool for the prediction, early diagnoses as well as timely interventions of hypertensive disorders of pregnancy.

Keywords: Hypertensive disorders of pregnancy, Gestational hypertension, Preeclampsia, Tigray, Ethiopia

* Correspondence: aidhbk@gmail.com
[1]School of Nursing, Mekelle University, P.O.Box:1871, Mekelle, Ethiopia
Full list of author information is available at the end of the article

Background

According to the American college of obstetricians and gynaecologists (ACOG), Hypertension in pregnancy is defined as: Systolic blood pressure greater than or equal to 140 mmHg and/or diastolic blood pressure greater than or equal to 90 mmHg in two occasions at least 6 h apart after fifth month of gestation for pregnancy induced hypertension or before pregnancy/before 20 weeks of gestation for chronic hypertension. Hypertensive disorders of pregnancy (HDP) refers to categories of conditions characterized by elevated blood pressure and classified as chronic hypertension (of any cause diagnosed before 20 weeks of gestation), gestational hypertension, chronic hypertension with superimposed preeclampsia and preeclampsia –eclampsia [1, 2].

Hypertensive disorder of pregnancy is one of the most common complications in pregnancy forming a triad together with hemorrhage and infection. It affects about 10% of pregnancies [3] and contributes for a significant maternal and perinatal mortality [4]. The World Health Organization (WHO) reported that 14.0% of global maternal deaths are attributed to hypertensive disorders of pregnancy [5]. In Latin-American and Caribbean countries 25.7% of maternal deaths were due to hypertensive disorders of pregnancy; in Asian and African countries, it contributed to 9.1% of maternal deaths and in fact about 16% in sub-Saharan African countries [5–7].

Hypertensive disorder of pregnancy is a global public health concern both in developed and developing countries. However, the risk that a woman in a developing country will die of the complications of hypertensive disorders of pregnancy is approximately 300 times higher than that for a woman in a developed country. A woman who develops pre-eclampsia is three times more likely to progress to eclampsia and if eclampsia is developed it is up to 14 times more likely to die of eclampsia [8].

The Ethiopian National Emergency Obstetric and Newborn Care (EMONC) study showed that pre-eclampsia/eclampsia complicated 1.2% of all institutional deliveries. Besides, 11% of all maternal deaths and 16% of direct maternal deaths were due to this obstetric complication [9] in another study in Ambo, Ethiopia maternal mortality due to hypertensive disorders of pregnancy was reported to be 12.3% [10] . The Ethiopian government has implemented different strategies to improve maternal health through increasing demand for services and easier access to emergency obstetric services. Expansion of health facilities, increased availability of supplies and deployment of appropriately skilled health professionals were among the strategies [11].

Despite the extensive research conducted the exact etiology of hypertensive disorders of pregnancy remained obscure. Thus, it is called a "disease of theories." It is a multisystem disease with a heterogeneous nature and variable progression [12]. It has been proposed that immunological, nutritional and genetic factors as well as vascular and inflammatory changes are contributing for the development of hypertensive disorders of pregnancy [4].

Cognizant that the disease has no definite cause, several studies focusing on risk factors have been conducted in different parts of the globe and identified various risk factors for hypertensive disorders of pregnancy. These risk factors include socio-demographic variables such, personal and lifestyle factors, obstetric related factors, familial factors and medical related variables [13–16]. Specifically, nulliparity, extreme ages, obesity, a family history of hypertension, previous history of hypertensive disorders of pregnancy in multipara women, personal/family history of chronic hypertension/diabetes mellitus, high energy diet, gestational diabetes, mental stress during pregnancy, long inter-pregnancy interval, lower socioeconomic status and inadequate antenatal supervision were found to be associated with higher risk of developing hypertensive disorders of pregnancy in most studies [17–22]. Studies identified rural residence as a risk factor [23] and taking fruit or vegetables during pregnancy were found to be protective of hypertensive disorders of pregnancy [19].

Generally, maternal mortality due to hypertensive disorders of pregnancy remained high in spite of all the efforts. Studies conducted in different parts of the globe reported a range of risk factors though findings were not conclusive showing variations among populations and ethno-geographic groups. Moreover, inconsistent findings prevail across literatures even for a particular risk factor. Besides, there is paucity of evidence regarding factors associated with hypertensive disorders of pregnancy in Ethiopia. Even the few published studies conducted in Ethiopia were based on a document review which might have introduced bias due to incompleteness and poor quality of the data at the health facility [24, 25]. Thus, the current study attempted to assess risk factors for hypertensive disorders of pregnancy in Tigray region to generate evidences which are most relevant to support health policies and strategies.

Methods

Study setting and period

This study was conducted in selected public hospitals in Tigray region. Seven hospitals were included in the study namely Ayder, Mekelle, Adigrat, St. Marry, Suhul, Lemlem Carl and Kahsay Abera hospital. The six hospitals are located at the centre of the six respective zones of Tigray region mainly serving the people of the zones. Ayder referral hospital is found in Mekelle city serving as a referral hospital for about 8 million people from the entire Tigray region and partly from Afar and Amhara regions. In Tigray region, there are 28 health facilities providing basic emergency obstetrics and newborn care (BEmONC) and 15 facilities providing comprehensive emergency obstetrics and newborn care respectively [26]. The selected hospitals provide services for substantial number of patients with and without obstetrics complications. These hospitals are selected in this study due to the fact that they are staffed by obstetricians who can correctly diagnosed hypertensive disorders of pregnancy and relatively equipped by diagnostic facilities. Data were collected from June 2017 to November 2017.

Study design

A facility based matched case control study was employed. These women were pregnant mothers attending antenatal care clinics in the study hospitals. Cases and control were matched in parity, time and site of the study. The case and control mothers were included after 20 weeks of gestation as per the diagnosis and the criteria set.

Study population

The study population were all pregnant mothers attending the maternity centers of the study hospitals. Mothers with a history of confirmed chronic hypertension or diagnosed before 20 weeks gestation which is greater than or equal to 140/90 mmHg and without superimposed preeclampsia were excluded from the study because chronic hypertension can be a risk factor for preeclampsia but not for gestational hypertension. Since we measured the different hypertensive disorders as a single outcome, chronic hypertension was excluded as it can be an outcome and a risk factor at the same time. Chronic hypertensive women superimposed with preeclampsia-eclampsia was included as an outcome because this category has common exposure as the rest of the categories.

A case was defined as a mother diagnosed to have hypertensive disorders of pregnancy by an obstetrician in the antenatal period (*international classification of disease*/ICD – 10 codes O13, O14 and O15 [27]). Hypertensive disorders of pregnancy included gestational hypertension, preecalampsia-eclampsia and preeclampsia/eclampsia superimposed on chronic hypertension.

A control was defined as a pregnant women enrolled in the antenatal care clinic of the hospital and who did not have a diagnosis of hypertensive disorders. For each case two controls were interviewed in the same day and the same facility where the case was identified. Besides, cases and controls were matched according to their parity category.

Sample size determination and sampling procedure

The sample size was calculated based on the comparison of proportions for matched case-control study using the following assumptions: Considering 95% CI, 80% power, case to control ratio of 1:2 and taking different sample size were produced for different risk factor for hypertensive disorders of pregnancy. Maximum sample size was obtained taking History of paternal hypertension as a risk factor from a previous study in Cameroon [28] where the proportion of exposure among cases to be 17.4% and among controls, 6%. Accordingly, these yields a maximum sample size of 100 cases and 200 controls. Adding a 10% non-response rate, the final sample size required for the study was 110 cases and 220 controls.

All cases who fulfil the defined criteria were consecutively included until the desired sample size was obtained. For every case included, two controls who best matched were identified.

Operational definitions [2]

Hypertensive disorders of pregnancy- mother diagnosed with gestational hypertension, preeclampsia-eclampsia, chronic hypertension with superimposed preeclampsia or chronic hypertension (of any cause).

Gestational hypertension- systolic blood pressure ≥ 140 mmHg and/or diastolic blood pressure ≥ 90 mmHg measured on two occasions at least 4 h apart after twenty weeks of gestation in the absence of proteinuria or other systemic symptoms.

Preeclampsia- characterized by new onset of hypertension after 20 weeks gestation (systolic blood pressure ≥ 140 mmHg and/or diastolic BP ≥90) mmHg and proteinuria. However, in the absence of proteinuria other manifestations such thrombocytopenia (platelet count less than 100,000/μl), impaired liver function (elevated blood levels of liver transaminases to twice the normal concentration), the new development of renal insufficiency (elevated serum creatinine greater than 1.1 mg/dl or a doubling of serum creatinine in the absence of other renal disease), pulmonary edema, or new onset cerebral or visual disturbances are used to diagnose the case.

Eclampsia- characterized by new onset grand mal seizures in a woman with preeclampsia.

Chronic hypertension- includes essential hypertension as well as hypertension secondary to a range of conditions which is characterized by a blood pressure greater than or equal to 140 mmHg systolic and/or 90 mmHg diastolic confirmed before pregnancy or before 20 completed weeks gestation.

Chronic hypertension superimposed with Preeclampsia - mothers known to have hypertension before pregnancy or before 20 weeks of gestation and who had developed signs of preeclampsia after 20 weeks of gestation.

Proteinuria- a dipstick result of 1+ and above in a qualitative measurement.

Data collection

Data collection was carried out in the maternity ward (antenatal care clinic and labor and delivery ward). It was collected by face to face interview technique using a pretested questionnaire. The questionnaire was developed following a thorough review of literatures from different sources and it included information related to socio-demographic condition, obstetrics and medical status, lifestyle and nutritional habits of the participants (Additional file 1). In addition to the questionnaire, patient medical records were reviewed to abstract relevant variables related with laboratory, clinical and obstetrics data. It was conducted by trained midwives and supervised by MPH professionals.

Measurement

Height was measured in standing position bare foot and expressed in centimetres while weight was recorded in killograms. Body mass index (BMI) was calculated as weight (pre-pregnancy weight in the preceding 3 months) divided by height in meter square (kg/m^2). For those who failed to remember their pre-pregnancy weight, the measured weight in the first trimester was taken as the weight gain during this time is low. In areas where women do not book early for antenatal care as the case in developing countries, pregnancy BMI is not recommended. Hence, in this case the pre-pregnancy weight was considered to calculate body mass index. In addition maternal mid-upper arm circumference (MUAC) was measured as it is considered to be relatively stable during pregnancy [29].

Maternal height category was made according to the calculated percentiles of the study participant and classified into four groups: ≥160 cm (25th percentile and lower); 161–162 cm (26th to 50th percentile); 163–165 cm (51th to 75th percentile); and ≥ 166 cm (76th percentile and higher). Body mass index (BMI) defined as pre-pregnancy weight in kilogrammes divided by height in meters squared, was categorised as follows: underweight (BMI < 18.5); normal weight (BMI = 18.5–24.9); overweight (BMI = 25–29.9); and obese (BMI ≥30). Likewise, monthly income was categorized into the lowest 25 percentile (below $91.9), between 25 and 75 percentile ($92–183.7), and above 75 percentile (greater than $183.8). Harvard university food frequency questionnaire [30] was used to assess the fruit and vegetables consumption status of mothers. Accordingly to the FFQ dietary assessment a list of fruits and vegetables were offered and asked how often they eat on average with in the last one year (ranging from never or less than once per month to 6+ per day). Those women who consumed fruits more than 2–4 times per week were considered as regular consumers of fruits or vegetables. For coffee consumption both frequency and volume were assessed.

Data quality control

The questionnaire was prepared in English and translated into Tigrigna and back to English by independent language experts for consistency. Pre-test was conducted ahead of the actual data collection to see the appropriateness of the tool. Three days training was given for data collectors and supervisors on the content of the questionnaire and its administration. In order to maintain data quality primary data were collected from participants prospectively. The supervisors and the principal investigator checked questionnaires for completeness and inconsistencies on a daily basis.

Analysis

Data entry was done in EPI-info 7 and exported to STATA Version 14 for cleaning and analysis; data cleaning was also done. Descriptive summary measures are reported. To identify factors associated with hypertensive disorders of pregnancy bivariate and matched analysis was done for the outcome of interest by comparing the cases with controls. Moreover, crude matched odds ratio and their 95% confidence intervals along with their p values in conditional logistic regression were calculated. In multivariable analysis, matched analysis was performed using conditional logistic regression to identify risk factors of hypertensive disorders. Adjusted odds ratio and their 95% confidence intervals were reported. Significance was declared at P-value ≤ 0.05. Multi-collinearity was checked among the independent variables by running the *regress* and *vif* syntaxes in the *stata* software. Accordingly, the variance inflation factor (*VIF*) was close to one and the tolerance which is the reciprocal of the variance inflation factor was also far above 0 which showed minimal collinearity. Post estimation command (Hosmer and Lemeshow test) in the logistic regression was run by using the *estat gof* to check the model fitness. Thus, the p-value for the Hosmer and Lemeshow chi-square was greater than 0.05 which indicated the fitness of the model. Overall findings were presented in texts and tables.

Ethical consideration

The study was approved by the institutional review board of the college of health sciences Addis Ababa University. Participants involved in the study voluntarily. There were no other risks for the participants to participate in the study, other than those encountered in day-to-day life. It was described that information obtained from this study may be of valuable to mothers and new-borns in general. The anonymity of the study was maintained by excluding personal identifiers from the data collection tool and the records of the study were kept strictly confidential. Finally Informed consent was sought from the participants.

Results

Socio-demographic characteristics

A total of 330 mothers were interviewed in the data collection period that was held from June to November, 2018. Overall 110 cases matched on parity, day of interviews and study site/hospital with 220 controls taken part in the study to identify risk factors of hypertensive disorders of pregnancy. Of the total cases, gestational hypertension, preeclampsia, eclampsia and preeclampsia/eclampsia superimposed on chronic hypertension comprised of 36(32.7%), 55(50%), 14(12.7%), and 5(4.5%) respectively. Respondents were predominantly married, Orthodox Christianity followers and Tigrian by ethnicity in both cases and controls (90% and above in all cases). Regarding the occupation, majority of the mothers were housewives and comparable proportions were reported among cases and controls (64.5% Vs 68.2%). The Mean ± (SD) age of cases and controls were 27.6 ± 5.6 and 26.7 ± 5.8 years respectively. The proportion of older age mothers (age ≥ 35) was found to be higher among cases as compared to controls (23.6% Vs 11.8%)($P = .006$). Besides, rural residents were higher among cases 71(64.5%) as compared to controls 76 (34.5%) ($P < .001$) (Table 1).

Dietary, familial and lifestyle factors

Twenty two (20%) of pregnant mother had family history of hypertension among cases while only 14(6.4%) pregnant women had family history of hypertension among controls. The mean pre-pregnancy weight of cases and controls were 53.6 ± 8.4 and 51.3 ± 6.8 Kg, respectively. The maximum BMI recorded was 29.9 kg/m^2; 65 (59.1%) and 147 (66.8%) of the respondents had BMI ranging from 18.5 to 25 kg/m^2 in cases and controls respectively. The mid-upper arm circumference of mothers was categorized below the mean and above the mean (≥22. 1 and > 22.1) centimeters and more than 60% of the cases and controls were measured less than or equal to the mean. On average, the pre-pregnancy BMI was higher in women with hypertensive disorders than in those with normal pregnancies (20.36 ± 3.0 Vs 19.8 ± 2.6) ($P = .05$). Vegetable and fruit use were found to be less frequent in hypertensive disorders of pregnancy as compared with the normotensive women (42.7% Vs 60.4 and 54.5% Vs 87.7%). Likewise, frequency and volume of coffee use was demonstrated to be higher among cases when compared with controls ($P=. 01$, $P=. 03$) (Table 2).

Obstetrics and medical factors

The proportion of multiple pregnancy was 16.4% among cases, while it was 4.5% among controls ($p = 0.001$). On the other hand, average age at menarche was reported to be 15 years, which were similar among

cases and controls. About 3% of study participants had gestational diabetes mellitus and the proportion was different between cases and controls. It was 3.63% in cases while in controls it was 1.4% ($P = 0.02$) (Table 3).

Risk factors of hypertensive disorders of pregnancy

Bivariate analysis was run in the conductional logistic regression considering the discordant pairs between cases and controls to check the association between dependent and independent variables. Accordingly, rural residence, age > = 35 years, family history of hypertension, infrequent use of vegetables/fruits, higher pre-pregnancy weight, body mass index, coffee use, gestational diabetes mellitus and pre-pregnancy oral contraceptive use were identified as risk factors. In contrast, There was no difference among cases and controls with regard to average age, marital status, religion, ethnicity, occupation, maternal educational level, husband's educational level, income, history of abortion, history of smoking, pre-pregnancy interval and age at menarche (Table 4).

Variables which were found to be associated with the outcome variable in the bivariate analysis ($P < =0.2$) were taken to the multivariable analysis. This is basically to compensate for the power of the test since negative findings (that is, $p > 0.05$) may be just because of inadequate power. After adjusting for possible confounding factors in the matched pair conditional logistic regression only residence, fruit use, pre-pregnancy BMI of mothers, types of pregnancy and gestational diabetes mellitus were found to be independent predictors of hypertensive disorders of pregnancy. Mothers who live in a rural area were at greater odds of having hypertensive disorders as compared to mothers who reside in urban area (OR = 3.7, 95% CI; 1.9, 7.1). Similarly, mothers who do not consume at all or consume less amount of fruits in their diet had 5 times higher odds of developing hypertensive disorders than those who consume fruits regularly (AOR = 5.1 95% CI; 2.4, 11.15). Overweight (BMI > 25 Kg/m^2) mothers were also at risk of developing hypertensive disorders of pregnancy as compared with the normal and underweight mothers (AOR = 5.5 95% CI; 1.12, 27.6). In addition, multiple pregnancy and presence of diabetes mellitus were independent risk factors for the development of hypertensive disorders of pregnancy; the risk of developing hypertensive disorders of pregnancy was 5.4 times higher among diabetic mothers compared with those who are free of the disease (AOR = 5.4, 95% CI; 1.1, 27.0). On the other hand, the effect of age, family history of hypertension, use of vegetables, and drinking coffee disappeared in the multivariable analysis when adjusted for possible confounders.

Table 1 Socio-demographic characteristics of mothers with and without hypertensive disorders of pregnancy in Tigray, 2018

variable	HDP/Cases $N = 110$, N (%)	No HDP/Controls $N = 220$, N (%)	COR (95% CI)	P-value
Age group				
≤ 18	7(6.4)	10(4.6)	1.5(0.58, 4.1)	0.378
19–34	77(70.0)	184(83.6)	1.0	
≥ 35	26(23.6)	26(11.8)	2.3(1.3, 4.2)	0.006
Residence				
rural	71(64.5)	76(34.5)	3.1 (1.9, 5.0)	< 0.001
urban	39(35.4)	144(65.4)	1.0	
Marital status				
married	104(94.5)	199(90.5)	1.0	
Unmarried	6(5.4)	21(9.5)	0.5 (0.2,1.4)	0.2
Partner change				
Yes	14(12.7)	26(11.8)	1.09 (0.5, 2.2)	0.8
No	96(87.2)	194(88.2)	1.0	
Religion				
orthodox	103(93.6)	199(90.5)	1.4 (0.5, 3.6)	0.49
Muslim	6(5.5)	16(7.3)	1.0	
Maternal education				
literate	74(67.3)	153(69.5)	1.0	
illiterate	36(32.7)	67(30.5)	1.12(0.7, 1.9)	0.65
Ethnicity				
Tigrian	105(95.5)	200(90.9)	1.0	
Amhara	4(3.6)	17(7.7)	0.4 (0.14, 1.36)	0.15
Occupation				
Housewife	71 (64.5)	150(68.2)	1.0	
Government employee	22(20.0)	33(15)	1.4(0.7, 2.7)	0.26
NGO employee	8(7.3)	7(3.2)	2.5(0.8, 7.7)	0.08
				0.17
Private employee	7(6.4)	28(12.7)	0.5(0.2,1.3)	
Husband education				
Illiterate	14(12.7)	31 (14.1)	0.9 (0.4, 1.9)	0.8
Read and write	14(12.7)	26(11.82)	1.1(0.5, 2.3)	0.7
Primary	23(20.9)	42(19.1)	1.1(0.6, 2.1)	0.6
Secondary and above	59(53.6)	122(55)	1.0	
Income category				
≤ 2500	37 (33.64)	62 (28.18)	0.8(0.4,1.5)	0.5
2501–4999	48 (43.64)	106 (48.18)	0.9 (0.5, 1.7)	0.8
≥ 5000	25 (22.73)	52 (23.64)	1.0	

Discussion

The current study result showed that rural residence was associated with the development of hypertensive disorder of pregnancy. This finding is consistent with a previous finding in an epidemiological study among pregnant mothers in Cairo, Egypt [23]. This could be due to the fact that mothers from rural areas book antenatal care later in pregnancy and have fewer ANC visits which could be associated with delay in health seeking behaviour. This delay in health care seeking could in turn be influenced by lack of awareness on pregnancy related problems, husband and

Table 2 Dietary, familial and lifestyle characteristics of mothers with/without hypertensive disorders of pregnancy in Tigray, 2018

variable	HDP/Cases $N = 110$, N (%)	No HDP/Controls $N = 220$, N (%)	COR (95% CI)	P-value
Family history of hypertension				
Yes	22(20)	14(6.4)	3.6(1.7,7.6)	0.001
No	88(80)	206 (93.6)	1.0	
Mean weight ± (SD)	63.2 (8.7)	60.8 (7.3)		0.01
Mean Height ± (SD)	1.61(.06)	1.62(.05)		0.09
MAUC				
≤ 22.1	69 (62.7)	140(63.6)	1.0	
> 22.1	41(37.3)	80 (36.4)	1.0(0.6, 2.0)	0.82
Pre-pregnancy mean weight ± (SD)	53.6 (8.4)	51.3 (6.8)		0.006
Pre-pregnancy mean BMI ± (SD	20.36(3.0)	19.8 (2.6)		0.05
Fruit use				
Yes	60(54.5)	193(87.7)	1.0	
No	50 (45.5)	27 (12.3)	5.3 (3.0, 9.4)	< 0.001
Vegetable use				
Yes	47(42.7)	133(60.4)	1.0	0.002
No	63(57.3)	87(39.6)	2.1(1.3, 3.3)	
BMI of mothers				
< 18.5	33 (30.0)	67 (30.5)	1.0	
18.5–24.9	65 (59.1)	147 (66.8)	0.9(0.6,1.6)	0.8
≥ 25	12 (10.9)	6 (2.7)	4.3(1.4,13.6)	0.01
Coffee use				
Yes	93(84.5)	149(67.7)	3.0(1.6, 5.9)	0.001
No	17(15.5)	71(32.3)	1.0	
Frequency of coffee use ($N = 242$)				
≥ once a day	76 (81.7)	104 (69.8)	3.2 (1.3, 8.3)	0.01
< once a day	17 (18.3)	45 (30.2)	1.0	
volume of coffee use ($N = 242$)				
< 3 cups	28(30.1)	69(46.3)	1.0	
≥ 3 cups	65(69.9)	80(53.7)	2.1(1.0, 4.1)	0.03

family influences, local cultural influence and bad experiences in health facilities.

Similarly fruit consumption was found to be important predictor in this study, mothers who consume less fruits in their diets were at higher risk of developing hypertensive disorders of pregnancy which is in line with previous findings reported from Bahrdar, Ethiopia ([19], Cairo, Egypt [23] and Norway [17]. This was also supported by a systematic review and meta-analysis of studies whereby calcium intake was found to be protective to hypertensive disorders of pregnancy in a multivariable analysis [31]. Fruits are rich in micronutrients and many of the vitamins and minerals play antioxidant role which could in turn help in the prevention of hypertensive disorders of pregnancy.

Pre-pregnancy body mass index was calculated and overweight mothers were at higher odds of developing hypertensive disorders of pregnancy as compared with low and normal body mass index which is in agreement with reports from USA [32, 33]. Likewise, multiple pregnancy has been reported as an independent predictor of hypertensive disorders of pregnancy from various studies in different parts of the globe [22, 34, 35]. The current finding is also in support of those previous reports which showed 4.2 times increased risk of developing hypertensive disorders of pregnancy compared with the singleton pregnancy.

Gestational diabetes mellitus was also found to be an independent predictor of hypertensive disorders of pregnancy that supported the existing knowledge; because literatures noted that pregnant mother who developed

Table 3 Obstetrics and medical characteristics of mothers with/without hypertensive disorders of pregnancy in Tigray, 2018

Variable	HDP/Cases N = 110, N (%)	No HDP/Controls N = 220, N (%)	COR (95% CI)	P-value
Pregnancy type				
Multiple	18 (16.4)	10 (4.5)	4.1(1.8, 9.6)	0.001
Single	92 (83.6)	210 (95.5)	1.0	
Gestational diabetes mellitus				
Yes	7 (6.36)	3 (1.4)	4.7(1.2,18.0)	0.02
No	103 (93.6)	217 (98.6)	1.0	
Pre-pregnancy oral contraceptive use				
Yes	42(38.2)	63 (28.6)	1.5 (0.9, 2.4)	0.08
No	68 (61.8)	157 (71.4)	1.0	
Presence of anemia at first visit				
Yes	94 (85.5)	194(88.2)	1.3 (0.6, 2.9)	
No	16(14.5)	26(11.8)	1.0	0.43
Age at menarche				
≤ 15 years	72 (65.4)	148 (67.3)	0.9(0.6, 1.5)	0.734
> 15 years	38 (34.6)	72 (32.7)	1.0	
Pre-pregnancy interval (N = 216)				
< 5 years	54 (83.08)	117 (77.5)	1.0	
≥ 5 years	11 (16.92)	34 (22.5)	0.9 (0.4, 2.2)	0.88
History of abortion				
Yes	25 (22.7)	39 (17.7)	1.0	0.263
No	85 (77.3)	181 (82.3)	0.7 (0.4,1.2)	

Table 4 Bivariate and multivariable analysis for the predictors of hypertensive disorders of pregnancy in Tigray, 2018

Variables	Matched unadjusted OR(95% CI)	Matched adjusted OR(95% CI)
Residence		
Rural	3.1 (1.9, 5.0)*	3.7(1.9, 7.1)**
Urban	1.0	1.0
Age		
Mean ± (SD)	1.02(0.9, 1.06)	0.96 (0.9, 1.02)
Marital status		
Married	1.0	1.0
Unmarried	0.5(0.2, 1.4)	0.44 (0.12, 1.5)
Family History of hypertension		
Yes	3.6 (1.7, 7.6)*	2.1 (0.7, 6.4)
No	1.0	1.0
Fruit use		
Yes	1.0	1.0
No	5.3 (3.0, 9.4)*	5.1 (2.4, 11.15)**
Vegetable use		
Yes	1.0	1.2(0.6, 2.3)
No	2.08 (1.3, 3.3)*	
History of smoking		
Yes	1.0	1.0
No	0.3 (0.07, 1.2)	0.6 (0.07, 5.2)
BMI of mothers (prepregnancy)		
< 18.5	1.0	1.0
18.5–24.9	0.95 (0.56, 1.6)	1.7 (0.8, 3.4)
25–29.9	4.3 (1.4, 13.6)*	5.5 (1.12, 27.6)*
Coffee use		
Yes	3.08 (1.6, 5.9)*	1.9 (0.8, 4.4)
No	1.0	1.0
Pregnancy type		
multiple	4.1 (1.8, 9.6)*	4.2 (1.3, 13.3)*
single	1.0	1.0
Presence of gestational diabetes mellitus		
Yes	4.6 (1.2, 18.0)*	5.4 (1.1, 27.0)*
No	1.0	1.0
Oral contraceptive use		
Yes	1.5 (0.9, 2.4)	1.2(0.6, 2.4)
No	1.0	1.0

*P-value <0.01, **P-value <0.001

diabetes mellitus would have higher predisposition to develop hypertensive disorders of pregnancy and it has been identified as the most common predictor in previous studies [22, 34, 36–38].

Family history of hypertension was a predictor in the bivariate analysis but its effect vanished in the adjusted model and this contradicts with previous reports. These studies reported an increased risk of hypertensive disorders with a positive family history of chronic hypertension [21, 28, 36, 39–41].

Similarly, drinking more than 3 cups of coffee per day was not a significant risk factor in this study which means it is in conformity with some studies showing no difference [42] and contradicted with others. For instance, a study in Bahrdar, Ethiopia showed that mothers who reported to have taken coffee during pregnancy had higher odds of developing preeclampsia [19]. However, another study in Rotterdam, the Netherlands reported the substantial protection of coffee against the development of pregnancy induced hypertension [42].

Extreme lower or higher ages in pregnancy (age < 20 and > 35 years) were reported as a risk factor for hypertensive disorders of pregnancy in previous

studies; *Tebeu PM et.al* reported that teenage mothers were at increased risk of developing hypertensive disorders [28] on the other hand, *Suzuki. S.* and *Igarashi M.* in their study revealed that age > = 35 was a significant factor for the development of preeclampsia [43] but in the current study though age > = 35 showed a significant risk in the first model, no difference was observed in the adjusted model. The difference may be due to the fact that majority of the respondents were within the age range of 19–34.

In many studies nulliparity was reported as a common risk factor for the development of hypertensive disorders of pregnancy [32–34, 41] but in this study its effect was not possible to measure as it was a matching variable. Unlike the current finding, partner change was reported as a risk factor for hypertensive disorders of pregnancy in other literatures [23]. The reason may be there were few mothers who changed their partner in the study and this in turn could make the difference invisible.

In previous studies illiteracy was reported to be a risk factor for hypertensive disorders of pregnancy [28] as it affects the age at marriage and pregnancy as well as health seeking behaviour but in the current study no association was reported. The continuous health education program provided by the health extension workers at the community and household levels might have helped to have similar level of awareness about the issue.

Some studies reported inter-pregnancy interval as a risk factor for hypertensive disorders of pregnancy. Longer inter-pregnancy interval had higher risk of developing hypertensive disorders of pregnancy [44] but in the current study no association was found.

The aforementioned findings should be viewed in light of the following limitations. Since cases were selected consecutively as soon as they were identified, selection bias might be introduced. Moreover, dietary assessment was self-reported and assessed at diagnosis which could have introduced recall bias.

Conclusion

The study assessed different risk factors of hypertensive disorders of pregnancy. Thus, rural residence, less fruit consumption, multiple pregnancy, presence of gestational diabetes mellitus and pre-pregnancy overweight were identified as independent risk factors. This highlights that there is a need to extend obstetric services to the grass root level in which rural residents can get all types of services in a closer distance. In addition, it necessitates strong nutritional education for the community during pregnancy and even the time preceding pregnancy including the routine supply of supplements. There is also a need to remind health professionals to properly identify and manage pregnant women having diabetes mellitus. It is recommended that these factors can be used as a screening tool for the prediction, early diagnoses as well as timely interventions of hypertensive disorders of pregnancy.

Abbreviations
ACOG: American College of Obstetricians and Gynaecologists; BEmONC: Basic Emergency Obstetrics and Newborn Care; BMI: Body Mass Index; EmONC: Emergency Obstetric and Newborn Care; HDP: Hypertensive Disorders of Pregnancy; ICD: International Classification of Disease; MPH: Master of Public Health; MUAC: Mid Upper Arm Circumference; WHO: World Health Organization

Acknowledgements
The authors would like to extend their gratitude to the study participants for their consensual participation. Likewise, the authors would like to thank data collectors and supervisors for their commitment throughout the data collection process. Finally, special gratitude goes to Mekelle and Addis Ababa universities for funding the study.

Funding
The study was funded by both Addis Ababa and Mekelle universities.

Authors' contributions
HBK is the primary author, participated in the conceptualization, design, acquisition, analysis and interpretation of the data and drafted the manuscript. FEG was the primary academic advisor, contributed for design, acquisition, analysis and interpretation of the data and critically revised the manuscript. WMA was co-advisor, contributed for design, acquisition, analysis and interpretation of the data and critically revised the manuscript for important intellectual content. All authors read and approved the final manuscript.

Competing interests
The authors declare that they have no competing interests.

Author details
[1]School of Nursing, Mekelle University, P.O.Box:1871, Mekelle, Ethiopia.
[2]School of Public Health, Addis Ababa University, Addis Ababa, Ethiopia.

References
1. Lowe SA, Bowyer L, Lust K, McMahon LP, Morton M, North RA. et al., SOMANZ guidelines for the management of hypertensive disorders of pregnancy 2014. Aust N Z J Obstet Gynaecol 55(5)e1-29.
2. American college of obstetricians and gynecologists (ACOG). Hypertension in Pregnancy (Report of the ACOG Task Force on Hypertension in Pregnancy). Obstet Gynecol. 2013;122(5):1122–31.
3. National Institute for Health and Clinical Excellence (NICE). Hypertension in pregnancy: the management of hypertensive disorders during pregnancy. In: National Collaborating Centre for Women's and Children's health; 2010.
4. Cunningham F, Leveno K, Bloom S, Hauth J, Rouse D, Spong C. Williams Obstetrics 22rd Edition. New York: McGraw Hill. Companies Inc; 2005. Chapter 34, Hypertensive disorders in pregnancy; p. 426–50.

5. Say L, Chou D, Gemmill A, Moller AB, Daniels J, Temmerman M ea. Global causes of maternal death: a WHO systematic analysis. Lancet Glob Health. 2014;2(6):e323–33.

6. Khan KS, Wojdyla D, Say L, Gülmezoglu M, Van Look P. WHO analysis of causes of maternal death: a systematic review. Lancet. 2006;367(9516):1066–74.

7. Steegers EA, Von Dadelszen P, Duvekot JJ, Pijnenborg R. Pre-eclampsia. Lancet. 376(9741):631–44.

8. EngenderHealth, Balancing the Scales Expanding Treatment for Pregnant Women with Life-Threatening Hypertensive Conditions in Developing Countries A Report on Barriers and Solutions to Treat Pre-eclampsia & Eclampsia New York. 2007.

9. Gaym A, Bailey P, Pearson L, Admasu K, Gebrehiwot Y. Disease burden due to preeclampsia/eclampsia and the Ethiopian health system's response. Int J Gynecol Obstet. 115(1):112–6.

10. Garomssa H, Dwivedi A. Maternal mortality in ambo hospital: a five year retrospective review. Ethiop J Reprod Health. 2008;2(1):1–13.

11. FDRE-MOH, Health sector transformation plan (HSTP) 2015/16–2019/20. 2015: p. 25 29.

12. Association of Ontario Midwives. Hypertensive disorders of pregnancy. (clinical practice guideline no. 15), 2012.

13. Wolde Z, Segni H, Woldie M. Hypertensive disorders of pregnancy in Jimma University Specialized Hospital. Ethiopian journal of health sciences. 2011; 21(3):147–54.

14. Kaaja R. Predictors and risk factors of pre-eclampsia. Minerva Ginecol. 2008; 60(5):421–9.

15. Kichou B, Henine N, Kichou L, Benbouabdellah M. Epidemiology of pre-eclampsia in Tizi-ouzou city (Algeria). in Annales de cardiologie et d'angeiologie.

16. Levenson JW, Skerrett PJ, Gaziano JM. Reducing the global burden of cardiovascular disease: the role of risk factors. Prev Cardiol. 2002;5(4):188–99.

17. Brantsæter AL, Haugen M, Samuelsenet SO, Torjusen H, Trogstad L, Alexander J. A dietary pattern characterized by high intake of vegetables, fruits, and vegetable oils is associated with reduced risk of preeclampsia in nulliparous pregnant Norwegian women. J Nutr. 2009;139(6):1162–8.

18. Atkinson JO, Mahomed KW, Michelle A, Woelk GB, Mudzamiri S. Weiss. Dietary risk factors for pre-eclampsia among women attending Harare maternity hospital, Zimbabwe. Cent Afr J Med. 1998;44(4):86–92.

19. Endeshaw M, Ambaw F, Aragaw A, Ayalew A. Effect of maternal nutrition and dietary habits on preeclampsia: a case-control study. International Journal of Clinical Medicine. 5(21):1405.

20. Guerrier G, Oluyide B, Keramarou M, Grais RF. Factors associated with severe preeclampsia and eclampsia in Jahun, Nigeria. Int J Women's Health. 2013;5:509.

21. Dalmáz CA, Dos Santos KG, Botton MR, Roisenberg I. Risk factors for hypertensive disorders of pregnancy in southern Brazil. Rev Assoc Med Bras. 57(6):692–6.

22. Conde AA, Belizan JM. Risk factors for preeclampsia in a large cohort of Latin American and Caribbean women. BJOG Int J Obstet Gynaecol. 2000; 107(1):75–83.

23. El-Moselhy EA, Khalifa HO, Soliman M, Mohammad KI, Abd El-Aal HM. Risk factors and impacts of pre-eclampsia: an epidemiological study among pregnant mothers in Cairo Egypt. Journal of American Science. 2011;7(5):311–23.

24. Gidey G, Bayray A, Gebrehiwot H. Patterns of maternal mortality and associated factors; a case-control study at public hospitals in Tigray region, Ethiopia, 2012. Int J Pharm Sci Res. 2013;4(5):1918.

25. Terefe W, Getachew Y, Hiruye A, Derbew M, Hailemariam D, Mammo D. et. al. Patterns of hypertensive disorders of pregnancy and associated factors at Debre Berhan Referral Hospital, North Shoa, Amhara Region. Ethiop Med J. 2015; supplement 2:57-65.

26. Ethiopia federal democratic republic, MOH. Health & health-related indicators 2016/2017, 2010.

27. WHO, the WHO Application of ICD-10 to deaths during pregnancy, childbirth and the puerperium: ICD-MM. 2012.

28. Tebeu P, Foumane P, Mbu R. Risk factors for hypertensive disorders in pregnancy: a report from the maroua regional hospital, cameroon. J Reprod Infertil. 2011;12(3):227–34.

29. WHO, maternal anthropometry and pregnancy outcomes. A WHO collaborative study. World Health Organization Supplement. 1995;73:32–7.

30. Harvard university Food frequency assessment questionnaire, Dietary assessment 2007.https://regepi.bwh.harvard.edu/health/nutrition.htm ctrc/Nutrition/Documents/Food_Frequency_Questionnaires.pdf.

31. Schoenaker DA, Soedamah-Muthu SS, Mishra GD. The association between dietary factors and gestational hypertension and pre-eclampsia: a systematic review and metaanalysis of observational studies. BMC Med. 2014;12(157):1–18.

32. Eskenazi BL, Fenster L, Sidney S. A multivariate analysis of risk factors for preeclampsia. JAMA. 1991;266(2):237–41.

33. Turzanski F, Shannon R. Modifiable risk factors for hypertensive disorders of pregnancy among Latina women; 2009.

34. Dawson LM, Parfrey PS, Hefferton D, Dicks EL, Cooper MJ, Young D. Familial risk of preeclampsia in Newfoundland: a population-based study. J Am Soc Nephrol. 2002;13(7):1901–6.

35. Duckitt K, Harrington D. Risk factors for pre-eclampsia at antenatal booking: systematic review of controlled studies. BMJ. 2005;330(7491):565.

36. Shamsi U, Hatcher J, Shamsi A, Zuberi N, Qadri Z, Saleem S. A multicentre matched case control study of risk factors for preeclampsia in healthy women in Pakistan. BMC Womens Health. 2010;10(14):1–7.

37. Ota E, Ganchimeg T, Mori R, Souza JP. Risk factors of pre-eclampsia/eclampsia and its adverse outcomes in low-and middle-income countries: a WHO secondary analysis. PLoS One. 2014;9(3):1–9.

38. Suleiman AK. Risk factors on hypertensive disorders among Jordanian pregnant women. Global J Health Sci. 2014;6(2):138–44.

39. Tessema GA, Tekeste A, Ayele TA. Preeclampsia and associated factors among pregnant women attending antenatal care in Dessie referral hospital, Northeast Ethiopia: a hospital-based study. BMC pregnancy and childbirth. 2015;15(73):1–7.

40. Nanjundan P, Bagga R, Kalra JK, Thakur JS, Raveendran A. Risk factors for early onset severe pre-eclampsia and eclampsia among north Indian women. J Obstet Gynaecol. 2011;31(5):384–9.

41. Sultana AJ, Aparna J. Risk factors for pre-eclampsia and its perinatal outcome. Annals of biological research. 2013;4(10):1–5.

42. van der Hoeven T, Browne JL, Uiterwaal C, et al. Antenatal coffee and tea consumption and the effect on birth outcome and hypertensive pregnancy disorders. PLoS One. 2017;12(5):1-12.

43. Suzuki S, Igarashi M. Risk factors for preeclampsia in Japanese twin pregnancies: comparison with those in singleton pregnancies. Arch Gynecol Obstet. 2009;280(3):389–93.

44. Harutyunyan A, Armenian H, Petrosyan V. Investigation of risk factors for preeclampsia development among reproductive age women living in Yerevan, Armenia: a case-control study. Yerevan: College of Health Sciences, American University of Armenia; 2009.

18

Towards more accurate measurement of edge to os distance in low-lying placenta using three dimensional transvaginal ultrasound: an innovative technique

Somayya M. Sadek[*], Reda A. Ahmad, Hytham Atia and Adel G. Abdullah

Abstract

Background: Measurement of edge to os distance (EOD) is essential to differentiate low-lying from normal placenta, and to plan for delivery. Till now, measurement by 2D TVS is the gold standard, however, its accuracy is questioned. In this study, we introduced an innovative technique for measurement of EOD using 3D TVS. Our aim was to compare EOD measurements of the standard 2D technique, to those of our innovative 3D technique, and to correlate the difference, if any, with placental site and internal os width.

Methods: This study was conducted in the ultrasound unit of obstetrics and gynecology department, Zagazig University Hospitals, during the period from June 2014 to August 2017. Seventy six cases in whom the lower placental edge didn't reach the internal os (IO), and the EOD was less than 35 mm, were included in the study. Placental location was identified by 2D transabdominal sonography then 2D TVS was used to measure the EOD in all cases. Our new technique was then applied to measure EOD by 3D TVS following stepwise manipulations of the orthogonal planes in multiplanar view. Width of IO was measured also in all cases.

Results: The mean EOD measured by 3D TVS was significantly shorter than that measured using the 2D TVS. Anterolateral/posterolateral and lateral placentas were associated with high discrepancy in measurements between both methods, being the highest with lateral group. There was significant positive correlation between the IO width and the degree of difference between the EOD measured by both methods.

Conclusions: Two dimensional TVS may not be accurate in EOD measurements in many cases of low-lying placentas, and 3D TVS may increase the accuracy of measurements in these cases. This new method is simple, precise and easily applied.

Keywords: Low-lying, Placenta, Distance, Three-dimensional, Ultrasound

Background

Placenta previa is a risky obstetric condition that often herald deleterious maternal and fetal outcomes. It is a relatively common problem complicating one of every 200 deliveries. This rate is prone for more increment with the rising cesarean delivery rate [1–3].

Most authors consider the diagnosis of previa when the lower placental edge is covering or reaching the internal os (IO), and it is defined as low-lying if the edge to os

distance (EOD) is 1–20 mm [2, 4, 5]. However, some still consider these cases as previa [6], while others suggest EOD of 35 or even 40 mm to define the low-lying placenta [7]. Placenta previa has been commonly classified into major (overlapping or reaching the IO) and minor (within 2 cm from IO) types, or into four groups according to the EOD measured by TVS; grade I (more than 2 cm from os), grade II (11–20 mm), grade III (0–10 mm) and grade IV (Overlapping the os by any distance) [8].

This unfinished debate regarding the definition of previa and low-lying placenta is basically raised in concern to the anticipated progressively increased risk of antepartum

* Correspondence: somayya74@gmail.com
Obstetrics and Gynecology Department, Faculty of Medicine, Zagazig
University, Zagazig, Egypt

bleeding as the placenta becomes closer to the IO, beside the need to define the relatively safe distance to allow vaginal delivery. It is agreed that cesarean delivery would be the ideal mode of delivery when the placenta is covering or within 10 mm from the IO. The majority still prefer cesarean delivery also when EOD is 11–20 mm [9], while some hypothesized the safety of vaginal delivery in such cases [8, 10, 11]. When the EOD is 20–35 mm, cases would deserve the attempt for vaginal delivery with caution after detailed counselling. Despite being safer than the previous 2 groups, they are still at increased risk of antepartum or postpartum hemorrhage [4, 12, 13].

When few millimeters may be critical in the diagnosis and management, there is a real need for a precise method to measure the EOD accurately. Two dimensional transvaginal sonography (2D TVS) is the routinely used and gold standard diagnostic method for evaluation of such cases with confirmed safety [14, 15], but its accuracy for such purpose was questioned by *Simon* et al. when significantly different measurements for the same EOD were reported by two sonographers. The three dimensional transvaginal sonography (3D TVS) evaluation was suggested as a more precise and objective method for EOD measurement [16].

In this study, we introduced an innovative technique for measurement of EOD using 3D TVS in cases with low-lying placenta. Our aim was to compare EOD measurements of the standard 2D technique, to those of our 3D technique, and to correlate the difference, if any, with placental site and IO width.

Methods

This prospective observational study was conducted in the ultrasound unit of obstetrics and gynecology department, Zagazig University Hospitals, during the period from June 2014 to August 2017. Cases were recruited from those referred to our unit for transvaginal ultrasound scan to confirm or exclude suspected placenta previa during antenatal care. After approval by the local ethical committee of Zagazig University Hospitals (ZU-IRB#4961-3-6-2014) and oral consent, ultrasound examination was carried out for all cases using C1-5D curved abdominal probe and RIC5–9D three-dimensional endovaginal probe (Voluson E6, GE Medical Systems, Zipf, Austria).

Transabdominal sonography (TAS) was performed for these cases to localize the placenta in relation to uterine walls. Placental location was classified as direct anterior/ posterior, anterolateral/ posterolateral and lateral. Then, 2D TVS examination followed, to determine the relation between the lower placental edge and the IO. The probe was introduced in the vagina gently and under sonographic live visualization till reaching the cervix without compressing it. Depth was adjusted to get the cervix together with a part of the lower uterine segment in which the lower placental edge was well visualized. A mid-sagittal view of the cervix was obtained by panning and rotational movements of the probe till the cervical canal was visualized from the IO (the upper point of the cervical canal) to the external os. In cases with placental edge not reaching the IO, the probe was rotated 90°to both sides, keeping the IO in view, then the shortest distance between the placental edge and the IO (EOD) was measured in millimeters using two points (straight line) [7]. All 2D sonographic examinations were performed by one expert sonographer (R.A.). All cases in whom the lower placental edge didn't reach the IO, and the EOD was less than 35 mm, were included in the study [7].

We used G*Power software (version 3.1.9.2, Heinrich-Heine-Universitat, Dusseldorf, Germany) to calculate the sample size. Given there is no previous studies suggesting mean difference in EOD measurements between 2D TVS and 3D TVS, we calculated the required sample

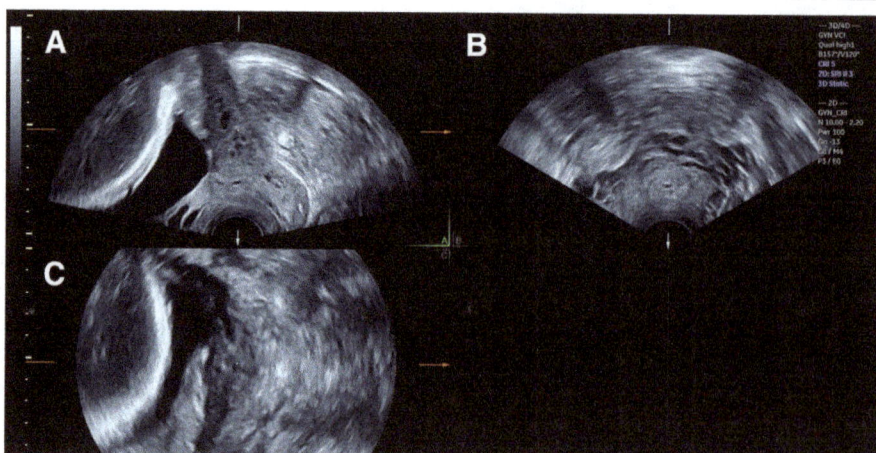

Fig. 1 The multiplanar view of the initial dataset. The reference plane is the mid-sagittal view of the cervix (A)

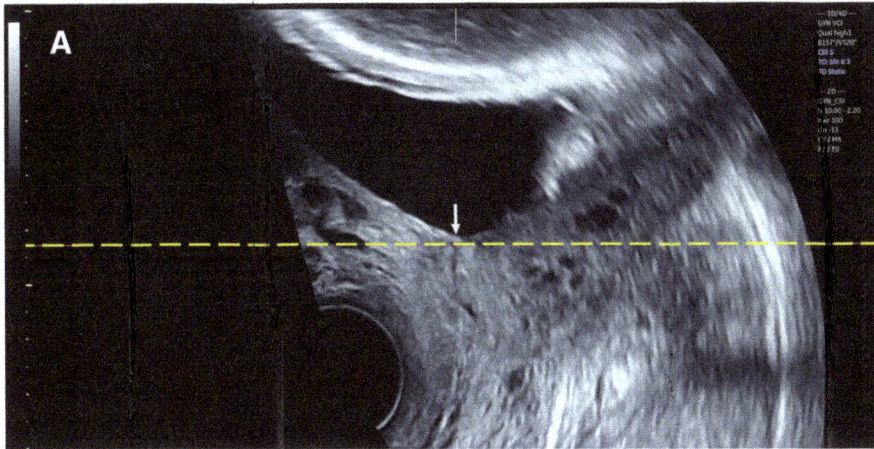

Fig. 2 Plane A (sagittal view of the cervix) after manipulations (The IO was centered in the plane, the reference point was positioned at the IO then rotation around the z-axis to make the IO (arrow) at the lowest level in the lower uterine segment)

size sufficient for effect size d 0.4, α error 0.05 and power 95%. Least required sample size was 70 cases.

Three-dimensional transvaginal sonography (3D TVS) was then performed for all cases included in the study by another expert sonographer (S.M.), who was blinded to the 2D TVS measurements. Before volume acquisition, a mid-sagittal view of the cervix was obtained, avoiding compression of the cervix or the lower segment. Examination was done in absence of uterine contractions and maternal and fetal movements. Volume was acquired with volume box and sweep angle adjusted to include at least the upper half of the cervix and the whole part of the lower uterine segment containing the lower placental edge (Quality: high 1). The multiplanar view of the initial dataset (Fig. 1) was manipulated in each case according to the following steps: (1) The IO was centered in Plane A, with magnification as needed. (2) The reference point was positioned at the IO in Plane A (upper point of the cervical canal). (3) Plane A was rotated around the z-axis to bring the reference point (i.e. IO) to the lowest level in the lower uterine segment (Fig. 2) (4) Plane B then represented the coronal view of the lower uterine segment and the upper part of the cervical canal, which appears as a rectangular hyperechogenic area. The reference point was repositioned in the middle of the upper edge of the cervical canal and the plane was rotated around the z-axis to bring the reference point to the lowest level in the lower segment (Fig. 3) (5) Plane C then represented the axial view of the cervix at the level of the IO, and for more confirmation, when the reference point was moved slightly above this level, the IO disappeared. In this plane, the cervical mucosa appeared nearly as an oval hyperechogenic area with a slit inside representing the IO. This slit was between the opposing anterior and posterior cervical walls at the upper end of the cervical canal (rectangular potential space). The reference point was repositioned in the

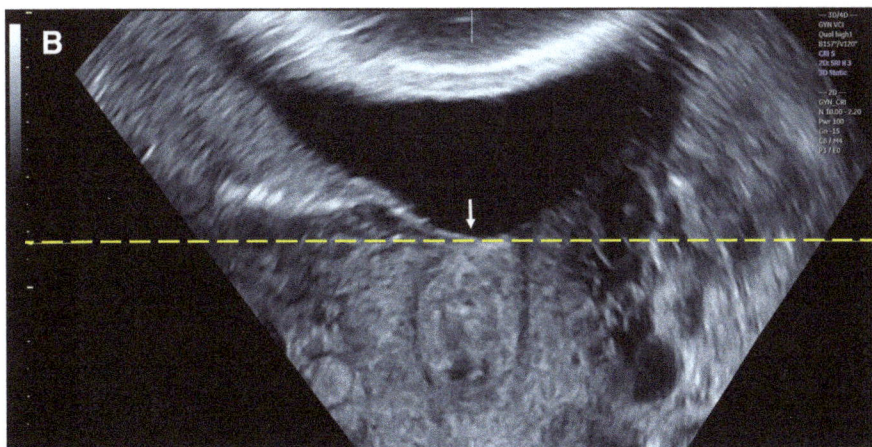

Fig. 3 Plane B (coronal view of the cervix) after manipulations (The reference point was positioned in the middle of the upper edge of the cervical canal, then rotation around the z-axis to make the IO (arrow) at the lowest level in the lower segment)

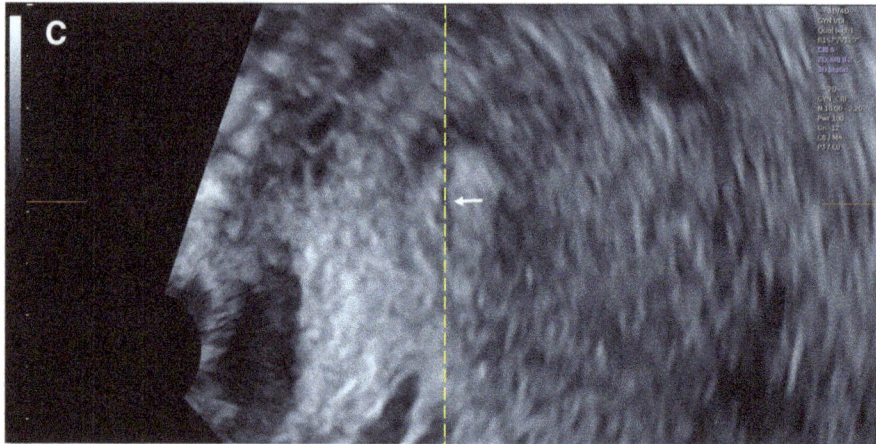

Fig. 4 Plane C (axial view of the cervix) after manipulations (The reference point was positioned in the middle of the IO (arrow), then rotation around the z-axis to get the IO parallel to the y-axis)

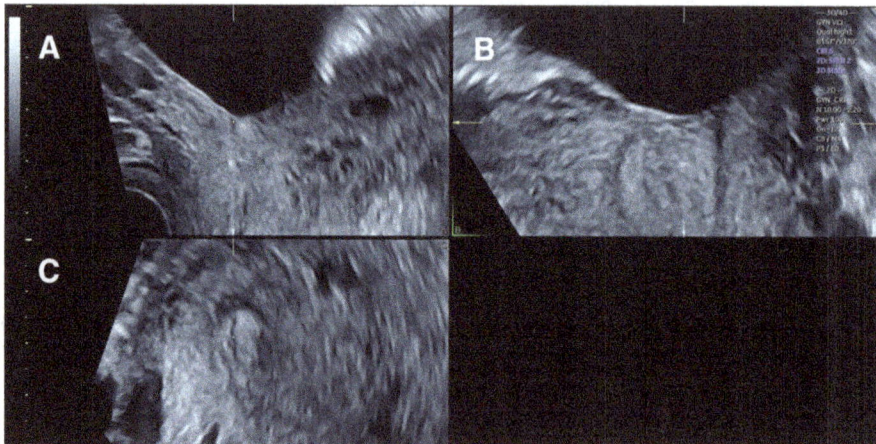

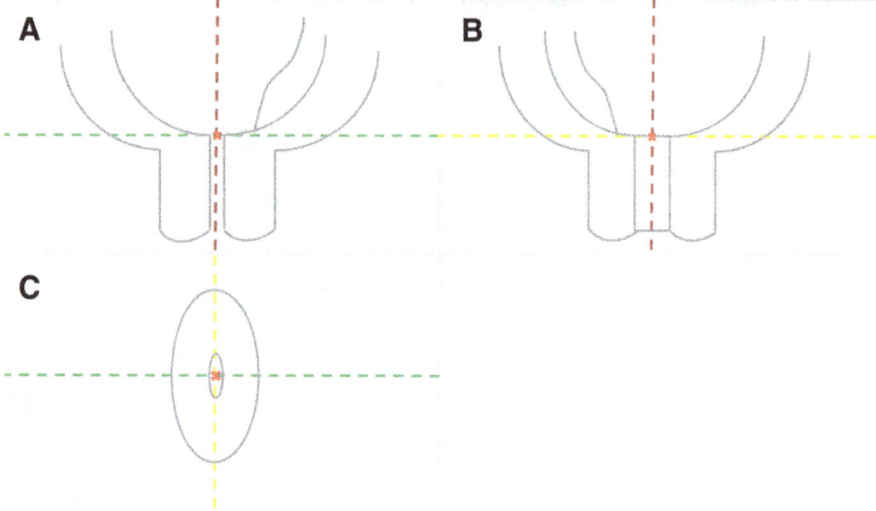

Fig. 5 The multiplanar view after manipulations of the three planes, with an illustrative diagram: In reference to Plane A, the red line is the y-axis, the green line is the x-axis and the yellow line is the z-axis

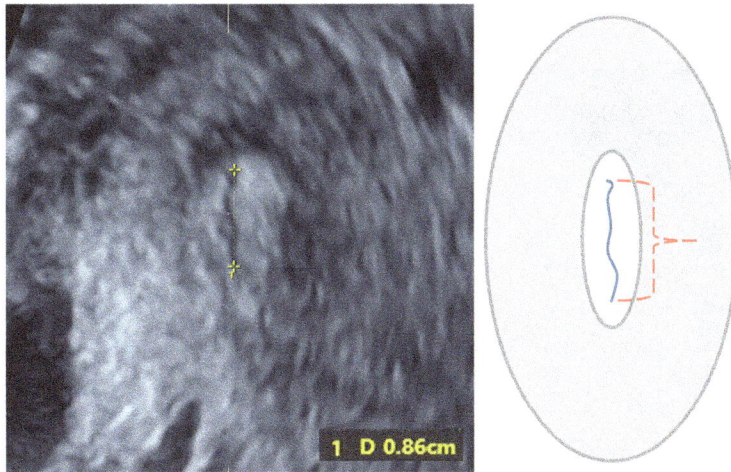

Fig. 6 Measurement of the IO width in Plane C, with an illustrative diagram. The cervical mucosa appears as an oval hyperechogenic area with a slit inside representing the IO

middle of the IO. The plane was rotated around the z-axis to get the slit shaped IO parallel to the y-axis (Figs. 4 and 5) (6) Width of the internal os was measured in millimeters in Plane C (Fig. 6) (7) Plane A was rotated 360° around the y-axis. During rotation the lower placental edge became nearer to the reference point then moved away again. The shortest distance between the lower placental edge and the reference point (center of IO) was measured (using two points) in millimeters as the EOD (Fig. 7). Measurement of EOD by 3D TVS is summarized in Table 1.

Statistical analysis was performed using the following software products: SPSS© version 21 [IBM© Corp., Armonk, NY]. Shapiro–Wilk test was used to examine the numerical data for normality of distribution. Skewed data

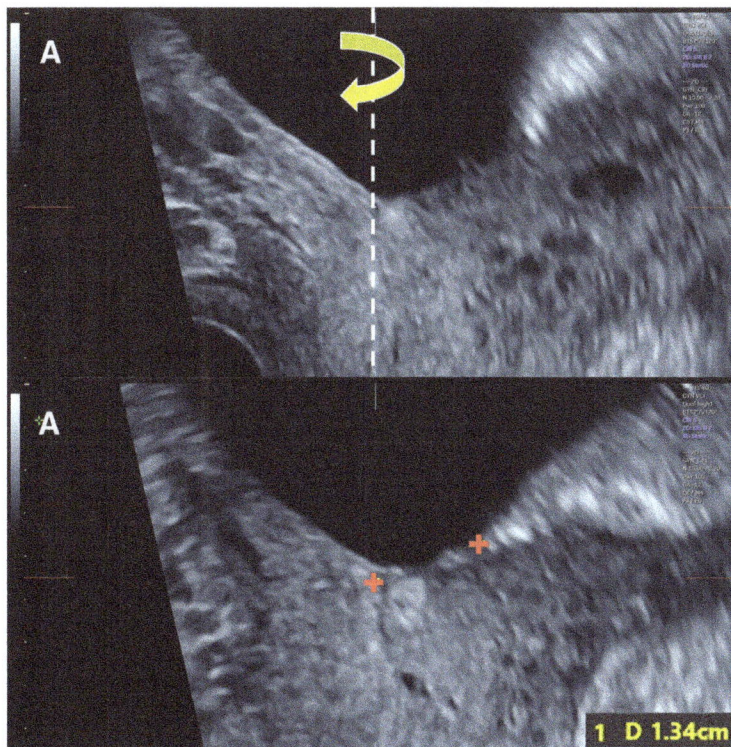

Fig. 7 Plane A: Rotation 360° around the y-axis (arrow), then the shortest distance between the lower placental edge and the reference point (center of IO) was measured

Table 1 Summary of EOD measurement by 3D TVS

Volume acquisition

1. Reference plane: The mid-sagittal view of the cervix.

2. Acquisition box and angle: adjusted to include the upper part of the cervix and the lower uterine segment containing the lower placental edge.

Volume display

1. Plane A:

a. The IO is centered in the plane.

b. The reference point is positioned at the IO.

c. Rotation around the z-axis to make the IO at the lowest level in the lower uterine segment.

2. Plane B:

a. The reference point is positioned in the middle of the upper edge of the cervical canal.

b. Rotation around the z-axis to make the IO at the lowest level in the lower segment.

3. Plane C:

a. The reference point is positioned in the middle of the IO.

b. Rotation around the z-axis to get the IO parallel to the y-axis.

4. Plane A:

a. Rotation 360° around the y-axis.

b. Measure the shortest distance between the lower placental edge and the reference point (center of IO).

were presented as median and interquartile range (IQR). Normally distributed data were presented as mean ± standard deviation (SD). Categorical data were presented as number and percentage (%). Paired sample t-test was done to compare EOD measurements between 2D TVS and 3D TVS. Chi-Square test was used to compare patients grouped according to the EOD measured by both

Table 2 Demographic data of the study group

Variable		Mean ± SD
Age (years)		29.7 ± 6.3
BMI (kg/m^{2})		26.1 ± 2.1
Gestational age at exam.(weeks)		32.7 ± 2.8
Variable		n (%)
Gestational age at exam.(weeks)	28- < 32	28 (36.8%)
	32- < 34	16 (21.1%)
	34- < 36	17 (22.4%)
	≥36	15 (19.7%)
Parity	0	6 (8%)
	1–2	35 (46%)
	≥3	35 (46%)
Previous cesarean	0	15 (19.7%)
	1–2	43 (56.7%)
	≥3	18 (23.6%)

Table 3 Placental location distribution

Placental location	n (%)
Anterior	3 (3.9%)
Anterior to the right	27 (35.5%)
Anterior to the left	14 (18.4%)
Posterior	3 (3.9%)
Posterior to the right	10 (13.2%)
Posterior to the left	10 (13.2%)
Right	7 (9.2%)
Left	2 (2.6%)

techniques. ANOVA was used to study the effect of placental location on the discrepancy in EOD measurements between both methods, Games- Howel Post Hoc test was used to test the degree of affection for every placental location. The relation between the same EOD discrepancy and internal os diameter measured by 3D TVS was tested by Pearson correlation coefficient.

Results

During the study period, 76 cases were eligible for the study. Demographic data of the study group are shown in Table 2. Placental location was direct anterior/posterior in 6 cases (7.9%), anterolateral/ posterolateral in 61 cases (80.3%) and lateral in 9 cases (11.8%) (Table 3) (see also Additional file 1). The mean internal os width ranged from 6 to 23 mm with mean ± SD of 13.9 ± 5.5 mm (Fig. 8).

Despite EOD measured by 3D TVS was slightly longer in 7 cases (mean difference = − 1.45 mm, SD = − 1.21), paired sample t test revealed that the mean EOD measured by 3D TVS ($M = 18.3$, SD = 6.30) was significantly shorter than that measured using the 2D TVS ($M = 24.26$, SD = 7.08). We can be 95% confident that the true

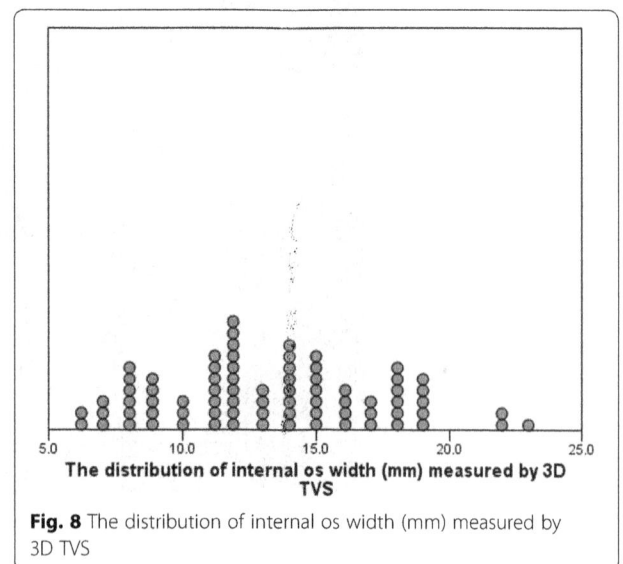

Fig. 8 The distribution of internal os width (mm) measured by 3D TVS

Table 4 Comparison of the mean EOD as measured by 2D and 3D TVS

		2D TVS	3D TVS	Paired sample t-test
Edge to os distance	Mean distance	24.26 ± 7.08	18.3 ± 6.30	0.000
	Groups	n (%)	n (%)	Chi-Square test
	≤ 10 mm	1 (1.3%)	8 (10.5%)	0.000
	11–20 mm	22 (28.9%)	42 (55.3%)	
	21–30 mm	34 (44.7%)	23 (30.3%)	
	31–35 mm	19 (25%)	3 (3.9%)	

Patients were stratified according to the EOD by both methods

difference between these means is CI = [4.62, 7.29]. Cohen's d was estimated 0.89, effect size = 0.4. This lead to dramatic increase in number of cases with EOD ≤ 10 mm [1 (1.3%) by 2D TVS vs 8 (10.5%) by 3D TVS], and cases with EOD 11–20 mm [22 (28.9%) by 2D TVS vs 42 (55.3%) by 3D TVS], $P = 0.000$ (Table 4).

The ANOVA revealed a main effect of placental location on the degree of difference in measurements of EOD between 3D and 2D TVS, $F(7, 68) = 4.122$, $P = 0.001$ (Table 5). Anterolateral/posterolateral and lateral placentas were associated with high discrepancy in measurements between both methods, being the highest with lateral group (Table 6).

Pearson correlation coefficient revealed a significant positive correlation between the IO width and the degree of difference between the EOD measured by both methods, r (74) = 0.345, $P = 0.001$ (Table 7).

Discussion

In our daily practice, 2D TVS is essential in defining the relation between the lower placental edge and the IO in cases of low-lying placenta and placenta previa. This relation is fundamental in differentiating these types and for decision-making regarding the mode of delivery in such risky cases [14, 15]. In a previous case report, different measurements for EOD were reported by two sonographers [16]. However, the reproducibility of EOD

Table 5 Relation between the location of the placenta and the mean difference between 2D and 3D TVS EOD measurements

Placental location	Mean difference (2D-3D estimate)	One way ANOVA	Games- Howel Post Hoc test
Anterior	1 mm	0.001	1
Anterior to the right	5.3 mm		0.028
Anterior to the left	4.7 mm		0.250
Posterior	0.7 mm		1
Posterior to the right	7.3 mm		0.073
Posterior to the left	4.3 mm		0.137
Right	13.4 mm		0.005
Left	14.4 mm		0.387

Table 6 Relation between groups of placental location and the mean difference between 2D and 3D TVS EOD measurements

Placental location groups	Mean difference (2D-3D estimate) (mean ± SD) mm	One way ANOVA	Games- Howell Post Hoc test
Direct Anterior/posterior	0.85 ± 0.82	0.000	1
Anterolateral/posterolateral	5.33 ± 5.29		0.001
Lateral	13.59 ± 4.56		0.000

measurement by 2D TVS and the inter-observer variability were not studied. Moreover, the conflicting results of the different studies about the cutoff EOD above which vaginal delivery can be attempted in these cases raises the suspicion of the inaccuracy of 2D TVS measurement of the EOD [10, 12, 13].

Theoretically, using 2D TVS, we localize the IO as the uppermost point of the cervical canal in the midsagittal view of the cervix. This would be the case if the cervical canal was tubular in shape and the IO has a pinhole appearance. However, in all cases, we found that the cervical canal and the internal os appeared as a slit, in the axial view of the cervix, surrounded by an oval hyperechogenic area representing the cervical mucosa (previously described by *Simon and his colleagues* as an "oval patch") [16]. So, it is impossible to guarantee that the view in 2D examination of the cervix is strictly midsagittal, which may lead to errors in measurement of EOD; being nearer or farther from the placental edge (Fig. 9). Moreover, upon rotation of the vaginal probe to get the shortest EOD, both the IO and the lower placental edge must be visualized all through the movement, which becomes impossible upon reaching 90° lateral rotation on both sides. This is specifically important in cases of laterally located placentas. Therefore, another method was needed for more accurate spatial localization of the midpoint of the IO, and for simultaneous visualization of the IO and the lower placental edge during the rotation all around the IO to get the shortest EOD accurately.

The new method of EOD measurement by 3D TVS in the current study has achieved these goals. We could accurately localize the midpoint of the IO, and by positioning the reference point at this location, we could rotate the volume all around the IO while visualizing the lower placental edge to measure the actual shortest EOD whatever the placental location was. From a technical point of view, the most important steps were to place the reference point midway in the slit shaped internal os in plane C, and in the lowest level of the lower uterine segment in planes

Table 7 Relation between the IO width and the difference in EOD measured by both 2D and 3D TVS

Pearson Correlation	Difference between 2D and 3D measurements	Sig. (one- tailed)
IO width	0.345	0.001

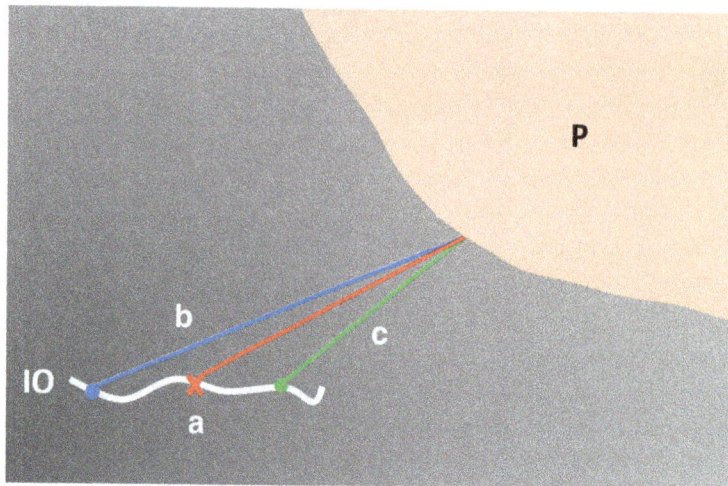

Fig. 9 Accurate measurement of EOD from the center of IO to the nearest point of lower placental edge (red line, a). When shifted farther from the placental edge, the EOD is longer (blue line, b). When shifted nearer to placental edge, the EOD is shorter (green line, c). P: Placenta; IO: Internal os

A and B. In plane B, the whole cervical canal was not visualized in all cases after manipulations, as this canal was curved in most cases and not always perpendicular to the lower uterine segment at the level of IO. However, this was not an essential prerequisite to complete the steps of measurement.

In the current study, the mean EOD measured by 3D TVS was significantly shorter than that measured using the 2D TVS, with dramatic increase in number of cases with EOD ≤ 10 mm and cases with EOD 11–20 mm measured by 3D TVS (Table 4). The most likely explanations of this difference are, firstly, the incorrect localization of the midpoint of the internal os (being *farther* from the placental edge) in 2D TVS and, secondly, the inability to simultaneously visualize the IO and the nearest point of the lower placental edge in a laterally located placenta.

As IO width ranged from 6 to 23 mm in this study, this can make a significant difference in measurement when there is marked shift from IO center. This was confirmed by the significant positive correlation between the IO width and the degree of difference between the EOD measured by both methods (Table 7). In seven cases, EOD measured by 3D TVS was longer than that measured by 2D TVS, mostly due to shift from the IO center *towards* the lower placental edge during 2D EOD measurement.

The difference in EOD measurement by 2D and 3D TVS was also related to the placental location. It was highly significant in anterolateral/posterolateral and lateral locations, being the highest with lateral group (Tables 5 and 6). This supports our hypothesis that the ability of 2D TVS to accurately measure the EOD decreases as the placenta is more lateral in location being almost impossible in directly lateral locations.

In their case report, *Simon* et al [16], described a different method of measuring EOD using 3D TVS, and the difference between 2D and 3D measurements was sufficient to shift from planned vaginal delivery to scheduled cesarean section for their case. They used multiplanar, omniView and surface rendered modes to accurately localize the center of the IO and to simultaneously visualize the whole lower placental edge and the IO.

Conclusions

Two dimensional TVS may not be accurate in measuring EOD in many cases of low-lying placentas, and 3D TVS may increase the accuracy of measurements in these cases. We believe that this new method is simple, precise and easily applied.

Further research is needed to assess the reproducibility of this method in comparison to the standard 2D method, and whether this innovative 3D technique will make difference in decision-making about mode of delivery in cases of low-lying placentas.

Additional file

Additional file 1: Demographic and ultrasonographic data for the study group. The file includes the relevant demographic data for study cases including age group, BMI, gestational age, parity and previous cesarean sections. Also, ultrasonographic parameters related to the study including placental locations, edge to OS diameters by both 2 D and 3 D US and internal os width. (XLS 39 kb)

Abbreviations

2D: Two dimensional; 3D: Three dimensional; EOD: Edge to os distance; IO: Internal os; TVS: Transvaginal sonography

Acknowledgements

Not applicable.

Funding

None.

Authors' contributions

SM: Conception, contributed in study design, data analysis and interpretation, manuscript drafting. *RA:* Acquisition and interpretation of data, and contributed in critical revision. *HA:* Contributed in data analysis and interpretation, manuscript writing. *AG:* contributed in design and critical revision. All authors read and approved the final manuscript.

Competing interests

The authors declare that they have no competing interests.

References

1. Cresswell JA, Ronsmans C, Calvert C, Filippi V. Prevalence of placenta praevia by world region: a systematic review and meta-analysis. Trop Med Int Heal. 2013;18:712–24.

2. Dashe JS. Toward consistent terminology of placental location. Semin Perinatol. 2013;37:375–9. https://doi.org/10.1053/j.semperi.2013.06.017.

3. Faiz AS, Ananth CV. Etiology and risk factors for placenta previa: an overview and meta-analysis of observational studies. J Matern Neonatal Med. 2003;13:175–90. https://doi.org/10.1080/jmf.13.3.175.190.

4. Hasegawa J, Nakamura M, Hamada S, Matsuoka R, Ichizuka K, Sekizawa A, et al. Prediction of hemorrhage in placenta previa. Taiwan J Obstet Gynecol. 2012;51:3–6. https://doi.org/10.1016/j.tjog.2012.01.002.

5. Gibbins KJ, Einerson BD, Varner MW, Silver RM. Placenta previa and maternal hemorrhagic morbidity. J Matern Neonatal Med. 2017;0:1–6. https://doi.org/10.1080/14767058.2017.1289163.

6. Young BC, Nadel a, Kaimal a. Does previa location matter? Surgical morbidity associated with location of a placenta previa. J Perinatol. 2014;34: 264–7. https://doi.org/10.1038/jp.2013.185.

7. Bhide A, Prefumo F, Moore J, Hollis B, Thilaganathan B. Placental edge to internal os distance in the late third trimester and mode of delivery in placenta praevia. BJOG An Int J Obstet Gynaecol. 2003;110:860–4.

8. Oppenheimer LW, Farine D. A new classification of placenta previa: measuring progress in obstetrics. Am J Obstet Gynecol. 2009;201:227–9. https://doi.org/10.1016/j.ajog.2009.06.010.

9. Royal College of Obstetricians and Gynaecologists (RCOG). Placenta praevia, placenta praevia accreta and vasa praevia: diagnosis and management - Green-top Guideline No.27. 2018. https://www.rcog.org.uk/en/guidelines-research-services/guidelines/gtg27a.

10. Vergani P, Ornaghi S, Pozzi I, Beretta P, Russo FM, Follesa I, et al. Placenta previa: distance to internal os and mode of delivery. Am J Obstet Gynecol. 2009;201:266.e1–5. https://doi.org/10.1016/j.ajog.2009.06.009.

11. Al Wadi K, Schneider C, Burym C, Reid G, Hunt J, Menticoglou S. Evaluating the safety of labour in women with a placental edge 11 to 20 mm from the internal cervical Os. J Obstet Gynecol Canada. 2014;36:674–7. https://doi.org/10.1016/S1701-2163(15)30508-9.

12. D'Antonio F, Bhide A. Ultrasound in placental disorders. Best Pract Res Clin Obstet Gynaecol. 2014;28:429–42. https://doi.org/10.1016/j.bpobgyn.2014.01.001.

13. Ghourab S. Third-trimester transvaginal ultrasonography in placenta previa: does the shape of the lower placental edge predict clinical outcome? Ultrasound Obstet Gynecol. 2001;18:103–8.

14. Leerentveld RA, Gilberts EC, Arnold MJ, Wladimiroff JW. Accuracy and safety of transvaginal sonographic placental localization. Obstet Gynecol. 1990;76(5 Pt 1):759–62 http://www.ncbi.nlm.nih.gov/pubmed/2216220.

15. Oppenheimer L, Armson A, Farine D, Keenan-Lindsay L, Morin V, Pressey T, et al. Diagnosis and Management of Placenta Previa. J Obstet Gynaecol Canada. 2007;29:261–6. https://doi.org/10.1016/S1701-2163(16)32401-X.

16. Simon EG, Fouche CJ, Perrotin F. Three-dimensional transvaginal sonography in third-trimester evaluation of placenta previa. Ultrasound Obstet Gynecol. 2013;41:465–8.

19

Determinants of client satisfaction to skilled antenatal care services at Southwest of Ethiopia: a cross-sectional facility based survey

Serawit Lakew[1*], Alaso Ankala[2] and Fozia Jemal[3]

Abstract

Background: Patient satisfaction to Antenatal care services has traditionally been linked to the quality of services given and the extent to which specific needs are met. Even though data in this area was limited in Ethiopia, improving quality of care was one of the strategies in health sector development program IV. This study, therefore, attempted to assess client satisfaction to skilled antenatal care services in the study area.

Methods and materials: A cross-sectional facility based survey was conducted among women who were attending antenatal care clinic, using quantitative method triangulated with qualitative data collection. Participants were selected using systematic sampling method according to the flow pregnant women to the antenatal care clinics. The study was carried out in all functional public health centers in the district. During the survey, 405 women were interviewed. A logistic regression model was applied to control for confounders.

Results: Out of the total respondents, overall satisfied to skilled antenatal care services were about 277(68%). The most common specific component of antenatal care that had good-satisfaction by the respondents was "Privacy" at examination (81.7%). Most satisfied health education session was "Diet and nutrition" session (82.2%). Absence of sonar test, no doctor and long waiting time were commonest causes of dissatisfaction. Respondents who have ≥ 2 previous antenatal care visit were 3 times more likely (AOR = 2.93; 95% CI, 1.21, 7.12) to have satisfaction to antenatal care services as compared to those with ≤ 1 visit. Women whose current visit fourth were 9 times more likely (AOR = 9.02, 95% CI; 1.76, 46.1) to be satisfied for antenatal services than those who were in the first visit. Women with family monthly income of $US 25–100 per month were 60% (AOR = 0.4, 95% CI; 0.2, 0.8) less likely to have satisfaction by skilled antenatal care services than those who had monthly household income below $US 25.

Conclusion and recommendation: Women who reported good-satisfaction to overall skilled antenatal care services were highest as compared to previous Ethiopian study findings. Demographic, economic, obstetric and distance factors were independent predictors of satisfaction to skilled antenatal care services. Non natives must be encouraged to seek satisfying services.

Keywords: Satisfaction, Skilled antenatal care, Women, Southwest of Ethiopia

* Correspondence: lserawit@yahoo.com
[1]Department of Nursing and Midwifery, Arbaminch University, Arba Minch, Ethiopia
Full list of author information is available at the end of the article

Background

Pregnancy is a very important event from both social and medical point of view. ANC is an opportunity to advice the women on how to prepare for complications and promote the benefit of skilled attendance at birth [1].

W.H.O recommends that pregnant women should feel welcome at clinics for ANC in that it should be user-friendly. Examinations and tests should be carried at times that suit the woman. The teamwork between professionals and the pregnant woman is decisive for the safety of the woman and her fetus [2]. Every woman has the right to obtain recommended services of ANC from a skilled attendant at her pregnancy. A skilled attendant is not only trained to attend to normal pregnancies but also to recognize and manage complications and make referrals to hospital if more advanced care is needed. Women in rural areas were most at risk of giving birth and ANC services in the absence of skilled attendant [3, 4].

Ratings of women satisfaction for ANC indicated higher across developing countries and vary from country to country [5–9]. Studies found that overall satisfaction was highest in Cameroon and Egypt. In Cameroon, it was about 96.9% satisfied [10]. In Egypt, more than 90% reported satisfied for waiting time in lab results, Staff help, trust the doctor followed by cleanness of the center, privacy, most of accessibility items, and most of physician performance items. Least satisfied (below 30%) for location of the center, health education program, and explanation of the problems by physicians [11].

In Riyadh, about 87.7% pregnant women attending ANC felt unhappy because they had to wait up to 1 hour before being seen by the physician. About 63.1% were satisfied with information regarding their treatment. Around 18.9% thought that information was not enough and 17.25% reported they did not receive any information about their treatment [12].

In Kenya, about 96% of women who attended FI ANC clinics and 97% who attended NI ANC clinics were either "satisfied" or "very satisfied" with their clinic visit. A 'very poor' grade of satisfaction was considered to be a weak area of antenatal services. The dissatisfaction expressed mainly related to the process of imparting health education (such as: commitment, availability of time and language barrier) and not to the availability of health education material [13].

In Nigeria, most respondents were satisfied by the services given at the clinic (81.1%). Sitting arrangement was most satisfied (97.9%). Toilet and bathroom facilities were least satisfied (39.3 and 38.1% respectively). About 91.6% respondents reported "diet and nutrition" more satisfied during the interactive session than others. Prevention of cervical cancer was least discussed topic (65.7%) [14]. Obafemi Awolowo University study findings added that about 55% of women attending ANC clinic were satisfied with the quality of health talk. Around 72.6% were satisfied by the opinion that the services of the hospital were good and met their needs. About 53.7% agreed with the competency of the hospital staff. About 39.1% agreed with timely response of the staff and 20.5% on the opinion that the staffs were friendly and polite [15].

In various African country, Continued utilization of ANC services in the future pregnancy was directly linked to the satisfaction of the clients ($p < 0.05$) [14]. Significant satisfaction was also observed for being attending in public centers over private in Cameroon and those who served in Mendera Kochi and Higher Two Centers over others at Jimma town of Ethiopia [10, 16]. Those who have no formal education, attended primary education, monthly income < 500 birr and between 750 and 1000 birr, planned pregnancy and no history of stillbirth had significant associations for satisfied ANC services over their counter parts at $p < 0.05$ [16].

In Cameroon, significant association was observed for good satisfaction at their first pregnancy, the sitting area comfort, and competence of staff as compared to its counterparts [10]. Pakistan qualitative discussants reported, distant location of facilities, lack of functional equipment, medicines and supplies as perceived poor satisfaction [17]. Previous Ethiopian studies focused on the relationship between women's satisfaction and the provision and utilization of health care services [18]. No data could have been found on specific component of services satisfaction in Ethiopia in general and the study area in particular. This study, therefore, attempted to place its contribution through its findings.

Conceptual frame work

As indicated by Fig. 1, this conceptual frame work was adopted from one systematic review on women satisfaction to maternity care services in developing world, since it matches with this local system [9]. ANC services satisfaction was one component with background characteristics, provider factors, obstetrics factors and amenities were independent predictors. The frame work was adjusted to local system for to make it more convenient (Fig. 1).

Methods
Study design and setting

Health facility based cross-sectional study was conducted from Jan 1 to March 12, 2016. Health Facility includes Hospitals, Health Centers, Health Posts and Private Clinics. Arba Minch Zuria was one of the districts in the southwest of Ethiopia. It was located in the Great Rift Valley. As per the report of district health department statistics office, it had 30 kebeles (kebele is the lowest administrative state in Ethiopia) and a total population of 202,495 of whom 100,842 are men and 101,653

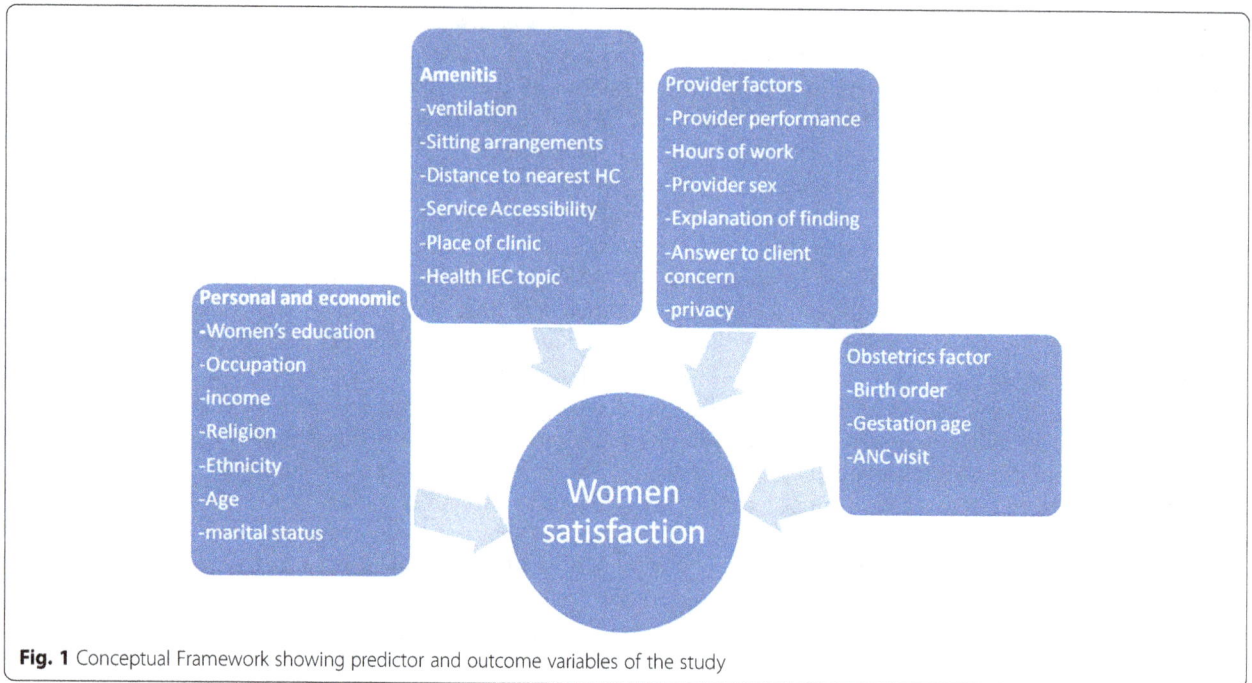

Fig. 1 Conceptual Framework showing predictor and outcome variables of the study

women. The district was located some 454kms south-west of Addis Ababa. The district had no any functional hospitals. But, it had five functional health centers and about thirty health posts (staffed by Health Extension Workers who are non-skilled providers) and private clinics together [19, 20]. The private clinics in the study region had no routine ANC services, since it had service fee and costly. Routine ANC services exist only in government health centers because services were free. In the district, skilled providers exist in the public health centers and private clinics only. Health Centers, therefore, were selected as study unit.

Sample size and sampling procedure

Sample size was determined by using single population proportion (SPP) formula based on the assumptions of 95% confidence level, 60.4% p-value (previous Rural Ethiopian study) and a 10% contingency. Accordingly, the total sample size was 405 women participant. Systematic sampling technique was used to select the study subjects. Number of Participants in each health centers was estimated based on three steps. First, total catchment population to each health centers were obtained from district health offices, department of statistics. Next, estimated proportion (N) of pregnancy in the catchment population of each health centers (using 4.5% of the whole population [21]) was obtained. Finally, the number of attendance for ANC (using 34% [22]) within the total estimated pregnancy was calculated in each health center. Respondents (n) who were registered for antenatal care during data collection at post-procedure

period were interviewed by systematic sampling technique until the required sample size was achieved in each health center. The Kth value was calculated based on number of registered for ANC of the day divided by expected sample a day (in each health center). From the first K^{th} values, one woman was selected by lottery method. The consecutive woman was selected by every k^{th} value. Also consider that ANC registration was performing in the morning for rural Ethiopian Health facility as tradition (Fig. 2).

For qualitative method, a convenience sampling technique was used to select pregnant women participant for the FGD by taking health center as homogeneity criteria. Accordingly, 10 FGDs were purposively selected with 2 FGDs in each of five active health centers. Selected respondents were not participant on quantitative. FGDs were conducted on two occasions with different days after the end of quantitative interview. It was accomplished by same data collectors under supervision.

Questionnaire development and measurement

Questionnaire was adapted from previous similar studies in the abroad [11] and adjusted in the local system. The questions and statements were grouped and arranged according to the particular that they can address. After extensive revision, the final version of the English questionnaire was developed. An individual who were expert for English and Amharic languages translated the English version into Amharic and the vice versa. For quantitative method: data were collected using face-to-face client interview questionnaires (by exit

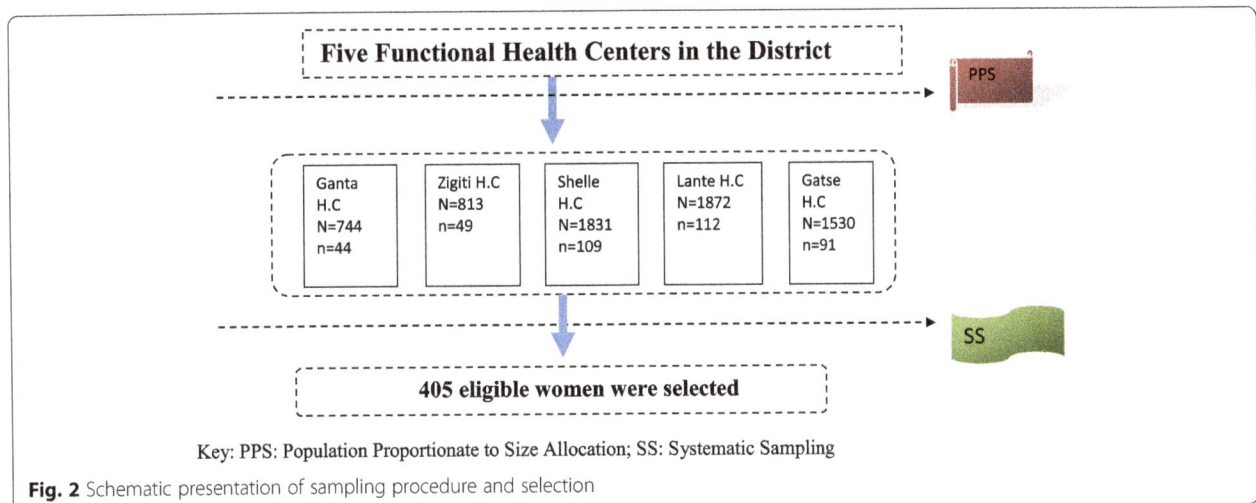

Fig. 2 Schematic presentation of sampling procedure and selection

interview). Having skilled Antenatal Care services were those participant who had ANC by skilled Health personnel, such as Nurse, Midwife, Health Officer and/ or Doctor at Health Facility. Having good satisfaction to Skilled Antenatal Care services were those women who answered 'good' to satisfaction questions in general and the vice versa for poor satisfaction. Predictor variables included in the data collection tool were demographic and Socio-economic variables; obstetrics variables; provider and staff variables; and amenities. For qualitative method: Focus group interview guideline was used to guide and probe the FGDs. The FGD interview guideline includes probing questions on areas of care clients satisfied and areas of care clients not satisfied. About 6–12 volunteered discussants were selected for each FGD session from each health centers. Every participant had given chance to talk as per the need to talk.

Statistical analysis

For quantitative method, after data collection each questionnaire was manually checked for completeness and then coded. After this validation, data were entered using EPI INFO version 3.5.2 and exported to SPSS statistical software package windows version 20 for analysis. Descriptive and summary statistics were used to describe the study population by variables of interest based on conceptual framework and for outliers. The degree of association between independent and dependent variables were described using crude and adjusted odds ratio. Bivariate analysis was applied to examine the association between each of the independent variables and satisfaction of ANC services. Multivariate statistical method used in the analysis was logistic regression model to control confounders. For qualitative methods, FGD data transcribed into English language verbatim, read critically and essential themes were identified. Ideas related to various themes were color coded and then organized into concepts and presented using narratives. The result was presented in tri-angulations with the quantitative data using subjects verbatim as illustrations.

Data quality control

Data Collection tool was adopted and pretested [11]. Three days Training was given to data collectors and supervisors. Every day, completed questionnaires were reviewed and checked for completeness and relevance by the supervisors. All the necessary feedback was offered to data collectors in the next morning before the actual procedure. Data checked for completeness, coded, entered into computer, cleaned, and frequency checked for outliers and missing values before analysis.

Ethical issues

Ethical clearance was obtained from Arba Minch College of Health Sciences Research and Publication core process (RPCP) and Southern National regional state Health Bureau. The study was commenced after letter of cooperation written to each catchment health facility administrators from Zonal administrators (ZHB). Informed written consent was secured to all study subjects. Each respondent was informed for the objective of the study and assurance of confidentiality, risks and benefits. List of Colleges Ethics committee includes: Alemayehu Bekele Kassahun, Addisu Alemayehu Gube, Tarekegn Tadesse Hunede, and Bereket Workalemahu Ayele.

Results
Socio-demographic and personal characteristics
Of the total 405 sample, the response rate was 100%. Of the age distribution of the women, about 315 (77.8%) of the participant were the dominant group of 20–34 years. The mean age of the participant was 27.6 years ± 5.6 SD.

Concerning woman education, more than half 203 (50.1%) had reported no history of formal education. Gamo ethnic group were the dominant 346 (85.4%) over others among the attendee participated. Except the few, most of women arrived the health facility traveling ≥ 1 km from their home, around 323 (79.8%) (Table 1).

Table 1 Independent variables used in the analysis categories and percentage distribution, Arba Minch Zuria district, Southwest Ethiopia, March 2016

Variable	Status of Satisfaction, (n = 405)	
	Good satisfaction, n (%)	Poor satisfaction, n (%)
Age		
< 20 yrs	26(6.4)	16(4.0)
20-34 yrs	212(52.3)	103(25.4)
≥ 35 yrs	39(9.6)	9(2.2)
Woman education		
No education	153(37.8)	50(12.3)
primary	81(20.0)	56(13.8)
Secondary+	43(10.6)	22(5.4)
Distance to the nearest HC		
< 1 km	42(10.4)	40(9.9)
≥ 1 km	235(58.0)	88(21.7)
Ethnicity		
Gamo	255(63.0)	91(22.5)
Welayta	16(4.0)	24(5.9)
Others[a]	6(1.5)	13(3.2)
Birth order (n = 318)[d]		
1	48(15.1)	32(10.1)
2–3	106(33.3)	47(14.8)
4–5	49(15.4)	14(4.4)
6+	19(6.0)	3(0.9)
Previous ANC visit		
< 2 visit	195(48.1)	110(27.2)
≥ 2 visit	82(20.2)	18(4.4)
Marital Status		
Married	274(67.7)	118(29.1)
Others[b]	3(0.7)	10(2.5)
Religion		
Orthodox	123(30.4)	67(16.5)
Protestant	129(31.9)	58(14.3)
Others[c]	25(6.2)	3(0.7)
Family Monthly Income (n = 360)[d] (in $US)		
< 25	85(23.6)	23(6.4)
25–50	105(29.2)	65(18.1)
> 50	53(14.7)	29(8.1)

N.B: [a] include Zayse and Amhara, [b] widowed, divorced & single, [c] Muslim, catholic, traditional, [d] had missing values

Regarding respondents religion, Ethiopian Orthodox and Protestant Christianity religion followers alone account for 377 (93.1%) of the respondents. This showed the two religion dominance in the study region. Birth order of majority of woman was between 2 to 5 among the study participants, about 67.9%. When observing income, net monthly income of the women as family income grouping was higher in middle income categories ($US 25–50), accounting 218 (53.8%) of respondents. The median monthly income of the family was $US 37.5 (Table 1).

Satisfaction by components of skilled ANC services

Overall satisfaction was classified as poor or good satisfaction. Most women were satisfied with the services offered, about 277(68%). Satisfaction among components of services range from 24 to 82% satisfied. More importantly, satisfaction status was specifically described based on main components of services for Skilled Antenatal Care. Regarding accessibility for services, more women satisfied for staff hours of work 247 (61%) and sitting arrangements 289 (71.4%). Half and more of the women were satisfied by cleanness of the Center 241 (59.5%) and Toilet facility 226 (55.8%) (Table 2 and Fig. 3).

Provider "examination time" client satisfied was far large 309 (76.3%) among others within "performance of provider" responses category as women report suggested and relatively lower responses observed in "explanation of results of investigation", about 241 (59.5%). Major 'poor satisfaction' response in this category was 'location of the center' among others, about 211 (52.1%). Regarding privacy, poor-satisfaction report was 74 (18.3%), which is the lowest of all and the vice versa was the highest (Table 2).

Only about a third of the women had good satisfaction to explanation of the problem, explanation of rationale of the investigation on provider performance component, and delivering of the information in staff performance component, about (33.1, 31.6, and 33.6%), respectively (Table 2).

Majority of FGD respondents also reported that most providers had no respect for working hour's punctuality. For that reason our waiting time was beyond expected time to wait. Most of wasting time occurs on either exit time end or entrance beginning. Once they start the procedure, time utilization was effective. One 21 years old lady said, now I decided to visit the facility not based on government working hours, but providers working hours.

Describing satisfaction by health education and communication session in the ANC clinic

The health education and communication session on women satisfaction during ANC visit observed that overall health education program was not-satisfied by the majorities, about 245 (60.5%) of the

Determinants of client satisfaction to skilled antenatal care services at Southwest...

147

Table 2 Percent distribution of level of women Satisfaction to different components of ANC services, Arba Minch Zuria district, Southwest Ethiopia, March 2016 (n = 405)

Aspects of Care	Status of Satisfaction			
	Good Satisfied		Poor satisfied	
	Number	%	Number	%
Overall satisfaction to ANC services	277	68.4	128	31.6
Amenities				
Location of the center	194	47.9%	211	52.1%
Hours of work	247	61%	158	39%
Ventilation	196	48.4%	219	51.6%
Sitting arrangement	289	71.4%	116	28.6%
Cleanness of the center	241	59.5%	164	40.5%
Cleanness of the Toilet	226	55.8%	179	44.2%
Performance of provider				
Answering questions	290	71.6%	115	28.4%
Taking history	255	63%	150	37%
Explanation of problem	271	66.9%	134	33.1%
Trusting the doctor	289	71.4%	116	28.7%
Examination time	309	76.3%	96	23.7%
Explanation of rational for investigation	277	68.4%	128	31.6%
Explanation of results of Investigation	241	59.5%	164	40.5%
Performance of staff				
Delivering of information	269	66.4%	136	33.6%
Maintaining Privacy	331	81.7%	74	18.3%

respondents. When specifically observing, cervical cancer prevention IEC session was not satisfied by nearly half of women, about 206 (50.9%). The 'no-satisfaction' respondents report were highest for STI prevention, about 268 (66.1%), malaria prevention 214 (52.9%), Physical exercise 212 (52.4%), and Breast self examinations 302 (74.6%) (Table 3).

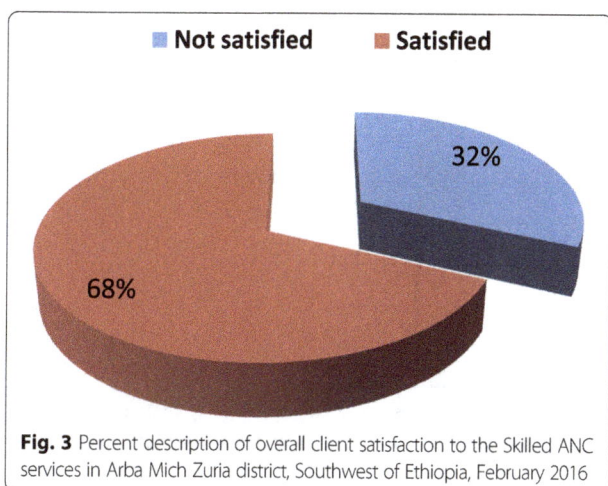

Fig. 3 Percent description of overall client satisfaction to the Skilled ANC services in Arba Mich Zuria district, Southwest of Ethiopia, February 2016

Highest client 'Good satisfaction' reports were observed as compared to "poor satisfaction" on some specific sessions. These included personal hygiene 284 (70.1%), tooth care 214 (52.8%), diet and nutrition 333 (82.2%), clothing 277 (68.4%), fetal movement monitoring 256 (63.2%), allowable medication 276 (68.1%), importance of breast feeding 247 (61%), basics of newborn care 211 (52.1%), follow-up for appointment 303 (74.8%), signs of labor 288 (71.1%), danger signs 286 (70.6%), and family planning and child spacing sessions 300 (74.1%) (Table 3). Majority discussants of focus group reported the major Health Education areas focused by the providers were diet at pregnancy and personal hygiene and its importance. We were happy with the sessions given. We identified healthier dietary selection for a pregnant woman. Providers also encouraged us to increase daily consumption of meal in that we have to have at least an additional two meal plan per a day over the routine. A single 34 years old respondent added "a provider told me to continue with the food that I was using even before pregnancy. Such as: vegetable diets, cereals and legumes that I get it from my farm land. Provider also addressed to balance my diet plan with my current weight and weight gain throughout the progress of pregnancy".

Table 3 Percent distribution of women satisfaction to health education and communication session on ANC clinic, Arba Minch Zuria district, Southwest Ethiopia, March 2016 (n = 405)

Health Education Topics	Status of Satisfaction			
	Good Satisfied		Poor satisfied	
	Number	%	Number	%
Overall Health education program	160	39.5%	245	60.5%
Prevention of Cervical Cancer	96	23.7%	309	76.3%
STI's prevention	137	33.8%	268	66.1%
Malaria prevention	191	47.2%	214	52.9%
Physical exercise	193	47.7%	212	52.4%
Personal hygiene	284	70.1%	121	29.8%
Teeth care	214	52.8%	191	47.2%
Diet and nutrition	333	82.2%	72	17.8%
Clothing	277	68.4%	128	31.6%
Fetal movement monitoring	256	63.2%	149	36.8%
Allowable medication	276	68.1%	129	31.9%
Breast feeding importance	247	61%	158	39%
Basics of newborn care	211	52.1%	194	47.9%
Follow-up appointment	303	74.8%	102	25.2%
Breast Self examination	103	25.4%	302	74.6%
Signs of labor	288	71.1%	117	28.8%
Danger signs of pregnancy	286	70.6%	119	29.4%
Family planning and child spacing	300	74.1%	105	25.9%

Describing satisfaction by number of current visit and gestational age

As observed, 'women satisfied' was increasing with frequently visiting for this pregnancy. Women satisfied were observed among the fourth and more visits of the respondents (88.6% Vs 66.7, 65.1, and 68.2%). Regarding gestational age, similar phenomena were observed in that in all trimester most women reported "good satisfaction" over that of "poor satisfaction". But, first trimester satisfaction and dissatisfaction was nearly closer each other (58.3 and 41.7% Vs 67.7 and 32.3%; 69.5 and 30.5%) as compared to second and third trimester. Third and second trimester satisfaction was huge over first, about (69.5 and 67.7% Vs 58.3%), respectively. The average gestational age at first visit of this pregnancy visit was 21.1 weeks ± 7.2 SD (Figs. 4 and 5).

Perceived main causes of dissatisfaction to skilled ANC services

A total of about 128 (32%) respondents had reported for having no satisfaction to Skilled Antenatal Care services in the facility of study district. Among this, reports of no sonar test (27.3%), unavailability of gynecologists (25%) and long waiting time in the clinic (20.3%) took the largest part. Even though they were lower 'no good laboratory services', 'not explaining about the clinic', 'overcrowding', and 'poor education session' reports also took proportions as the causes of dissatisfaction for overall Skilled Antenatal Care services (Fig. 6). In addition to this some of the discussants forwarded 'up on shortage of some medical instruments, providers usually used to refer us to the distant located hospital. Because of this, most of women did not go because of transportation and accommodation cost problem that we encounter at urban hospital and also hospital service was inconvenient than that of rural Health Centers'. A single 28 years old woman among the discussants of Gatse Health Center said 'I was not happy on the centers timely examination. There is long waiting and now I waited for long time'.

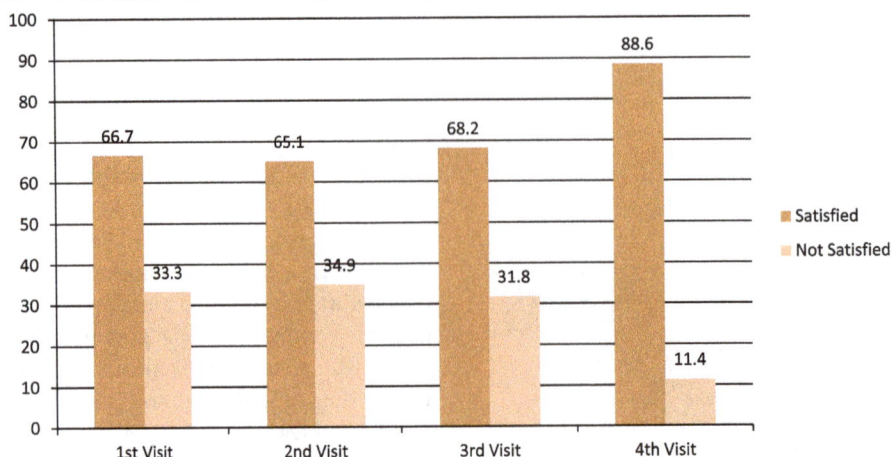

Fig. 4 Percent description of women current ANC visit by satisfaction status to ANC services, Arba Minch Zuria district, Southwest Ethiopia, March 2016 (n = 405)

Determinants of client satisfaction to skilled antenatal care services at Southwest...

149

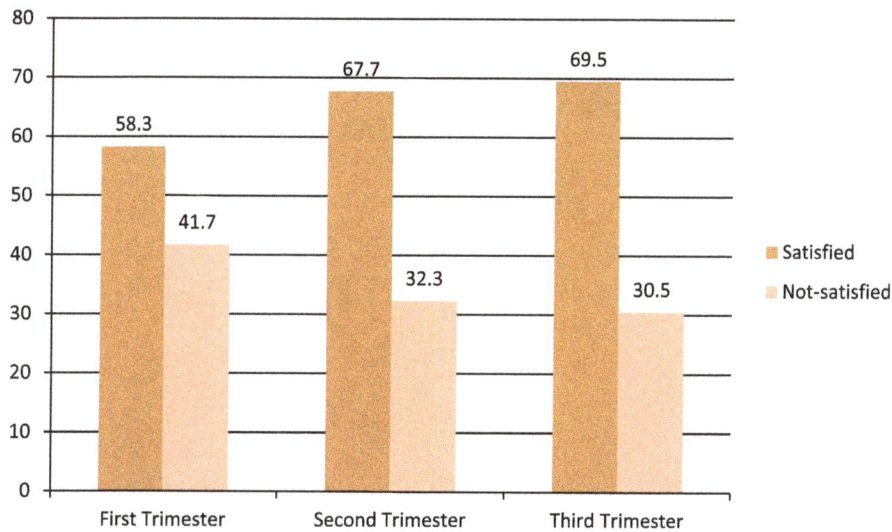

Fig. 5 Percent description of women gestational age of current pregnancy visit by satisfaction status to ANC services, Arba Minch Zuria district, Southwest Ethiopia, March 2016 (n = 405)

Factors associated with satisfaction to skilled ANC services

Bivariate and multivariable logistic regression analysis was used to calculate odds ratios and corresponding 95% confidence intervals for the predictors of satisfaction to Skilled Antenatal Care services. Concerning predictors of satisfaction in the bivariate analysis, having satisfaction to Skilled Antenatal Care services was associated with having birth order, distance to the nearest health center, previous ANC visit, family monthly income, marital status, ethnicity, and current visit type (Table 4).

When adjusted for other confounders in multivariable logistic regression analyses, only six variables, distance to the nearest health center, previous ANC visit, family monthly income, marital status, ethnicity, and current visit type were the potent predictors of women satisfaction to Skilled Antenatal Care services. Woman who arrived from 1 km or more distance to the center were 2.27 times more likely (AOR = 2.27; 95% CI, 1.27, 4.06) to have satisfied to Skilled Antenatal Care than those who are from below 1 km distance (Table 4).

Respondents who had 2 or more previous ANC visits were three times (AOR = 2.93; 95% CI, 1.21, 7.12) more likely to be satisfied to ANC services as compared to those with less or equal to one visit. Those women with family monthly income of $US 25–100 per month were

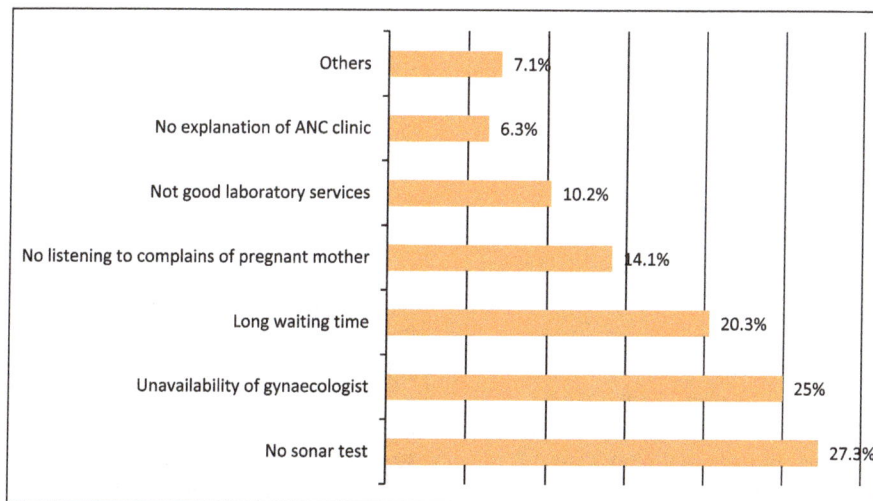

N.B. others include: Poor health education session and crowding clinic in the morning

Fig. 6 Percent distribution of women by main causes of dissatisfaction to skilled ANC services, Arba Minch Zuria district, Southwest Ethiopia, March 2016 (n = 128)

Table 4 Adjusted and unadjusted odds ratio of logistic regression model showing effects of predictor variables on the likely hood of client satisfaction for skilled ANC services, Arba Minch Zuria District, South West Ethiopia, March 2016

Predictor variables		Had satisfaction							
		Yes $n = 277$, 68.4%	No $n = 128$, 31.6%	COR	95% CI		AOR	95% CI	
					lower	upper		lower	upper
Birth Order ($n = 318$)	1	15.1%	10.1%	1.0+			1.0+		
	2–3	33.3%	14.8%	1.5	0.85	2.64	1.14	0.58	2.26
	4–5	15.4%	4.4%	2.33*	1.11	4.91	1.55	0.66	3.63
	6+	6%	0.9%	4.22*	1.15	15.4	3.45	0.38	31.4
Distance to the nearest HC[a]	< 1 km	9.9%	10.4%	1.0+			1.0+		
	≥ 1 km	21.7%	58%	2.54*	1.55	4.18	2.27**	1.27	4.06
Previous ANC visit	≤ 1	48.1%	27.2%	1.0+			1.0+		
	≥ 2	4.4%	20.2%	2.57*	1.47	4.5	2.93**	1.21	7.12
Family monthly income ($US)	< 25	23.6%	6.4%	1.0+			1.0+		
	25–50	29.2%	18.1%	0.44*	0.25	0.76	0.4**	0.2	0.8
	> 50	14.7%	8.1%	0.49*	0.26	0.94	0.67	0.27	1.67
Marital Status	Married	67.7%	29.1%	7.74*	2.09	28.6	8.17**	1.43	46.5
	Others[b]	0.7%	2.5%	1.0+			1.0+		
Ethnicity	Gamo	63%	22.5%	1.0+			1.0+		
	Welayta	4%	5.9%	0.24*	0.12	0.47	0.26**	0.13	0.54
	Others[c]	1.5%	3.2%	0.16*	0.06	0.45	0.2**	0.07	0.61
Current Visit	First	25.2%	12.6%	1.0+			1.0+		
	Second	20.7%	11.1%	0.93	0.57	1.53	1.09	0.57	2.08
	Third	14.8%	6.%	1.07	0.61	1.88	1.23	0.55	2.73
	Fourth and more	7.7%	1%	3.87*	1.3	11.57	9.02**	1.76	46.1

N.B: **Statistically Significant Association ($p < 0.05$), *significant by binary analysis, [1.0+] Reference category, [a]Health Center, [b]Singe, divorced, widowed, [c]Zeyse, Amhara

60% (AOR = 0.4, 95% CI; 0.2, 0.8) less likely to be satisfied by Skilled Antenatal Care services than those who had monthly household income below $US 25 (Table 4).

Compared to unmarried/divorced/widowed, married women were 8.17 times (AOR = 8.17, 95% CI; 1.43, 46.5) more likely to be satisfied to Skilled Antenatal Care. Non-native (Amhara, Zayse) ethnic groups were 80% (AOR = 0.2, 95% CI; 0.07, 0.61) decreased to have satisfied as compared to the native (Gamo) ethnic groups. And, women who come for fourth ANC visit were 9 times (AOR = 9.02, 95% CI; 1.76, 46.1) more likely to be satisfied than those who were in the first visit (Table 4).

Discussion

This health institution based cross-sectional study was attempted to assess the satisfaction status of women to Skilled Antenatal Care services in the district of Arba Minch Zuria, Southwest of Ethiopia. Findings of this study showed Skilled Antenatal Care services satisfaction were associated with demographic, economic, obstetric and accessibility factors of the respondents.

Accordingly, high number of respondents had reported they had good-satisfaction to the services. Many studies suggested that satisfaction of clients to ANC services varied from country to country [5–8]. This was inconsistent and higher finding as compared to Oman and previous Ethiopian (68% Vs 59% & 60%) [13, 16] and lower than Nigerian, Kenyan and Cameroons (68% Vs 81.1, 95, 96.4%) [10, 14, 23]. The highest finding could be an indication in Ethiopia for the ever-growing health sector development program for quality services so that it could be contributed to this comparative greater satisfaction. Conversely, the lower finding could be related to still the existence of comparative quality shortages in the study area of Ethiopia.

Satisfaction regarding location of the center, health education program and provider explanation of the problems on women ranges from about one-third to two-third, such as 39.5 to 66.9%. This was higher than Peruvian, Pakistan, European, and two African findings (39.5 to 66.9% Vs < 30%) [5–8, 17]. This higher finding of Ethiopia could be related to minimum surface area of the center due to few departments and buildings. This could give the center location closer to the roadside. Ethiopian provider usually had few minutes session for health education and explanation of the problem to the client. Greater satisfaction in this regard could be due to this short duration in the absence of intervention or treatment process that satisfies most of busy Ethiopian women to go to their home for home based work.

This study showed more than half women had satisfaction by 'hours of work' (61%). It was lower finding as compared to African Egyptian study finding (61% Vs 77.9%) [11]. This difference could be due to minimal working hours passed on work by providers in the facility of Ethiopia as per 24 h a day and 7 days a week. Shortage of skilled provider was also another issue to be considered in Ethiopia. Existence of these two facts alone were reported by Ethiopian HSDP-IV of 2012 report [24]. This comparative lower finding was also strengthened by majority of discussants that "..........every health professionals within the department on which they were in-charge had not found at government work hours that as we know, we mean at early 2:30 to 3:00hrs morning and 8:00 hrs to 8:30 hrs afternoon. Some exist in the facility compound, but not availed in the department on time. Some others totally not availed, but come late. Others, but not all, exit the facility early, before exit time (exit time: 6:30 morning or 11:30 after noon). It is most disappointing to all of us.............thanks to opportunity to talk".

In this study, good satisfaction to sitting arrangements, ventilation and cleanness of the toilet reported were nearly ¾[th] (71.4%), below half (48.4%), and more than half (55.8%) of the respondents, respectively. These were still lower from the highest findings of Nigeria (71.4, 48.4, 59.5% Vs 97.5, 84.1, 60.7%) [14]. This could show still insufficient arrangements for the three variables here in Ethiopia in the extent of its proper functioning to until it brings highest good satisfaction as compared to Nigeria's center with-in the continent of Africa.

Regarding performance of the provider and staff, all the findings of 'good satisfaction' in the current study were more than average as reported, such as: answering questions (71.6%), taking history (63%), trusting the provider (71.4%), examination time (76.3%), explanation of rational for investigation (68.4%), explanation of results of Investigations (59.5%) delivering information (66.4%) and maintaining privacy (81.7%). All of the mentioned components of services were comparatively lower from the Shawa Village Egyptian finding [11]. The probable explanation in this regard could be shortage of professional ethics, availability of non-women friendly services, and performance negligence's by professionals were dominating here in Ethiopian as compared to outside higher satisfaction countries. As it is mentioned in various studies (such as: Bangladesh and India) [25–27], high satisfaction was also related to Maintenance of privacy via a separate room or screen for examination.

This study assessed 'poor- satisfaction' health education and communication sessions as components of services. These included: Prevention of Cervical cancer, STI's prevention, Malaria prevention, Physical exercise, and Breast Self examination. On the other hand, more than average women reported for each of major HE sessions as 'good-satisfaction' included: Personal hygiene, Teeth care, Diet and nutrition, Clothing, Fetal movement monitoring, Allowable medications, Breast feeding, Basics of newborn care, Follow-up appointment, Signs of labor, Danger signs of pregnancy, and Family planning and child spacing. The poor satisfaction was contrary to Nigerian finding [14]. This could be due to not addressing these specific tasks on HE session here in Ethiopia by majorities of providers as contrasted by Nigeria. The good satisfaction components was in-line with Nigerian and Cameroon findings [10, 14]. The positive relationship could be due to increasing health sector development program for education session development here and there.

More than average women reported for each of major HE sessions as 'good-satisfaction' included: Personal hygiene, Teeth care, Diet and nutrition, Clothing, Fetal movement monitoring, Allowable medications, Breast feeding, Basics of newborn care, Follow-up appointment, Signs of labor, Danger signs of pregnancy, and family planning and child spacing. This was in-line with Nigerian and Cameroon findings [10, 14]. This positive relation could be due to increasing health sector development program for education session development here and there. Focus group discussants also supported positive finding in that "........ohhh, it was good and interesting. Health education session focusing on personal hygiene, diet and nutrition, and communicable disease prevention were clear to all of us. After education we have got special things to ourselves and our life. Our child can be protected from future infections, especially diarrhea and vomiting problems. One 38yrs old woman said: Now I will breast feed only for six months exclusively. Vaccinating baby is beneficial to me and to him".

Causes of dissatisfaction as client reported in the facility were: absence of sonar test, no doctor and long waiting time in the clinic. Other studies (Ghana, Nigeria and Ethiopia) also supported this as causes of dissatisfaction with services [16, 28, 29]. But, in this study, sonar test was the pioneer that reported by the majority of respondents as compared to other findings.

This study observed that having satisfied to Skilled Antenatal Care services was statistically significantly associated (AOR = 2.27; 95% CI, 1.27, 4.06) with distance ≥ 1 km that women traveled to arrive to the nearest Health Center. This was inconsistent with Pakistan qualitative finding [17] as far distance was one of the factors for dissatisfaction. This difference could be due to reduced expectations of women from outside village that she could get adequate services of her need. As suggested by developing countries study, women with low expectations with more services could result in good satisfaction of services and the vice versa [9].

Women Satisfied to SANC services was significantly associated (AOR = 2.93; 95% CI, 1.21, 7.12) with frequent (> 1times) previous ANC visits that women had. This was directly linked to Ibadan, Nigerian finding [14] and Riyadh [12] in which patient satisfaction was significantly higher among women in the highest visit groups. The positive association in this regard could be due to developing awareness on its importance by repeated visiting, increasing client need and effective response to this need by the health care workers here and there. Moreover, satisfied woman are more likely to increase the compliance with ANC visits [30]. Therefore, majority of subsequently visiting women could probably be satisfied groups in the current study and others.

In this study, having satisfied to Skilled Antenatal Care services was significantly associated (AOR = 0.4, 95% CI; 0.2, 0.8) with respondents who had monthly family income of $U.S 25–50/month. This was in line with previous home study [16] in that better satisfaction observed in lower income groups. Outside home, Malaysia, it was also positively linked as having no cost or low spending money for the ANC services had better services satisfaction [30]. The synonymous finding could probably indicate that low costly services are more satisfying to the poor ANC clients here and there.

Women in married marital status were significantly associated (AOR = 8.17, 95% CI; 1.43, 46.5) for having satisfied to Skilled Antenatal Care services. No other studies before could have observed this association directly. In this study, we could explain that this significant association could probably be related to existence of high number of married women among the study participants. This was because, married marital status and ANC service utilization had significant association in Ethiopia [31, 32].

This study revealed that having satisfied to Skilled Antenatal Care services were statistically significantly associated with being from Welayta (AOR = 0.26, 95% CI; 0.13, 0.54) and other (other includes: Amhara and Zayse) ethnic group (AOR = 0.2, 95% CI; 0.07, 0.61) respondents. This ethnic association with maternal Skilled Antenatal Care services satisfaction was also linked by Kenyan, Sri Lanka and Nigerian studies [33–35]. This particular ethnic discrimination could probably be related with non-native ethnic group's perception as being discriminated for services quality. This was because there was no one from minor ethnic group reported for ethnic related discrimination in FGDs. Concerned bodies needed to make specific interventions to poorly satisfied ethnic groups and further study is required.

This study shows that respondents who were in the fourth ANC visit were significantly associated (AOR = 9.02, 95% CI; 1.76, 46.1) for good-satisfaction to Skilled Antenatal Care services. This was supported by finding of Riyadh [12]. High good-satisfaction with highest visit gives the women opportunity to ask her concerns and this could increase her good feeling towards the services. Besides this, high number visit could possibly enhance positive relationship between providers and client, making maximum good feelings or satisfaction towards the women. This probable explanations were also supported by Tanzanian finding [36]. As satisfaction can be one of the effect for quality, perceived good quality services was also associated to that of subsequent ANC visit by a woman, as one home study suggested [37].

Strengths of the study

Being facility based is an advantage for better representing of the study district on the outcome variable as compared to being community based house to house survey. This was because it included respondents in the most recent service use. So, recall bias was highly minimized. Being triangulated design was also the strength. Moreover, being professional data collectors (nurse) used was an advantage for effective collection of obstetrics related information from the respondent's as it is difficult for non-health professionals.

Limitations of the study

Design related cause-effect relationship for all significant associations may not be established. Being facility based interviews could be disadvantageous in that it inhibits criticism of medical care by some of respondents even if it had weighted advantage over recall bias minimizations. The woman could depend on a single satisfying service for decisions of overall satisfaction, even though her self-report was the primary option for capturing customer satisfaction data. Social desirability bias could have affected the quality of data collected because study subjects might get difficulty to answer dissatisfaction in the presence of an interviewer. This bias was minimized via interviewing in a separate room by non-staff members' enumerator without wearing gown. Being non-scale based satisfaction measurement data collection tool could be the disadvantage for better observation of concentrated area in a scale of satisfaction. Moreover, women who were on a first visit could not be able to judge quality of some components of services accurately. This bias was reduced by clarification of components of services and allowing her to observe some amenities back again during the interview. Selection of questions and indicators could also have lead to a skewed interpretation.

Conclusion and recommendations

Women who reported having good-satisfaction to overall Skilled Antenatal Care services were highest. The most common specific component of ANC that had good-satisfaction by the respondents was maintaining "Privacy" during examination (81.7%). The most common health education topic during ANC services which was satisfied by the respondents was "Diet and nutrition" (82.2%). Absence of sonar test, no doctor, and long waiting time in the center were commonest causes of dissatisfaction by client report. Woman birth order, distance to the nearest health center, previous ANC visit, family monthly income, marital status, ethnicity, and current ANC visit type were independent predictors of satisfaction to Skilled Antenatal Care services. Providers must re-plan and improve their performances in the district for another highest satisfaction in the future. Especial attention must be given to those ethnics other than Gamo in the district regarding overall ANC services, since dissatisfaction was highest among them. Policy makers and other stake holders should give attention to increase ANC visit coverage in the country by developing strategies with the aim of maximum satisfaction to Skilled Antenatal Care services. Government officials should be engaged in development of middle income economy for women through women economy development strategy and intervention throughout the country. Early ANC visitors should also be given attention by providers to increase chance for return visit through maximizing client satisfaction in every component of services.

Abbreviations
ANC: Antenatal Care; FGD: Focus Group Discussion; HE: Health Education; IEC: Information, Education and Communication

Acknowledgements
Our special gratitude and appreciation goes to Arba Minch Health Sciences college research and publication core process for budgeting this research project. We were also grateful to Arba Minch Zuria administrators, Regional Health Bureau, data collectors, respondents and supervisors for their unreserved effort to the success of this work.

Funding
This study was undertaken by the grant from Arbaminch College of Health Sciences Office of Research and Publication Core Process. Funding includes for Data collection, entry and writing-up. Publication fee had not been funded from the college.

Authors' contributions
SL: Developed design and Conceptualization, performed statistical analysis and sequence alignment, and drafted the manuscript. AA: Participated on Design development, performed statistical analysis, participated drafting the manuscript. FJ: Coordinated the study, developed design, statistical analysis and participated manuscript draft development. All these authors read and approved the final manuscript.

Competing interests
We declare that we authors do not have any competing interests.

Author details
[1]Department of Nursing and Midwifery, Arbaminch University, Arba Minch, Ethiopia. [2]Department of Nursing and Midwifery, Arba Minch College of Health Sciences, Arba Minch, Ethiopia. [3]Department of Obstetrics and Gynecology, Tikur Anbesa Specialized Hospital, Addis Ababa University, Addis Ababa, Ethiopia.

References
1. Ethiopian Updated management protocol on selected obstetrics topics, Federal Democratic Republic of Ethiopia Ministry of Health.pdf. January 2010.
2. Holan S, Mathiesen M, Petersen K. A national clinical guideline for antenatal care. Oslo: Short version, Directorate for Health and Social Affairs; 2005.
3. Mafubelu D, Islam M. WHO, dept of making pregnancy safer annual report of 2006, P 6 of 56; 2007.
4. United Nations, author. The millenium development goals report. 2012.
5. Seclen-Palacin JA, Benavides B, Jacoby E, Velasquez A, Watanabe E. Is there a link between continuous quality improvement programs and health service users' satisfaction with prenatal care? An experience in Peruvian hospitals. Rev Panam Salud Public. 2004;16:149–57.
6. Luyben AG, Fleming VE. Women's needs from antenatal care in three European countries. Midwifery. 2005;21:212–23.
7. Bronfman-Pertzovsky MN, Lopez-Moreno S, Magis-Rodriguez C, Moreno-Altamirano A, Rutstein S. Prenatal care at the first level of care: characteristics of providers that affect users' satisfaction. Salud Publica Mex. 2003;45:445–54.
8. Uzochukwu BS, Onwujekwe OE, Akpala CO. Community satisfaction with the quality of maternal and child health services in Southeast Nigeria. East Afr Med J. 2004;81:293–9.
9. Srivastava A, Avan BI, Rajbangshi P, Bhattacharyya S. Determinants of women's satisfaction with maternal health care: a review of literature from developing countries. BMC Pregnancy Childbirth. 2015;15(97):p1–12.
10. Edie GEHE, Obinchemti TE, Tamufor EN, Njie MM, Njamen TN, Achidi EA. Perceptions of antenatal care services by pregnant women attending government health centres in the Buea Health District, Cameroon: a cross sectional study. Pan Afr Med J. 2015;21(45):1937–8688.
11. Montasser NAE-H, Helal RM, Megahed WM, Amin SK, Saad AM, Ibrahim TR, et al. Egyptian Women's satisfaction and perception of antenatal care. Int J Trop Dis Health. 2012;2(2):145–56.
12. Kamil A, Khorshid E. Maternal perceptions of antenatal care provision at a tertiary level hospital, Riyadh. Oman Med J. 2013;28(1):33–5.
13. Ghobashi M, Khandekar R. Satisfaction among expectant mothers with antenatal Care Services in the Musandam Region of Oman. Sultan Qaboos Univ Med J. 2008;8(3):325–32.
14. Nwaeze IL, Enabor OO, Oluwasola TAO, Aimakhu CO. PERCEPTION AND SATISFACTION WITH QUALITY OF ANTENATAL CARE SERVICES AMONG PREGNANT WOMEN AT THE UNIVERSITY COLLEGE HOSPITAL, IBADAN, NIGERIA. Ann Ib Postgrad Med. 2013;11(1):22–8.
15. Esimai O, Omoniyi-Esan G. Wait time and service satisfaction at antenatal clinic, Obafemi Awolowo University Ile-Ife. East Afr J Public Health. 2009;6(3):309–11.
16. Chemir F, Alemseged F, Workneh D. Satisfaction with focused antenatal care service and associated factors among pregnant women attending focused antenatal care at health centers in Jimma town, Jimma zone, South West Ethiopia; a facility based cross-sectional study triangulated with qualitative study. BMC Res Notes http://wwwbiomedcentralcom/1756-0500/7/164. 2014;7:164.
17. Majrooh MA, Hasnain S, Akram J, Siddiqui A, Memon ZA. Coverage and Quality of Antenatal Care Provided at Primary Health Care Facilities in the 'Punjab' Province of 'Pakistan'. PLoS One. 2014;9(11):e113390. https://doi.org/10.1371/journal.pone.0113390

18. Biro MA, Waldenstrom U, Brown S. Satisfaction with team midwifery Care for low- and High-Risk Women: a randomized controlled trial. Birth. 2003;30:1–10.

19. SNNPR, Gamo Gofa Zone, Arba Minch Zuria Woreda Health Office Report, 2013.

20. Ethiopian Housing and population Census of 2007 : Southern Peoples, Nations and Nationalities Region of Ethiopia. https://en.wikipedia.org/wiki/Southern_Nations,_Nationalities,_and_Peoples%27_Region.retrived.

21. Addisse M. Ethiopia public health training initiative, the Carter Center, the Ethiopia Ministry of Health, and the Ethiopia ministry of education, University of Gondar; 2003.

22. Central Statistical Agency [Ethiopia] and ICF International, Ethiopia Demographic and Health Survey (EDHS) 2011. Central Statistical Agency and ICF International, Addis Ababa, Ethiopia and Calverton, Maryland, USA. 2012.

23. Baotran N, Craig CR, Rachel SM, Elizabeth BA, Maricianah O, Katie D, et al. PATIENT SATISFACTION WITH INTEGRATED HIV AND ANTENATAL CARE SERVICES IN RURAL KENYA. AIDS Care. 2012;24(11):1442–7.

24. Ethiopia Health Sector Development Programme (HSDP) IV of 2010. MOH, Ethiopia. VERSION 19. ethiopia_hsdp_iv_final_draft_2010_-2015.pdf.

25. Aldana JM, Piechulek H, Al-Sabir A. Client satisfaction and quality of health care in rural Bangladesh. Bull World Health Organ. 2001;79:512–7.

26. George A. Quality of reproductive care in private hospitals in Andhra Pradesh. Women's perception. Econ Polit Wkly. 2002;37:1686–92.

27. Das P, Basu M, Tikadar T, Biswas GC, Mirdha P, Pal R. Client satisfaction on maternal and child health services in rural Bengal. Indian J Community Med. 2010;35:478–81.

28. Fawole AO, Okunlola MA, Adekunle AO. Client's perceptions of the quality of antenatal care. J Nat Med Assoc. 2008;100:1052–8.

29. D'Ambruoso L, Abbey M, Hussein J. Please understand when I cry out in pain: women's accounts of maternity services during labour and delivery in Ghana. BMC Public Health. 2005;5:140.

30. Rahman MM, Ngadan DP, Arif MT. Factors affecting satisfaction on antenatal care services in Sarawak, Malaysia, evidence from a cross sectional study. Springerplus. 2016;5:725.

31. Mekonnen Y, Mekonnen A. Utilization of maternal health Care Services in Ethiopia. Calverton, Maryland: ORC Macro; 2002.

32. Kwast BE, Liff JM. Factors associated with maternal mortality in Addis Ababa, Ethiopia. Int J Epidemiol. 1998;17(1):115–21.

33. Senarath U, Fernando DN, Rodrigo I. Factors determining client satisfaction with hospital-based perinatal care in Sri Lanka. Tropical Med Int Health. 2006;11:1442–51.

34. Oladapo OT, Osiberu MO. Do sociodemographic characteristics of pregnant women determine their perception of antenatal care quality? Matern Child Health J. 2009;13:505–11.

35. Bazant ES, Koenig MA. Women's satisfaction with delivery care in Nairobi's informal settlements. Int J Qual Health Care. 2009;21:79–86.

36. Gupta S, Yamada G, Mpembeni R, Frumence G, Callaghan-Koru JA, et al. Factors Associated with Four or More Antenatal Care Visits and Its Decline among Pregnant Women in Tanzania between 1999 and 2010. PLoS ONE. 2014;9(7):e101893. https://doi.org/10.1371/journal.pone.0101893.

37. Fesseha G, Alemayehu M, Etana B, Haileslassie K, Zemene A. Perceived quality of antenatal care service by pregnant women in public and private health facilities in Northern Ethiopia. Am J Health Res. 2014;2(4):146–51.

Successful preterm pregnancy in a rare variation of Herlyn-Werner-Wunderlich syndrome

Stefania Cappello[1]* [iD], Eleonora Piccolo[1], Francesco Cucinelli[2], Luisa Casadei[1], Emilio Piccione[1] and Maria Giovanna Salerno[2]

Abstract

Background: Herlyn–Werner-Wunderlich syndrome (HWWS) is an uncommon congenital anomaly of the female urogenital tract, characterised by uterus didelphys, obstructed hemivagina, and ipsilateral renal agenesis. We reported the difficult pregnancy course complicated by an extremely rare and unique case of this syndrome associated with ectrodactyly, a clinical combination never described in literature.

Case presentation: A 28- year-old nulliparous woman previously diagnosed for HWWS associated with ectrodactyly of the right foot and with a history of abdominal left hemi-hysterectomy, ipsilateral salpingectomy, vaginal reconstruction when she was an adolescent. She suffered from threats of abortion in the first trimester, recurrent urinary tract infections during all pregnancy. At 33 weeks + 5 days of gestational age, she was hospitalized for premature rupture of the membranes and uterine contractions and a caesarean section was performed because of breech presentation. Postpartum period was complicated by a pelvic abscess resolved with parental antibiotic therapies.

Conclusions: Our literature review shows an unusual aspect in our case: HWWS is not classically associated with skeletal anomalies. Moreover, the most frequent urogenital side affected is the right, not left side as in this woman. Preterm spontaneous rupture of membranes and fetal abnormal presentation represent frequent complications and probably post-caesarean infections are related to pregnancies in the context of this syndrome.

Keywords: Herlyn-Werner-Wunderlich syndrome (HWWS), OHVIRA syndrome, Müllerian duct anomalies, Ectrodactyly, Renal agenesis, Utero didelphys, Obstructed hemivagina, Pregnancy

Background

Herlyn –Werner-Wunderlich syndrome (HWWS) is a rare congenital anomaly of the female genital tract, characterised by the triad of uterus didelphys, blind hemivagina, and ipsilateral renal agenesis [1, 2]. It is even called OHVIRA syndrome (obstructed hemivagina, ipsilateral renal anomaly) and it is a result of the arrest of the midline fusion of the Müllerian ducts. This condition was first described in 70's and the incidence is low and probably underestimated [3]. Usually the diagnosis comes during adolescence due to hematocolpos, the frequent urinary tract infections or the presence of a pelvic mass

[4, 5]. Although all the Müllerian anomalies are related to infertility, frequent miscarriage, obstetric complications including abnormal fetal presentation, intrauterine growth restriction, and increased rate of caesarean section as well as abruptio placentae, premature rupture of membranes, retained placenta, postpartum haemorrhage, and increased fetal mortality [6, 7]. We presented a case of an unusual variant of HWWS associated with ectrodactyly [8] of the right foot, a combination never described [9], and the difficult course of her first preterm pregnancy with a particular postpartum complication. We are not sure if the ectrodactyly is an incidental finding or there is a causal effect with the disease, because it was not described by literature before.

* Correspondence: steficappello@gmail.com
[1]Department of Biomedicine and Prevention, Obstetrics and Gynecological Clinic, University of Rome "Tor Vergata", via Montpellier 1, 00133 Rome, Italy
Full list of author information is available at the end of the article

Case Presentation

A 28 year-old nulliparous woman, previously diagnosed for HWWS, was referred to San Camillo-Forlanini Hospital during her third spontaneous pregnancy. The clinical history of our patient began when at her birth, the ectrodactyly of the right foot (absence of the 2 medial rays), immediately became apparent. The karyotype analysis was normal 46 XX. At age 1, she underwent a surgical correction of this anomaly with consequent partial improvement of a functional deficiency. An upper abdominal ultrasound, performed after a history of recurrent urinary tract infections and pyelonephritis, revealed the absence of the left kidney and the right megaureter. At 12 years, after 2 months from menarche, due to severe acute pelvic pain, a pelvic ultrasound and a magnetic resonance imaging (MRI) were performed. MRI showed a left blind hemivagina with hematocolpos, uterus didelphys with hematometra in the left hemiuterus and ipsilateral hematosalpinx. These imaging findings were later confirmed by the diagnostic laparoscopy which showed normal right uterus, right fallopian tube and both regular ovaries. Consequently, she underwent a surgical reconstruction of the vagina consisting in the drainage of hematocolpos and the removal of the vaginal septum, whereas an abdominal left hemi- hysterectomy and ipsilateral salpingectomy were performed through a Pfannenstiel incision. Her obstetric history was significant for two spontaneous abortion at the age of 26, occurred at 7th and 12th weeks respectively. She had no problem of fertility in anamnesis. The woman came to our observation for the first time at 15 weeks of pregnancy for abortion threats resolved with vaginal progesterone. Singleton fetus was anatomically in the norm. The patient had a moderate protenuria of 1400 mg in 24 hours, so she started a proper diet and a monitor of urine proteins. Close and regular surveillance (clinical, laboratory, and ultrasound) was initiated. The obstetric ultrasound controls revealed adequate growth of a fetus without major malformations, and normal Doppler indices of the fetal, feto-maternal and utero-placental vessels. During the three trimesters, frequent urinary infections occurred that were appropriately treated after urine culture and antibiogram test. At 33 weeks + 5 days of gestational age she was admitted to our hospital for premature spontaneous rupture of membranes (pPROM): she reported light amniotic fluid leak one hour before our observation. The admission assessment detected a reduced amniotic fluid index, a regular fetal growth and posterior placenta in the norm; the umbilical artery Doppler values were in the range, the fetal cardiac monitoring was regular and uterine contractions were present. The vaginal examination revealed a soft cervix, 80% effaced, dilated about 2 cm, and the fetus was in breech at station -3. The ultrasound cervical length was 24 mm. A single course of antenatal corticosteroid therapy for fetal lungs maturity induction and tocolytic drugs were

administered. On the second day of hospitalization, an emergency caesarean section was performed because the cervix was modified (dilatation about 4 cm), uterine contractility increased while persisting breech presentation (Fig. 1). A female infant was born weighing 2278 gr, with Apgar scores 8/9/9 at 1, 5, and 10 minutes respectively; the umbilical artery ph was 7.35. The placenta weighed 380 grams. The mother and the newborn, made an uncomplicated post-surgical/postnatal course and were discharged on day 3 and 15 respectively. Seventeen days after caesarean section, the woman came back again to our institution for a complaint of asthenia and fever (> 38°C), resistant to paracetamol for five days. On physical examination, she had abdominal tenderness in the lower quadrants and physiological vaginal lochia. Blood exams showed increased leukocyte and inflammatory markers: white blood cells (WBC) were $14,2 \times 10^3$/ml (range $4,0-10,0 \times 10^3$/ml); C-reactive protein (CRP) was 19.98 mg/l (range 0,01-1 mg/dl) and procalcitonin was 0.22 ng/ml (negative: <0,05 ng/ml). The pelvic ultrasound and the computerized tomography (CT) demonstrated a pelvic abscess neighboring to the lower anterior wall of the uterus with dimensions of 53 x 47 mm (Fig. 2). The treatment started immediately and consisted in intravenous antibiotic therapy with Meropenem 500 mg three times a day and low-molecular weight heparin (LMWH), Enoxaparin 4000 UI subcutaneous daily. Six days after the hospital admission with the right therapy, the inflammatory indices reduced: WBC were $9,8 \times 10^3$/ml, PCR was 4.37 mg/l and procalcitonin was 0.12 ng/ml. After discharge, we started a follow-up to assess the clinical conditions of our patient: she was

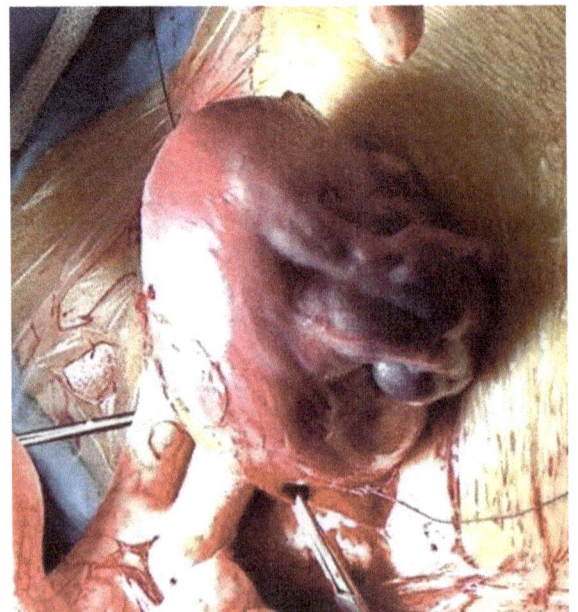

Fig. 1 Uterus at the time of caesarean delivery

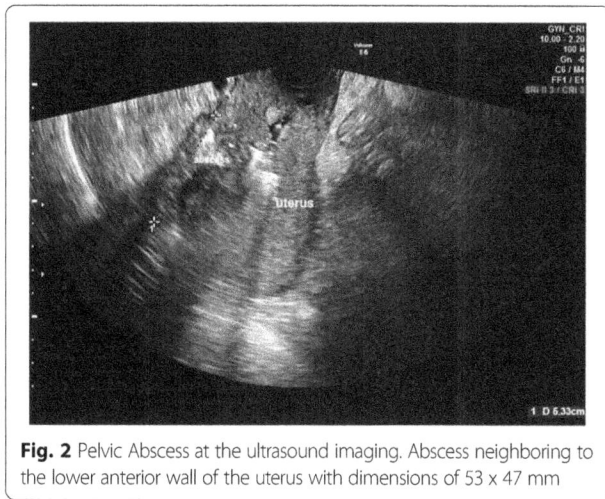

Fig. 2 Pelvic Abscess at the ultrasound imaging. Abscess neighboring to the lower anterior wall of the uterus with dimensions of 53 x 47 mm

asymptomatic, her blood exams were within normal ranges and the pelvic abscess was significantly decreased. Histopathologic examination of the placenta and umbilical cord obtained after about 40 days, not identified signs of chorioamnionitis and/or funisitis.

Discussion

Müllerian duct anomalies affect 2-3% of women [10]. The combination of uterus didelphys -class III of American Fertility Society –AFS- classification [11] and obstructed hemivagina was described the first time in 1922 [12], then in 70's Herlyn, Werner and Wunderlich reported other similar cases associated with renal anomalies [1, 2]. In 1983 this condition was identified as a syndrome characterised by the triad of uterus didelphys, blind hemivagina and ipsilateral renal agenesis [13]. Since 2007 this syndrome was named with the acronym of OHVIRA syndrome (obstructed hemivagina, ipsilateral renal anomaly), including two of the three of defects of the HWWS, which consists of different uterus anomalies (uterus didelphys or uterus septum) and renal anomalies as well as renal agenesis or polycystic kidney [14–16]. The occurrence of the HWWS seems to be 0.1-3.8%, and it is probably underestimated [3]. HWWS was included in the class U3B uterine anomaly, class C2 cervix anomaly, and class V3 vaginal anomaly according to the classification of ESHRE/ESGE [17]. The exact etiology of HWWS is still unclear, but it may be related to an abnormal development of the para- and mesonephric ducts. Didelphys uterus results from the failure of the fusion and differentiation of the Müllerian ducts during the eight week, which should give rise to cervix and uterus [18]. The Wolffian ducts give rise to ureters and kidneys, so when one of these is absent, the ureter and the kidney cannot fuse and the ipsilateral Müllerian duct is lateralized moving away from the urogenital sinus, causing the formation of a blind sac that will correspond to the blind or obstructed hemivagina. The distal portion of the

vagina originating from the urogenital sinus is not affected and develops normally. Patients affected by HWWS have no specific symptoms until puberty [5], then they typically present acute pelvic pain, dysmenorrhea, presence of pelvic mass, recurrent urinary tract infections and urinary retention. The diagnosis usually comes in the adolescence, a few years after the menarche, rarely at the birth or during pregnancy [19, 20]. In fact there is only a case described in literature by Wu et al. of a neonate diagnosed for HWWS presenting as a mass prolapsing per vaginum [21]. Clinical suspicion and early diagnosis are imperative to making a timely treatment to prevent complications such as infertility, endometriosis, pelvic adhesions, pyosalpinx, hemato or pyocolpos, and other obstetrics problems [22]. MRI was considered the gold standard for the diagnosis, but the 3d ultrasound plays always a major role for the identification of uterine anomalies [23]. Diagnostic laparoscopy in HWWS should performed only when the diagnosis by imaging is not clear or when MRI is not available [5, 24]. Twenty-five percent of women affected by Müllerian ducts anomalies presents obstetric complications such as recurrent miscarriage, abnormal fetal presentation, postpartum hemorrhage, retained placenta, fetal mortality, fetal growth restriction, premature rupture of membranes [7]. Obstetric outcome of HWWS women was studied after different surgical treatments. These may consist of conservative treatments like the desobstruction of hemivagina, the therapeutic drainage of hematocolpos, the vaginal septotomy and marsupialization; or less conservative interventions like laparoscopic hemi-hysterectomy associated or not with ipsilateral salpingectomy [25–28]. The best treatment of HWWS is controversial but most of the authors conclude that an explorative laparoscopy with vaginal septotomy and drainage of hematocolpos is enough to restore the functionality of both part of the uterus, avoiding hemi-hysterectomy [29, 30]. However, HWWS has good obstetric prognosis: 87% of pregnancy rate [27], approximately 62% positive obstetric outcomes without complications during delivery [5, 7]. Haddad reported the reproductive performance of 42 patients with obstructed hemivagina, 9 of whom had 20 pregnancies with 69% of live births [31]. Heinonen reported the reproductive performance and obstetric complications of 49 patients affected by didelphys uterus finding that the incidence of primary infertility was not significantly increased in these women. The rate of spontaneous miscarriage was 21%, not significantly different from the general population (15-20%). Preterm birth took place in 24% of all parts. This rate is higher than that of the general population (9-10%). Instead the caesarean sections rate is 84% and it reflects the high incidence of the breech presentation (51%) [29, 32]. In the presentation of this case we drew attention to its rarity because it involves the left part of the body, while usually is the right side affected [28, 33, 34] and the association with a malformation of the skeleton of the lower limbs, ectrodactyly of the right foot, was not ever been reported in literature; we found only a case report which described the combination of HWWS and lumbar scoliosis [35] and we are not sure if the skeletal involvement could be only an incidental finding. However, not all authors agree that it is a rarity the involvement of the left side: Yavuz et al. presented a case series of 13 women affected by HWWS and 6 of them had anomalies on the left side of the uro-genital tract [36]. According to the classification proposed by Zhun et al, this case belonged to class 1.1 of HWWS with a complete vaginal obstruction for a blind hemivagina [37] and she had no fertility problems following surgery.

In our experience, we focused on the course and management of the pregnancy complicated of this disorder. The pregnancy we described was at high-risk and the surgical treatment performed during adolescence was the least recommended by literature, however the obstetric outcome was positive thanks to a straight maternal-fetal follow-up. Our case was characterized by two complications of the pregnancy: preterm labour with pPROM and breech presentation, which are frequent in HWWS in literature. Additionally, pPROM was related to uterine anomaly and probably promoted by the frequent infections of urinary tract [38] that may be present in this syndrome, [39], mostly in the pregnant female. The infection occurred post the cesarean section may be caused by the pPROM, the elongate surgery time, the numerous adhesions of the previous surgery, which are known risk factors in post-operative infections [40].

Conclusions

HWWS is an unusual congenital anomaly with clinical significance and different options for surgical management. An early correct diagnosis and treatment are the goal to relieve symptoms and prevent complications to preserve sexual and reproductive abilities. Despite this, the pregnancies of these women are at an increased risk for unfavorable obstetric outcomes and can be characterized more frequently by complications that must be managed promptly by an accurate and regular maternal and fetal follow-up.

Abbreviations
AFS: American Fertility Society; CRP: C-reactive protein; CT: Computed Computed tomographic; ESGE: European Society of Gynecological Endoscopy; ESHRE: European Society of Human Reproduction and Embryology; HWWS: Herlyn-Werner-Wunderlich syndrome; LMWH: Low Low molecular weight heparin; MRI: Magnetic Magnetic resonance imaging; OVHIRA: Obstructed Obstructed hemivagina ipsilateral renal anomaly; pPROM: Premature Premature rupture of membranes; WBC: White White blood cells

Acknowledgements
We thank Cinzia Bartolelli M.D and Linda Pirollo M.D for their contribution to the ultrasound imaging; Valeria Lucantoni M.D. and Flavia Pierucci M.D. for the intraoperative documentation.

Funding
Not applicable

Authors' contributions
SC, FC and MGS were involved in the management of the pregnancy of the patient. EP1 and LC collected data for the report. SC and EP1 wrote the manuscript. EP2 and MGS were involved in planning and supervised the work. All authors read and approved the final manuscript.

Competing interests
The authors declare that they have no competing interests.

Author details
[1]Department of Biomedicine and Prevention, Obstetrics and Gynecological Clinic, University of Rome "Tor Vergata", via Montpellier 1, 00133 Rome, Italy. [2]Department of Woman's and Child's Health, Obstetrics and Gynecological Unit, San Camillo-Forlanini Hospital, Circonvallazione Gianicolense 87, 00152 Rome, Italy.

References
1. Herlyn U, Werner H. Simultaneous occurrence of an open Gartner-duct cyst, a homolateral aplasia of the kidney and a double uterus as atypical syndrome of abnormalities. Geburtshilfe Frauenheilkd. 1971;31:340–7.
2. Wunderlich M. Unusual form of genital malformation with aplasia of the right kidney. Zentralbl Gynakol. 1976;98(9):559–62.
3. Burgis J. Obstructive Müllerian anomalies: case report, diagnosis, and management. AM J Obstet Gynaecol. 2001;185(2):338–44.
4. Orazi C, Lucchetti MC, Schingo PM, Marchetti P, Ferro F. Herlyn-Werner-Wunderlich syndrome: uterus didelphys, blind hemivagina and ipsilateral renal agenesis. Sonographic and MR findings in 11 cases. Pediatr Radiol. 2007;37(7):657–65.
5. Del Vescovo R, Battisti S, Di Paola V, Piccolo CL, Cazzato L, Sansoni I, Grasso RF, Beomonte Zobel B. Herlyn –Werner-Wunderlich syndrome: MRI findings, radiological guide (two cases and literature review), and differential diagnosis. BMC Med Imaging. 2012;12:4.
6. Shavell VL, Montgomery SE, Johnson SC, Diamond MP, Berman JM. Complete septate uterus, obstructed hemivagina, and ipsilateral renal anomaly: pregnancy course complicated by a rare urogenital anomaly. Arch Gynaecol Obstet. 2009;280:449–52.
7. Afrashtehfar CD, Pigña-García A, Afrashtehfar KI. Müllerian anomalies. Obstructed hemivagina and ipsilateral renal anomaly syndrome (OHVIRA). Cir Cir. 2014;82(4):460–71.
8. Jindal G, Parmar VR, Gupta VK. Ectrodactyly/split hand feet malformation. Indian J Hum Genet. 2009;15(3):140–2.
9. Hydir Z, Beale V, O'Connor R, Clayton-Smith J. Genitourinary malformations: an under-recognized feature of ectrodactyly, ectodermal dysplasia and cleft lip/palate syndrome. Clin Dysmorphol. 2017;26(2):78–82.
10. Lin PC, Bhatnagar KP, Nettleton S, Nakajima ST. Female genital anomalies affecting reproduction. Fert Steril. 2002;78(5):899–915.
11. American Fertility Society. The American Fertility Society classification of adnexal adhesions, distal tubal occlusion, tubal occlusion secondary to tubal

ligation, tubal pregnancies. Müllerian duct anomalies and intrauterine adhesions. Fert Steril. 1988;49:944–55.

12. Purslow CE. A case of unilateral haematocolpos, hematometra and haematosalpinx. J Obstet Gynaecol Br Emp. 1922;29:643.

13. Karag'ozov I. Herlyn –Werner-Wunderlich syndrome. Akush Ginekol (Sofiia). 1983;22(1):70–6.

14. Smith NA, Laufer MR. Obstructed hemivagina and ipsilateral renal anomaly (OHVIRA) syndrome: management and follow-up. Fert Steril. 2007;87(4):918–22.

15. Živković K, Prka M, Živković N, Bucko A, Habek D. Unusual case of OHVIRA syndrome with a single uterus, unrecognized before labor and followed by an intrapartum rupture of obstructed hemivagina. Arch Gynaecol Obstet. 2014;290:855–8.

16. Han B, Herndon CN, Rosen MP, Wang ZJ, Daldrup-Link H. Uterine didelphys associated with obstructed hemivagina and ipsilateral renal anomaly (OHVIRA) syndrome. Radiol Case Rep. 2015;5(1):327.

17. Grimbizis GF, Gordts S, Di Spiezio Sardo A, Brucker S, De Angelis C, Gergolet M, Li TC, Tanos V, Brölmann H, Gianaroli L, Campo R. The ESHRE-ESGE consensus on the classification of female genital tract congenital anomalies. Gynecol Surg. 2013;10(3):199–212.

18. Vercellini P, Daguati R, Somigliana E, Viganò P, Lanzani A, Fedele L. Asymmetric lateral distribution of obstructed hemivagina and renal agenesis in women with uterus didelphys institutional case series and a systematic literature review. Fert Steril. 2007;87(4):719–24.

19. Muraoka A, Tsuda H, Kotani T, Kikkawa F. Severe hemoperitoneum during pregnancy with obstructed hemivagina and ipsilateral renal anomaly syndrome: a case report. J Reprod Med. 2016;61:290–4.

20. Reis MI, Vicente AP, Cominho J, Gomes AS, Martins L, Nunes F. Pyometra and pregnancy with Herlyn –Werner-Wunderlich syndrome. Rev Bras Ginecol Obstet. 2016;38(12):623–8.

21. Wu T-H, Wu T-T, Ng Y-Y, et al. Herlyn-Werner-Wunderlich syndrome consisting of uterine didelphys, obstructed hemivagina and ipsilateral renal agenesis in a newborn. Pediatr Neonatol. 2012;53:68–71.

22. Bhoil R, Ahluwalia A, Chauhan N. Herlin Werner Wunderlich syndrome with hematocolpos: an unusual case report of full diagnostic approach and treatment. Int J Fert Steril. 2016;10(1):136–40.

23. Gungor Ugurlucan F, Bastu E, Gulsen G, Kurek Eken M, Akhan SE. OHVIRA syndrome presenting with acute abdomen: a case report and review of the literature. Clin Imaging. 2014;38(3):357–9.

24. Jeong J-H, Kim YJ, Chang C-H, Choi H-I. A case of Herlyn- Werner-Wunderlich syndrome with recurrent hematopyometra. J Women's Med. 2009;2(2):76–80.

25. Stassart JP, Nagel TC, Prem KA, Phipps WR. Uterus didelphys, obstructed hemivagina, and ipsilateral renal agenesis: the University of Minnesota experience. Fert Steril. 1992;57(4):756–61.

26. Monks P. Uterus didelphys associated with unilateral cervical atresia and renal agenesis. Aust N Z J Obstet Gynaecol. 1979;19(4):245–6.

27. Candiani GB, Fedele L, Candiani M. Double uterus, blind hemivagina, and ipsilateral renal agenesis:36 cases and long-term follow-up. Obstet Gynaecol. 1997;90(1):26–32.

28. Chen FP, Ng KK. Term pregnancy at the site of atresia following vaginal canalization in a case of uterus didelphys with hemivaginal atresia and ipsilateral renal agenesis. Taiwan J Obstet Gynaecol. 2006;45(4):366–8.

29. Cozzolino M, Corioni S, Magro Malosso ER, Sorbi F, Mecacci F. Two successful pregnancies in Herlyn –Werner-Wunderlich syndrome. J Obstet and Gynaecol. 2014;34(6):534–5.

30. Altchek A, Paciuc J. Successful pregnancy following surgery in the obstructed uterus in a uterus didelphys with unilateral distal vaginal agenesis and ipsilateral renal agenesis: case report and literature review. J Pediatr Adolesc Gynaecol. 2009;22(5):e159–62.

31. Haddad B, Barranger E, Paniel BJ. Blind hemivagina: long-term follow -up and reproductive performance in 42 cases. Hum Reprod. 1999;14(8):1962–4.

32. Heinonen PK. Clinical implications of the didelphic uterus: long-term follow-up of 49 cases. Eur J Obstet Gynecol Reprod Biol. 2000;91(2):183–90.

33. Adair L 2nd, Georgiades M, Osborne R, Ng T. Uterus didelphys with unilateral distal vaginal agenesis and ipsilateral renal agenesis: common presentation of an unusual variation. J Radiol Case Rep. 2011;5(1):1–8.

34. Singh K, Thakur S, Soni A, Verma A. Herlyn-Werner-Wunderlich syndrome/ OHVIRA syndrome; a rare urogenital anomaly with unusual presentation in two case with review of literature. Clinics Mother Child Health. 2016;13(1):1–4.

35. Li Z, Yu X, Shen J, Liang J. Scoliosis in Herlyn-Werner-Wunderlich syndrome: a case report and literature review. Medicine (Baltimore). 2014;93(28):e185.

36. Yavuz A, Bora A, Kurdoğlu M, Goya C, Kurdoğlu Z, Beyazal M, Akdemir Z. Herlyn-Werner-Wunderlich syndrome: merits of sonographic and magnetic resonance imaging for accurate diagnosis and patient management in 13 cases. J Pediatr Adolesc Gynecol. 2015;28(1):47–52.

37. Zhun L, Chen N, Tong JL, Wang W, Zhang L, Lang JH. New classification of Herlyn –Werner-Wunderlich syndrome. Chin Med J (Engl). 2015;128(2):222–5.

38. Karat C, Madhivanan P, Krupp K, Poornima S, Jayanthi NV, Suguna JS, Mathai E. The clinical and microbiological correlates of premature rupture of membranes. Indian J Med Microbiol. 2006;24(4):283–5.

39. Tsai JL, Tsai SF. Case Report: A Rare Cause of Complicated Urinary Tract Infection in a Woman with Herlyn-Werner-Wunderlich Syndrome. Iran Red Crescent Med J. 2016;18(11):e40267.

40. Kawakita T, Landy HJ. Surgical site infection after cesarean delivery: epidemiology, prevention and treatment. Maternal Health Neonatol Perinatol. 2017;3:12.

21

Male involvement in the maternal health care system: implication towards decreasing the high burden of maternal mortality

Amanual Getnet Mersha

Abstract

Background: One of the essential components of antenatal care (ANC) is birth preparedness and complication readiness (BP/CR). Strengthening BP/CR measures is one of the principal strategies to reduce maternal mortality and morbidity. The current study aimed at determining the level of men's knowledge about obstetric danger signs, and their involvement in BP/CR among community of Northwest Ethiopia.

Method: A cross-sectional community based survey was conducted in Northwest Ethiopia from May 2016 to July 2016. Data was analyzed by the Statistical Package for the Social Sciences software Version 21.0 for Windows. Participants' socio-demographic characteristics, knowledge of obstetric danger signs, and level of involvement in BP/CR were described using frequencies and percentages. Bivariate and multivariable logistic regressions were employed to explore the associated factors and P-value of 0.05 was used as a cut-off point to declare significant association.

Result: From 856 men who were invited for the study, 824 men agreed for the interview giving a response rate of 96. 2%. Half of the men stated one danger sign that may occur during pregnancy 407(49.4%); one third during delivery 271(32.9%); and 213(25.8%) during postpartum period. Among all participants, 256(31.1%) had not made any preparations; 363(44.1%) made one step; 116(14.1%) made two steps; 82(9.9%) made three steps; 5(0.6%) made four steps; 2(0.24%) made five steps; and no one made all the birth preparation steps during the birth of their last child. BP/CR was significantly association with knowledge of at least one danger sign during pregnancy (AOR = 3.3, 95% CI: 3.1, 3.9); during delivery (AOR = 2.2, 95% CI: 1.1, 2.8); and post partum period (AOR = 1.8, 95% CI: 1.1, 2.4). Furthermore, BP/CR was found to be positively associated with being married, completing college education, escorting wife to antenatal care, and urban residence.

Conclusions: Men's level of knowledge about obstetric danger signs, and their involvement in BP/CR was found to be very poor. Considering the importance of male involvement in the maternal health care, it is recommended to advocate policies and strategies that can improve awareness of men and enhance their engagement in the maternal care.

Keywords: Ethiopia, Birth preparedness, Complication readiness

Correspondence: amanuelget16@gmail.com
Department of Gynecology and Obstetrics, School of Medicine, College of Medicine and Health Sciences, University of Gondar, P.O. Box: 196, Gondar, Ethiopia

Background

Globally, an estimated number of 303,000 maternal deaths occur annually from causes related to pregnancy and childbirth. Around 99% of these deaths occur in developing countries and sub-Saharan African accounts for almost half of the maternal deaths (44%) [1, 2]. Maternal death may occur from complications that may occur while a woman is pregnant, during labor or after delivery. Preparing for birth and related complications ahead of time markedly reduce the number of women dying from such preventable causes [3].

One of the essential components of antenatal care (ANC) is birth preparedness and complication readiness (BP/CR). Birth preparedness and complication readiness (BP/CR) includes detection of danger signs, a plan for a birth attendant, a plan for the place of delivery, preparing potential blood donor and saving money for transport or other [4]. Some of the obstetric complications such as hemorrhage are difficult to precisely predict which mother will develop the complications, therefore every pregnant woman and spouse should make the necessary birth plans [5]. After the International Conference on Population and Development (ICPD) and 4th World Conference on Women held at Cairo [6] and Beijing [7] respectively, men's involvement in maternal health care system is being advocated. Studies had shown the helpful impact of male participation in maternal health in developing countries by improving maternal access to antenatal and postnatal services [8, 9].

The 2015 World Health Organization (WHO) recommendation on maternal and newborn health promotion interventions included active involvement of men during pregnancy, child birth and post partum period as an effective intervention to improve maternal as well as newborn health outcomes. However, male involvement is recommended provided only that women's autonomy in making their own decisions is respected [8].

A systematic review that included 13 studies aimed at assessing the effect of male partner involvement in low and middle income countries as an intervention to improve maternal health outcomes was published in 2018. The review demonstrated that male engagement as an intervention improves antenatal care utilization, postpartum care utilization, delivery at health facilities, child birth by a skilled attendant, and birth preparation and complication readiness [9].

Social norms, beliefs and values affect the types and extent of support that a pregnant woman can receive from her husband or other family members. For instance, a study conducted in Bangladesh showed low level of facility delivery service utilization among women whose husbands believed childbirth is a natural physiologic process that does not require a medical care; and women whose husbands were pressurized by other family members about appropriate place of delivery [10].

In societies where social norms, beliefs and values weaken women's rights, men have social as well as economical supremacy over their partners. Hence, in such patriarchal societies men make a decision regarding sexual affairs, family size, women's access to economic resources and health care service utilization. Achieving sustainable development goals (SDGs) requires alleviating gender based inequalities as well as improving male partner participation in the maternal health care system [11]. Male involvement should be continuously monitored so that it will not worsen gender inequality and affect women's reproductive rights [8].

A study conducted in Oromia regional state of Ethiopia showed that 89% of males were involved in deciding home as their spouses place of deliver [12]. In Patriarchal societies social norms, values and low attitude towards empowering women affects a women's level of maternal health service utilization. Hence, a careful engagement of male partners in the maternal health service in such communities may be an effective strategy to improve maternal health service utilization and reduce maternal morbidity as well as mortality. It is essential to assess men's current level of awareness and involvement in the maternal health care system in order to plan an effective intervention strategy to improve their involvement. Therefore, the current study aimed at assessing men's level of knowledge concerning obstetric danger signs, their level of birth preparedness and complication readiness (BP/CR) in Northwest Ethiopia.

Methods

Study design and setting

A cross-sectional descriptive community survey was conducted in North Gondar Zone, Northwest Ethiopia from May 3, 2016 to July 5, 2016. This zone has 19 districts; the zone has a total population of 2,903,165, of this 14.1% being urban residents.

Sample size and sampling technique

The sample size was calculated by using single population proportion formula by taking 5% desired precision, 95% confidence interval, assuming 42% men awareness of danger signs [21], design effect of 2 for cluster sampling and 10% non response rate, which results in sample size of 710. A multi stage cluster sampling procedure was employed to select four districts out of 19 districts of North Gondar zone. Firstly four districts, three rural districts and one urban district were randomly selected. All households within the catchment areas having men whose wife had given birth within the last 2 years were invited to interview. A total of 856 men were invited to participate in the study.

Data collection and management

A self administered questionnaire was adopted for our setting from Johns Hopkins Program for International Education in Gynecology and Obstetrics (JHPIEGO) [13]. The questionnaire has three sections: The first section is regarding socio demographic characteristics of the participants. The second section assesses participant's knowledge of obstetric danger signs during pregnancy, labor and post partum periods. The final section assesses birth preparedness and complication readiness among participants during the birth of their last baby. The data collection process had taken 2 months (from May 3, 2016 to July 5, 2016). Data was collected by five properly trained research assistants with previous experiences in survey data collection. So as to maintain the quality of the data the researcher reviewed collected data daily and sent feedbacks to the data collectors continuously. BP/CR practice was considered "well prepared" for BP/CR when at least three of the following six practices were reported to have been made in the birth of the last baby: prepared birth kit, identified a skilled attendant, saved money, knew where to go in case of emergency, contacted a blood donor in advance and prepared transportation in advance. Men who reported less than half of the above stated steps were considered to be less prepared. If at least three steps were reported as having been made, the respondent was labeled as well prepared. The three out six was chosen because previous studies have used 50% and above to determine who was well prepared [14]. The questionnaire, originally written in English, was translated to local language (Amharic) and back to English in order to ensure that the translated version gives the proper meaning. The content validity of the questionnaire was confirmed by local experts, including reproductive health experts. (Additional file 1) The questionnaire was pretested on 5% of the sample size prior to the real data collection, which was excluded from the final study. Considering the high burden of puerperal sepsis in this community, which is common in the first 10 days of postpartum period and accounts for 13% of maternal deaths in Ethiopia [15], The time frame of first 2 days in the questionnaire used by Johns Hopkins Program for International Education in Gynecology and Obstetrics (JHPIEGO) was amended to cover maternal health problems in the first 10 days of the post partum period. Once data were collected, each questionnaire was checked for completeness.

Operational definitions

Male partner

Male who has/had a spouse by means of formal marriage or informal union.

Birth preparedness and complication readiness (BP/CR)

Is a process of planning for normal birth and anticipating the actions needed in cases of an emergency.

Level of birth preparedness and complication readiness (BP/CR)

The steps made to have a normal birth outcome during the previous child birth.

Well prepared for birth

If at least three of the following steps have been made in the childbirth process of the last baby: prepared birth kit, identified a skilled attendant, saved money, knew where to go in cases of emergency, contacted a blood donor in advance and prepared transportation in advance.

Statistical analysis

The final data collection tool was checked for completeness, and responses were entered into and analyzed by the Statistical Package for the Social Sciences software Version 21.0 for Windows. Participants' socio-demographic characteristics, knowledge of obstetric danger signs, and level of BP/CR were described using frequencies and percentages in tables. Bivariate logistic regression was conducted to explore factors associated with BP/CR and factors that were found to have a p value of less than 0.2 were entered in to multivariable logistic regression. To declare significant association P-value 0.05 was used as a cut-off point and results expressed by using odds ratio (OR) with 95% confidence interval (CI).

Ethical considerations

This study was approved by the Institutional review board of University of Gondar. Informed written consent was obtained from each participant before starting the interview and participants were also told their right to stop the interview at anytime. The participants were also told that participation is based on their willingness. The obtained information was kept anonymous and recorded in such a way that the respondent could never be known.

Results

Socio-demographic characteristics of participants and their spouses

From 856 men who were invited for participation, 824 men agreed to the interview giving a response rate of 96.2%. A total of 721(87.5%) of the participants were found to be married and half of them have 3–4 children 403(48.9%). One third of the respondents 288(34.9%) did not go to school or did not complete their primary education. Participants from the rural areas accounts for the majority of respondents 637(77.3%). Participants who had escorted their wives to ANC follow up in previous pregnancy accounted for 334(40.5%) of the total participants and a quarter 201(24.4%) of the participants' spouses had delivered in a health facility. A total of 118(14.3%) participants' spouses had obstetric complication in their last pregnancy. (Table 1).

Knowledge of obstetric danger signs

Half of the participants had stated at least one danger sign during pregnancy 407(49.4%); 271(32.9%) of the participants stated at least one danger sign during delivery 271(32.9%) and fewer, 213(25.8%), of the participants stated at least one danger sign during the postpartum period. The commonest mentioned danger sign during pregnancy was high fever 105(12.7%) and excessive vaginal bleeding accounts for the majority of responses during childbirth as well as during the post partum

period. 85(10.3%) participants mentioned prolonged labor as a danger sign. There were also other signs mentioned which were not stated in the table such as anemia, dizziness, palpitation that accounted for 10.1% during pregnancy, 3.2% during delivery and 2.7% during postpartum period. (Table 2).

Level of BP/CR in spouses' previous pregnancy

As illustrated in table three, the most common preparations made during the birth of their last child were getting birth kit 309(37.5%) followed by saving money 218(26.5%). (Table 3) Furthermore, 91(11%) of the participants had arranged transportation, 25(3%) had identified which health facility to visit in case of emergency, 67(8.1%) had identified a skilled birth attendant, 3(0.4%) prepared possible blood donor during the birth of their last baby. Two hundred and fifty six men

Table 1 Socio-demographic characteristics of men and spouse's obstetric characteristics

Characteristic	N (%)
Age	
18–24	154(18.7%)
25–34	198(24%)
35–44	353(42.8%)
> 44	119(14.4%)
Marital status	
Single/divorced/widowed	103(12.5%)
Married	721(87.5%)
Number of children	
1–2	173(21%)
3–4	403(48.9%)
More than 4	248(30.1%)
Education	
No education	150(18.2%)
Primary Incomplete	138(16.7%)
Primary Complete	311(37.7%)
Secondary	124(15%)
College and above	101(12.3%)
Residence	
Rural	637(77.3%)
Urban	187(22.7%)
Escorted wife to ANC previous pregnancy	
Yes	334(40.5%)
No	490(59.5%)
Obstetric complication in previous pregnancy	
Yes	118(14.3%)
No	706(85.7%)
Place of delivery previous pregnancy	
Home	623(75.6%)
Health facility	201(24.4%)

Table 2 Men's knowledge of danger signs during pregnancy, labor and postpartum

Obstetric danger sign	N (%)
During Pregnancy	
High fever	105(12.7%)
Severe abdominal pain	97(11.8%)
Excessive vaginal bleeding	94(11.4%)
Abnormal body movements	61(7.4%)
Severe headache	70(8.5%)
Swollen hands/face	59(7.2%)
Loss of consciousness	33(4%)
Blurred vision	13(1.6%)
Knowledge of at least one sign	407(49.4%)
During Childbirth	
Excessive vaginal bleeding	102(12.4%)
Abnormal body movements	54(6.5%)
Retained placenta	37(4.5%)
High fever	98(11.9%)
Prolonged labor	85(10.3%)
Severe headache	64(7.8%)
Loss of consciousness	29(3.5%)
Knowledge of at least one sign	271(32.9%)
During postpartum	
Excessive vaginal bleeding	105(12.7%)
High fever	99(12%)
Abnormal body movements	56(6.8%)
Loss of consciousness	31(3.8%)
Foul smelling discharge	74(8.9%)
Severe headache	78(9.5%)
Knowledge at least one sign	213(25.8%)

Multiple responses possible

Table 3 BP/CR among men in previous pregnancy

BP/CR	N (%)
Identified birth kit	309(37.5%)
Saved money	218(26.5%)
Identified transport	91(11%)
Identified a blood donor in advance	3(0.4%)
Identified where to go for emergency	25(3%)
Identified skilled attendant	67(8.1%)
Made at least 3 steps	82(9.9%)

Multiple responses possible

(31.1%) had not done any preparations; 363(44.1%) had made one of the six birth preparing steps assessed; 116(14.1%) made two preparations; 82(9.9%) made three preparations; 5(0.6%) made four preparations; 2(0.24%) had made five preparations; furthermore, no one made all the six preparations assessed in the current study. (Fig. 1).

Factors associated with BP/CR

Place of residency, current marital status, escorting wife to antenatal care in previous pregnancy, number of children, level of education, knowledge of at least one danger sign during pregnancy, knowledge of at least one danger sign during delivery and knowledge of at least one danger sign during the postpartum period were associated with BP/CR in the bivariate logistic regression analysis. Further analysis by using multivariable logistic regression demonstrates that completing college education have a significant positive association with the steps taken for birth preparation and complication readiness (AOR = 3.2, 95% CI: 2.8, 4.6). Being married, escorting

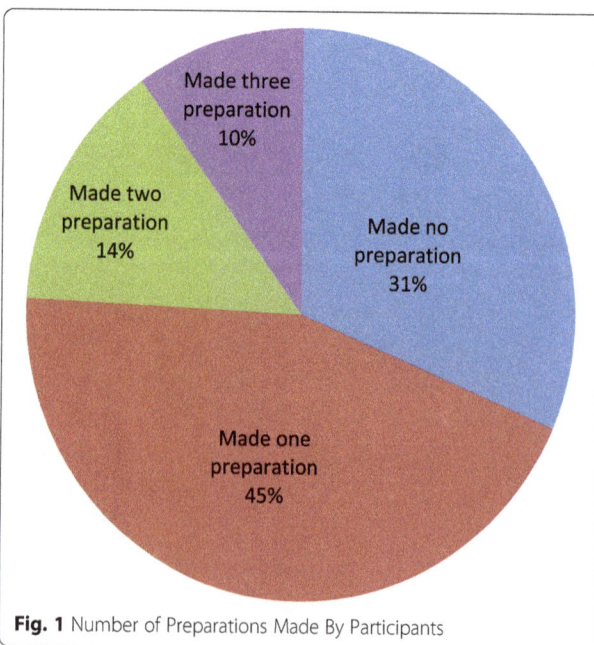

Fig. 1 Number of Preparations Made By Participants

wife to antenatal care, and urban residence were also found to be significantly associated with the steps taken for birth preparation and complication readiness. Furthermore, the steps made towards birth preparation and complication readiness were found to have significant associations with knowledge of at least one danger sign during pregnancy (AOR = 3.3, 95% CI: 3.1, 3.9), during delivery (AOR = 2.2, 95% CI: 1.1, 2.8) and post partum period (AOR = 1.8, 95% CI: 1.1, 2.4). (Table 4).

Discussion

As part of a comprehensive antenatal care provision a pregnant woman and her family should be provided with detailed information about pregnancy, child birth, and obstetric danger signs that may occur in the process of child birth [4]. Antenatal care creates a good opportunity for the service providers to develop a birth plan with a women and her spouse. Involving men on the maternal health care system improves health service utilization, decrease rate of maternal depression, raise maternal self-esteem, and decreased possibility of childbirth complications [16–20].

Male residents in Northwest Ethiopia were found to have inadequate awareness regarding obstetric danger signs. This could be due to the low percentage of participants who had accompanied their spouses to antenatal care during previous pregnancy (40.5%) and low percentage of facility delivery rate (24.4%). It could also be due to deficiencies in community health education programs in the country. The findings of this research are similar with a study conducted in Southern Ethiopia which reported that only 42.2% of men were found to be aware of the obstetric danger signs [21]. Similarly, other studies conducted in different countries also reported men's inadequate knowledge concerning the obstetric danger signs. However, our findings are in contrast with one study that assessed Kenyan men's awareness of obstetric danger signs in which the median knowledge score was reported to be 9 out of 10 selected danger signs. This discrepancy may relate to differences in study method; in the Kenyan study men were asked to say yes or no after 10 danger signs were read to them by the interviewer [22].

Although majority of maternal morbidities and mortalities occur in the immediate postpartum period [23], men in this community were able to state fewer possible danger signs in the postpartum period as compared to other periods (ante partum and delivery). This may be due to low level of postnatal care utilization (20.2%) in communities of Northwest Ethiopia [24] and/or the cultural practice in rural parts of Ethiopia that postpartum women spend their postpartum period with their mothers. This result is in line with a study conducted in

Table 4 Association between selected socio-demographic characteristics, obstetric characteristics, knowledge of danger signs and BP/CR

Characteristic	Prepared N (%)	Less prepared N (%)	Bivariate Analysis Unadjusted OR (95%CI)	Multivariable Analysis AOR (95%CI)
Age				
18–24	12(7.8%)	142(92.2%)	1	
25–34	15(7.6%)	183(92.4%)	0.4 (0.3–1.2)	
35–44	43(12.2%)	310(87.8%)	1.7 (0.6–6.2)	
> 44	12(10.1%)	107(89.9%)	0.5 (0.2–2.8)	
Number of children				
1–2	18(10.4%)	155(89.6%)	1	
3–4	39(9.7%)	364(90.3%)	0.4 (0.2–5.4)	
More than 4	25(10.1%)	223(89.9%)	1.4 (1.3–2.1)	
Education				
No education	9(6%)	141(94%)	1	
Primary Incomplete	11(7.9%)	127(92.1%)	1.5 (0.3–6.2)	
Primary complete	20(6.4%)	291(93.6%)	1.7 (0.8–3.9)	
Secondary	17(13.7%)	107(86.3%)	1.3 (1.2–2.5)	
College and above	25(24.7%)	76(75.3%)	3.8 (2.9–5.1)	3.2(2.8–4.6)*
Marital status				
Married	78(10.8%)	643(89.2%)	3.1 (2.8–3.6)	2.3(1.6–3.5)*
Single/divorced/widowed	4(3.8%)	99(96.2%)	1	
Residence				
Urban	46(24.6%)	141(75.4%)	5.8 (4.3–6.3)	4.2(2.9–5.6)*
Rural	36(5.7%)	601(94.3%)	1	
Escorted Wife to ANC in the previous pregnancy				
Yes	43(12.9%)	291(87.1%)	2.7 (1.8–3.2)	1.7(1.6–2.9)*
No	39 (8%)	451 (92%)	1	
Knowledge of at least one danger sign during pregnancy				
Yes	61(15)	346(85)	3.1 (2.5–3.4)	3.3(3.1–3.9)*
No	21(5.1)	396(94.9)	1	
Knowledge of at least one danger sign during labor				
Yes	39(14.4)	232(85.6)	3.7 (2.3–3.8)	2.2(1.1–2.8)*
No	43(7.8)	510(92.2)	1	
Knowledge of at least one danger sign postpartum				
Yes	37(17.4%)	176(82.6%)	2.6 (1.5–2.7)	1.8(1.1–2.4)*
No	45(7.4%)	566(92.6%)	1	

*p value< 0.05, in the table the number "1" indicates the reference variable

rural Tanzania that reported higher numbers of danger signs stated in the ante partum period [14].

We found discrepancies between men's knowledge and the common causes of maternal complications. The most common obstetric danger signs men reported in relation to pregnancy were high fever (12.7%), severe abdominal pain (11.8%), and vaginal bleeding (11.4%). The finding of this study is in agreement with a study conducted in Southern Ethiopia that reported vaginal bleeding and severe abdominal pain as the most stated

danger sign that may occur in the ante partum period [21]. In a Tanzanian study high fever, abdominal pain and vaginal bleeding were also commonly mentioned danger signs in the ante partum period [14]. A review conducted in 2014 reported that among all maternal deaths in Ethiopia obstructed labor and sepsis accounts for 29 and 13% respectively [15]. In a study conducted in Southwest Ethiopia, the incidence of obstructed labor was reported to be 12.2% [25]. However, prolonged labor as a danger sign during delivery was mentioned only by

10.3% of participants. Only 12% of participants mentioned fever as a danger sign in the postpartum period. Hence, awareness creation interventions are recommended in order to reduce major causes of maternal mortality and morbidity in this community.

Men's involvement in birth preparedness and complication readiness in this community was found to be scarce. Only 82(9.9%) participants reported making at least three of the six assessed steps during the birth of their last baby. A southern Ethiopian study also reported a low level (9.4%) of male involvement in BP/CR issues [21]. Moreover, the finding of this study is also in line with studies from other countries like Tanzania and Uganda [14, 26]. The low level of involvement in BP/CR may be explained by the low antenatal service utilization in this area, the poor quality of the service, mostly husbands did not accompany their wives during antenatal visit and even if they come there are also failures from the service providers to invite husbands to join the counseling process [26–29].

Higher level of education, being married, escorting wife to antenatal care, urban residence were found to have positive significant association with birth preparation and complication readiness. This may be due to the fact that those who have higher level of education have good level of understanding of the complications and importance of having a birth plan. In addition to that urban dwellers will access information as well as birth kits easily as compared to rural dwellers. Most of the educated ones have urban residency which can also explain the low level of birth preparation and complication readiness among rural residents. Escorting wife to antenatal care will increase exposure with health professionals that may improve the probability of being prepared for complications and childbirth. These factors were also found to be associated with men's involvement in BP/CR in studies conducted among other African countries like Tanzania and Uganda [30–32].

In the current study men's level of involvement in BP/CR was found to have a significant association with knowledge of obstetric danger signs during pregnancy, labor and postpartum. This may be due to the fact that knowledge of danger signs leads to greater anticipation and preparation to lessen effects of pregnancy and childbirth complications by reducing the first two delays (delay in decision making and delay in transportation) to tackle obstetric complications. The norms and values of the community towards women may have affected their interest of engaging in the maternal health issues. This finding is similar with a study conducted among male residents of southern Ethiopia which reported that awareness of danger signs doubles involvement [21].

Limitations and strengths of the study

As this is a cross sectional study, it is not possible to provide a causal relationship between being well-prepared and other variables. Moreover, the participants were required to remember things happened in the past 2 years so there is a possibility of recall bias. Although, all the necessary precautions were followed to maintain the quality of the data, it is not possible to avoid the effect of data collector's attitude on the quality of the data. These limitations mean that caution is required when generalizing the results to other settings. Despite these limitations our study demonstrates a lot of strengths. One of the strengths of this study was the large number of participate in the study and men's knowledge of danger signs and BP/CR were not assessed in this area previously.

Conclusions and recommendations

The current study demonstrated men's low level of knowledge concerning obstetrical danger signs as well as their involvement in birth preparedness and complication readiness in Northwest Ethiopia. This study also showed a strong association between BP/CR and men's level of awareness concerning obstetric danger signs. Additionally, BP/CR was also found to have a significant association with higher educational level, being married, escorting wife to antenatal care in their spouses' previous pregnancy, and being an urban resident. In patriarchal communities like Ethiopia so as to improve the maternal health service utilization, involving men in the maternal health care system without worsening the already existing gender inequalities is an essential strategy. Hence, it is recommended to advocate policies and strategies that can improve men's level of awareness and their engagement in the maternal care through health education and incentives. Community based awareness creation by utilizing mass media and campaigning is recommended. It is recommended to give special emphasis to improving utilization of postnatal care to improve the low level of knowledge in the post partum period, were most of maternal mortalities occur, as compared to the ante-partum and intra-partum period.

Abbreviations
ANC: Antenatal care; BP/CR: Birth preparedness and complication readiness

Acknowledgements
The author acknowledges the Support of University of Gondar, data analyst and data collectors. The author is very thankful for all the participants.

Funding

No financial support was gained to conduct this study.

Competing interests

The author declares that there are no competing interests.

References

1. Trends in maternal mortality. 1990 to 2015: estimates by WHO, UNICEF, UNFPA, World Bank Group and the United Nations Population Division. Geneva: World Health Organization. p. 2015.

2. Hogan MC, Foreman KJ, Naghavi M, Ahn SY, Wang M, Makela SM, et al. Maternal mortality for 181 countries, 1980-2008: a systematic analysis of progress towards millennium development goal 5. Lancet (London, England). 2010;375(9726):1609–23.

3. McPherson RA, Khadka N, Moore JM, Sharma M. Are birth-preparedness programmes effective? Results from a field trial in Siraha district, Nepal. J Health Popul Nutr. 2006;24(4):479–88.

4. Carroli G, Piaggio G, Khan-Neelofur D. WHO systematic review of randomised controlled trials of routine antenatal care. Lancet. 2001; 357(9268):1565–70. https://doi.org/10.1016/S0140-6736(00)04723-1.

5. Tura G, Afework MF, Yalew AW. The effect of birth preparedness and complication readiness on skilled care use: a prospective follow-up study in Southwest Ethiopia. Reprod Health. 2014;11:60.

6. Alison McIntosh C, L. Finkle J. The Cairo Conference on Population and Development: A New Paradigm? 1995. 223 p.

7. Larson EL.,"United Nations Fourth World Conference on Women: Action for Equality, Development, and Peace (Beijing, China: September 1995)",Emory Int'l L Rev,vol. 10, pp.1996. Accessed at http://www.un.org/womenwatch/daw/beijing/pdf/Beijing%20full%20report%20E.pdf.

8. Davis J, Luchters S and Holmes W. Men and maternal and newborn health: benefits, harms, challenges and potential strategies for engaging men. Melbourne: Centre for International Health, Burnet Institute; 2012 (http://www.comminit.com/hiv-aids/content/men-and-maternal-and-newborn-health-benefits-harms-challenges-and-potential-strategies-e. Accessed 12 Jan 2015).

9. Tokhi M, Comrie-Thomson L, Davis J, Portela A, Chersich M, Luchters S. Involving men to improve maternal and newborn health: a systematic review of the effectiveness of interventions. PLoS One. 2018;13(1):e0191620.

10. Story, et al. Husbands' involvement in delivery care utilization in rural Bangladesh: a qualitative study. BMC Pregnancy Childbirth. 2012;12:28. https://doi.org/10.1186/1471-2393-12-28.

11. Amnesty International. Women, Violence and health. London: Amnesty International; 2005. Accessed at https://www.amnestyusa.org/pdfs/mazeofinjustice.pdf.

12. Wassie L, Bekele A, Ismael A, Tariku N, Heran A, Getnet M, et al. Magnitude and factors that affect males' involvement in deciding partners' place of delivery in Tiyo District of Oromia region, Ethiopia. Ethiop J Heal Dev. 2014;28:1–43.

13. JHPIEGO (2004) Monitoring Birth Preparedness and Complication Readiness: Tools and Indicators for Maternal and Newborn Health. Baltimore: JHPIEGO;. Available: https://pdf.usaid.gov/pdf_docs/pnada619.pdf.

14. August F, Pembe AB, Mpembeni R, Axemo P, Darj E. Men's knowledge of obstetric danger signs, birth preparedness and complication readiness in rural Tanzania. PLoS One. 2015;10(5):e0125978.

15. Berhan Y, Berhan A. Causes of maternal mortality in Ethiopia: a significant decline in abortion related death. Ethiop J Health Sci. 2014;24(Suppl):15–28.

16. Schaffer MA, Lia-Hoagberg B. Effects of social support on prenatal care and health behaviors of low-income women. J Obstet Gynecol Neonatal Nurs. 1997;26:433–40.

17. Yargawa J, Leonardi-Bee J. Male involvement and maternal health outcomes: systematic review and meta-analysis. J Epidemiol Community Health. 2015;69(6):604–12.

18. Berhane Y. Male involvement in reproductive health. Ethiop J Health Dev. 2006;20(3):135–6.

19. Lewis G. Beyond the numbers: reviewing maternal deaths and complications to make pregnancy safer. Br Med Bull. 2003;67:27–37.

20. Koblinsky MA. Beyond maternal mortality--magnitude, interrelationship, and consequences of women's health, pregnancy-related complications and nutritional status on pregnancy outcomes. Int J Gynaecol Obstet. 1995; 48(Suppl):S21–32.

21. Debiso AT, Gello BM, Malaju MT. Factors Associated with Men's Awareness of Danger Signs of Obstetric Complications and Its Effect on Men's Involvement in Birth Preparedness Practice in Southern Ethiopia, 2014. Adv Public Health. 2015;2015:9.

22. Dunn A, Haque S, Innes M. Rural Kenyan men's awareness of danger signs of obstetric complications. Pan Afr Med J. 2011;10:39.

23. Khan KS, Wojdyla D, Say L, Gulmezoglu AM, Van Look PF. WHO analysis of causes of maternal death: a systematic review. Lancet. 2006;367:1066–74.

24. Workineh YG, Hailu DA. Factors Affecting Utilization of Postnatal Care Service in Amhara Region, Jabitena District, Ethiopia. Sci J Public Health. 2014;2(3):169–76. https://doi.org/10.11648/j.sjph.20140203.15.

25. Fantu S, Segni H, Alemseged F. Incidence, causes and outcome of obstructed labor in jimma university specialized hospital. Ethiop J Health Sci. 2010;20(3):145–51.

26. Kabakyenga JK, Ostergren PO, Turyakira E, Pettersson KO. Knowledge of obstetric danger signs and birth preparedness practices among women in rural Uganda. Reprod Health. 2011;8:33.

27. Sekoni OO, Owoaje ET. Male knowledge of danger signs of obstetric complications in an urban city in South west Nigeria. Annals of Ibadan postgraduate medicine. 2014;12(2):89–95.

28. Pembe AB, Urassa DP, Carlstedt A, Lindmark G, Nystrom L, Darj E. Rural Tanzanian women's awareness of danger signs of obstetric complications. BMC Pregnancy Childbirth. 2009;9:12.

29. Rashad WM, Essa R. Women's Awareness of Danger Signs of Obstetrics Complications; 2010. p. 1299–306.

30. Kakaire O, Kaye DK, Osinde MO. Male involvement in birth preparedness and complication readiness for emergency obstetric referrals in rural Uganda. Reprod Health. 2011;8(1):12.

31. Tweheyo R, Konde-Lule J, Tumwesigye NM, Sekandi JN. Male partner attendance of skilled antenatal care in peri-urban Gulu district, Northern Uganda. BMC Pregnancy Childbirth. 2010;10:53.

32. Redshaw M, Henderson J. Fathers' engagement in pregnancy and childbirth: evidence from a national survey. BMC Pregnancy Childbirth. 2013;13:70.

22

Risk factors associated with the development of postpartum diabetes in Japanese women with gestational diabetes

Yukari Kugishima, Ichiro Yasuhi[*] (iD), Hiroshi Yamashita, So Sugimi, Yasushi Umezaki, Sachie Suga, Masashi Fukuda and Nobuko Kusuda

Abstract

Background: Although the onset of gestational diabetes (GDM) is known to be a significant risk factor for the future development of type 2 diabetes, this risk specifically in women with GDM diagnosed by the International Association of Diabetes and Pregnancy Study Group (IADPSG) criteria has not yet been thoroughly investigated. This study was performed to investigate the risk factors associated with the development of postpartum diabetes in Japanese women with a history of GDM, and the effects of the differences in the previous Japanese criteria and the IADPSG criteria.

Methods: This retrospective cohort study included Japanese women with GDM who underwent at least one postpartum oral glucose tolerance test (OGTT) between 2003 and 2014. Cases with overt diabetes in pregnancy were excluded. We investigated the risk factors including maternal baseline and pregnancy characteristics associated with the development of postpartum diabetes.

Results: Among 354 women diagnosed with GDM during the study period, 306 (86%) (116/136 [85.3%] and 190/218 [87.2%] under the previous criteria and the IADPSG criteria, respectively) who underwent at least 1 follow-up OGTT were included in the study. Thirty-two women (10.1%) developed diabetes within a median follow-up period of 57 weeks (range, 6–292 weeks). Eleven (9.5%) and 21 (11.1%) were diagnosed as GDM during pregnancy based on the previous Japanese criteria and the IADPSG criteria, respectively, which did not significantly differ between those criteria. A multivariate logistic regression analysis revealed that HbA1c and 2-h plasma glucose (PG) at the time of the diagnostic OGTT during pregnancy were independent predictors of the development of diabetes after adjusting for confounders. The adjusted relative risk of HbA1c ≥5.6% for the development of diabetes was 4.67 (95% confidence interval, 1.53-16.73), while that of 2-h PG ≥183 mg/dl was 7.02 (2.51-20.72).

Conclusions: A modest elevation of the HbA1c and 2-h PG values at the time of the diagnosis of GDM during pregnancy are independent predictors of the development of diabetes during the postpartum period in Japanese women with a history of GDM. The diagnostic criteria did not affect the incidence of postpartum diabetes.

Keywords: Diagnostic criteria, Gestational diabetes, HbA1c, Predictive factors, Postpartum diabetes

* Correspondence: yasuhi@nagasaki-mc.com
Department of Obstetrics and Gynecology, NHO Nagasaki Medical Center,
1001-1 2-chome Kubara, Omura City, Nagasaki 856-8562, Japan

Background

The onset of gestational diabetes (GDM) during pregnancy is known to be a significant risk factor for the future development of type 2 diabetes. The odds ratio, in comparison to patients who are normoglycemic during pregnancy, is 7.43 [1]. Although evidence to support this was already published in 1978 [2], it has received much more attention in the background of the recent worldwide pandemic of diabetes and obesity [3]. In this background, women with a history of GDM have been becoming a key target population in efforts to prevent the future development of diabetes.

In 2010, new international diagnostic criteria for GDM were published [4]. The criteria were based on evidence of the perinatal outcomes. Thus, it has not been well investigated whether women with GDM who are diagnosed according to the IADPSG criteria are at a similarly high risk of developing postpartum diabetes. We previously reported that there was no significant difference in the effect of the early postpartum development of impaired glucose tolerance between the IADPSG criteria and the previous Japanese criteria [5]. However, it is still not clear whether the differences in the diagnostic criteria affect the risk of the future development of diabetes.

The introduction of the IADPSG criteria has resulted in a 3-fold increase in the prevalence of GDM in the Japanese population [6]. Thus, a more efficient follow-up system is necessary for screening for postpartum diabetes. The triage of high-risk women to more intensive follow-up protocols seems to be more relevant. There seem to be a large number of risk factors, including maternal characteristics and pregnancy factors that are linked to the future development of type 2 diabetes in women with a history of GDM [7]. The maternal characteristics include maternal obesity, a family history of diabetes, ethnicity, advanced maternal age. The pregnancy factors include, but are not limited to, an early diagnosis of GDM, fasting hyperglycemia, an elevated HbA1c value, and insulin use [7]. In our previous study, we aimed to demonstrate the risk factors associated with

abnormal glucose tolerance at 6–8 weeks postpartum [5]. However, thus far, no studies of Japanese subjects that followed up patients beyond the early postpartum period have been reported.

In this current study, we aimed to identify the risk factors associated with the development of diabetes in Japanese women with a history of GDM over a longer postpartum period, and to investigate whether the differences between the previous Japanese criteria and the IADPSG criteria influence the risk of the development of postpartum diabetes.

Methods

In this retrospective cohort study of a single perinatal care center in Japan, we obtained data for women with GDM who underwent postpartum 75-g oral glucose tolerance tests (OGTT) at the National Hospital Organization Nagasaki Medical Center (Omura, Japan) between January, 2003 and December, 2014. We used two different diagnostic criteria during this period: the Japan Society of Obstetrics and Gynecology (JSOG) criteria [8], which were used until June 2010; and the IADPSG criteria, which were used from July 2010 (Table 1). Because of the possibility of pregestational diabetes, we excluded women who were diagnosed with overt diabetes during pregnancy according to the IADPSG criteria [4], including those with a fasting plasma glucose level of ≥126 mg/dl or an HbA1c level of ≥6.5% on an OGTT during pregnancy. We only included women of Japanese ethnicity in the present study. In both of the study periods with different diagnostic criteria, to screen for GDM during pregnancy, we performed universal screening of all pregnant women using a 50-g glucose challenge test around 24 weeks' gestation; those with values of ≥135 mg/dL underwent a diagnostic 75-g oral glucose tolerance test (OGTT) after overnight fasting. We also measured the HbA1c values at the time of the diagnostic OGTT.

We used the standard treatment practices for women with GDM, including diet and insulin therapy based on the results of the self-monitored blood glucose (SMBG) level. Insulin therapy was prescribed if the patient achieved less than 80% of the target blood glucose levels,

Table 1 The diagnostic criteria using the 75-g 2-h OGTT in Japan

	GDM		Postpartum diabetes
Diagnostic criteria	JSOG criteria [2]	IADPSG criteria [1]	WHO criteria [3]
Glucose load	75 g	75 g	75 g
Time of the diagnosis	Until June 2010	From June 2010	
Fasting PG	≥100 mg/dl	≥92 mg/dl	≥126
1-h PG	≥180 mg/dl	≥180 mg/dl	N/A
2-h PG	≥150 mg/dl	≥153 mg/dl	≥200
Required to diagnose GDM	Two or more abnormal values	One abnormal value or more	One abnormal value or more

OGTT oral glucose tolerance test, *GDM* gestational diabetes, *JSOG* Japan Society of Obstetrics and Gynecology, *IADPSG* Internal Association of Diabetes and Pregnancy Study Group, *WHO* World Health Organization, *PG* plasma glucose, *N/A*, not addressed

including fasting and 2-h postprandial blood glucose levels of <95 mg/dl and <120 mg/dl, respectively. We did not prescribe any oral hypoglycemic agents during pregnancy or the postpartum period.

Women with a history of GDM underwent the first follow-up OGTT at 6–8 weeks postpartum; thereafter, the test was then repeated every 6–12 months. We defined postpartum diabetes according to the WHO criteria [9] (Table 1).

We obtained the patients' basic maternal characteristics including their age, pre-pregnancy body mass index (BMI), and family history of diabetes (defined as unspecified diabetes among first- and second-degree relatives). We also obtained data related to their pregnancy, including the gestational age (GA) at the time of the diagnostic OGTT, the plasma glucose (PG) and HbA1c levels at the time of the diagnostic OGTT, the requirement of insulin therapy, and weight gain throughout pregnancy.

The primary outcome measure was postpartum development of diabetes. We investigated the association between the primary outcome measure and the risk factors, including the basic maternal and perinatal characteristics. We first used a univariate logistic regression analysis to test the association between each risk factor and the postpartum development of diabetes. Factors with a p value of <0.05 on the univariate analysis were included in a multivariate logistic regression analysis. The multivariate logistic regression analysis was used to test for independent associations between risk factors and the development of diabetes. In the multivariate analysis, we converted the factors that were numerically associated with the development of postpartum diabetes into categorical variables as a clinical viewpoint. A receiver operator characteristic (ROC) curve was used to identify the optimum cut-off values for those variables. We also used Student's t-test and a chi-squared test to compare numerical variables and the difference in ratios between groups, respectively. P values of <0.05 were considered to indicate statistical significance. This study was conducted with the approval of the Institution Review Board of Nagasaki Medical Center to collect the clinical data with informed consent.

Results

We included 306 women who underwent at least one postpartum follow-up OGTT. In the same period, 354 women were diagnosed with GDM, including 136 and 218 by the JSOG and the IADPSG criteria, respectively. Among the patients who underwent at least 1 postpartum OGTT, 116 (38%) and 190 (62%) women were diagnosed according to the JSOG and IADPSG criteria, respectively. Thus, the follow-up rate (defined by the performance of at least 1 postpartum OGTT) was 86%

(306/354) in total subjects and 85.3% (116/136) and 87.2% (190/218) in the JSOG and the IADPSG criteria, respectively. The maternal characteristics of the patients in each group and the results of their diagnostic OGTTs during pregnancy are shown in Table 2. The PG levels during the diagnostic OGTT were significantly higher in women during the JSOG period (JSOG group) than they were during the IADPSG period (IADPSG group). The rates of women who underwent two or more follow-up OGTTs in the JSOG and IADPSG periods were 70% and 78%, respectively, and did not differ to a statistically significant extent. More than half of the women underwent an OGTT at more than one year postpartum. There was a significant difference in the length of the follow-up period between the two groups (Table 2).

During the mean follow-up period of 68 ± 61 weeks (median, 57 weeks; range, 7–292 weeks), 32 (10.5%) women developed diabetes within a follow-up period of 59 ± 53 weeks (median, 47 weeks; range, 7–230 weeks). This rate was not significantly different from that of the women who did not develop diabetes (mean, 69 ± 62 weeks; median, 58 weeks; range 7–292 weeks). Eleven (9.5%) and 21 (11.1%) women with diabetes were included in the JSOG and IADPSG groups, respectively (Table 2); the incidence was not different between the different diagnostic criteria group even after adjusting for the follow-up period. Regarding the time period from the index delivery to the onset of diabetes in those who developed diabetes, women diagnosed under the IADPSG criteria developed diabetes significantly sooner than those diagnosed under the JSOG criteria (44 ± 26 vs. 88 ± 78 weeks, $p = 0.024$).

The women who developed postpartum diabetes were more obese before pregnancy ($p = 0.0032$), showed elevated 2-h PG ($p = 0.016$) and HbA1c ($p < 0.0001$) levels at the time of the diagnostic OGTT, and required more insulin therapy during pregnancy ($p = 0.0031$) in comparison to those who did not develop diabetes during the study period (Table 3). A univariate logistic regression analysis revealed that a higher pre-pregnancy BMI ($p = 0.0044$), 2-h PG ($p = 0.016$), HbA1c ($p < 0.0001$), and the requirement of insulin therapy ($p = 0.0031$) were significant risk factors for the postpartum development of diabetes (Table 4). In multivariate regression models that used the variables that were identified as significant in the univariate analysis, we found that only the 2-h PG and HbA1c levels were independent predictors of the development of diabetes during the postpartum period (Table 5). The association remained significant after controlling for maternal age, parity, a family history of diabetes, the GA and fasting and 1-h PG at the OGTT, weight gain during pregnancy, and the follow-up period (Table 5). Because fasting and the 1-h PG showed near-significance in the univariate analysis (Table 4), we also

Table 2 The maternal characteristics and 75-g OGTT results during pregnancy in terms of the different diagnostic criteria

Variables	All subjects (n = 306)	Postpartum OGTT		
		JSOG criteria (n = 116)	IADPSG Criteria (n = 190)	P value *
Maternal age (years)	33.0 ± 5.1	33.2 ± 4.8	32.9 ± 5.2	0.52
Nulliparous (%)	136 (44%)	46 (40%)	90 (47%)	0.19
Family history of diabetes (%)	124 (41%)	47 (41%)	77 (41%)	1.0
Pre-pregnancy BMI (kg/m^2)	23.5 ± 4.8	24.0 ± 4.9	23.2 ± 4.8	0.14
Pre-pregnancy BMI ≥25 kg/m^2	92 (30%)	41 (35%)	52 (27%)	0.14
GA at OGTT (weeks)	24.2 ± 6.7	23.9 ± 7.6	24.4 ± 6.1	0.60
OGTT results during pregnancy				
Fasting PG (mg/dl)	86 ± 10	88 ± 11	85 ± 10	0.0046
1-h PG (mg/dl)	186 ± 27	197 ± 23	179 ± 26	<0.0001
2-h PG (mg/dl)	161 ± 26	168 ± 22	156 ± 27	0.0001
HbA1c (%)	5.5 ± 0.4 (n = 269)	5.5 ± 0.4 (n = 108)	5.5 ± 0.4 (n = 158)	0.94
Insulin therapy during pregnancy (%)	162 (53%)	54 (47%)	108 (58%)	0.057
Weight gain during pregnancy (kg)	7.3 ± 5.1	6.9 ± 5.8	7.5 ± 4.6	0.37
Mean follow-up period (weeks) (median, range)	68 ± 61 (57, 7–292)	83 ± 81 (58, 7–292)	59 ± 43 (57, 7–164)	0.0006
At least two follow-up OGTTs (%)	229 (75%)	81 (70%)	148 (78%)	0.079
More than 12 months of follow-up OGTTs (%)	165 (54%)	61 (53%)	104 (55%)	0.19
Women who developed diabetes (%)	32 (10.5%)	11 (9.5%)	21 (11.1%)	0.66

* P values represent comparisons between the JSOG and IADPSG criteria using Student's t-test or a chi-squared test

OGTT oral glucose tolerance test, JSOG Japan Society of Obstetrics and Gynecology, IADPSG Internal Association of Diabetes and Pregnancy Study Group, BMI body mass index, GA gestational age, PG plasma glucose

examined the association between those two variables and the development of diabetes by a multivariate analysis including these two variables in addition to the four significant variables and found that neither fasting nor the 1-h PG was significantly associated with the postpartum disorder.

From the clinical point of view, we converted these numerical variables to categorical variables (Table 6). We used cutoff values of 183 mg/dl (area under the curve [AUC] 0.64) and 5.6% (AUC 0.74) for 2-h PG and HbA1c, respectively, which were derived from the ROC. A 2-h PG value of ≥183 mg/dl and an HbA1c value of ≥5.6% were significantly associated with the development of postpartum diabetes with an adjusted relative risk (RR) of 7.02 (95% confidence interval [CI] 2.51–20.72, p = 0.0002) and 4.67 (95% CI 1.53–16.73, p = 0.0061), respectively (Table 6).

Discussion

In this retrospective Japanese cohort study, 10.5% of women with a history of GDM developed diabetes during a median follow-up period of 57 weeks within up to 5 years. We also found that the 2-h PG and HbA1c values during the diagnostic 75-g OGTT in pregnancy were significant independent predictors of the postpartum development of diabetes, with an RR of 7.02 and 4.67, respectively, if a 2-h PG level of ≥183 mg/dl and an

HbA1c value of ≥5.6% were used as cutoff values, after adjusting for the considerable confounders. With regard to the diagnostic criteria, there was no significant difference in the prevalence of the development of postpartum diabetes between the women who were diagnosed by the JSOG criteria (9.5%) and those who were diagnosed by the IADPSG criteria (11.1%).

To the best of our knowledge, this is the first report regarding the development of diabetes at more than one year postpartum in Japanese women with a history of GDM. In addition, among many follow-up studies of GDM patients, few studies have reported the prevalence of postpartum diabetes in women with a history of GDM who were diagnosed according to the IADPSG criteria. We found that the prevalence of postpartum diabetes in the IADPSG group was not significantly different to that in the JSOG group, although the mean follow-up period was significantly longer in the JSOG group (Table 2). In addition, in women diagnosed with postpartum diabetes, the duration from the index delivery to the development of diabetes was significantly shorter in the IADPSG group than in the JSOG group. Thus, in comparison to the previous criteria, the IADPSG criteria seemed to recognize more women who develop postpartum diabetes earlier. Assaf-Balut et al. [10] reported that the change in diagnostic criteria from the Carpenters-Coustan (CC) criteria to the IADPSG

Table 3 The maternal characteristics and 75-g OGTT results during pregnancy: The difference between women who developed postpartum diabetes and those who did not

	Diabetes ($n = 32$)	Non-diabetes ($n = 274$)	P value[*]
Maternal age (years)	34.3 ± 4.6	32.9 ± 5.1	0.14
Nulliparous (%)	11 (34%)	125 (46%)	0.22
Family history of diabetes (%)	13 (41%)	110 (41%)	1.0
Pre-pregnancy BMI (kg/m^2)	25.9 ± 5.7	23.2 ± 4.7	0.0032
Pre-pregnancy BMI $\geq$25 kg/m^2	17 (53%)	76 (28%)	0.0031
GA at OGTT (weeks)	23.8 ± 7.9	24.3 ± 6.6	0.71
JSOG criteria period	11 (34%)	105 (38%)	0.66
OGTT results during pregnancy			
Fasting PG (mg/dl)	89 ± 11	86 ± 10	0.091
1-h PG (mg/dl)	195 ± 25	185 ± 27	0.056
2-h PG (mg/dl)	172 ± 32	160 ± 25	0.016
HbA1c (%) ($n = 269$)	5.8 ± 0.4 ($n = 29$)	5.5 ± 0.4 ($n = 240$)	<0.001
Insulin therapy during pregnancy (%)	25 (78%)	137 (51%)	0.0031
Weight gain during pregnancy (kg)	7.6 ± 3.9	7.2 ± 5.2	0.72
Follow-up period (weeks) (median, range)	59 ± 53 (47, 7–230)	69 ± 62 (58, 7–291)	0.39
At least two follow-up OGTT (%)	26 (81%)	203 (74%)	0.63
More than 12 months follow-up OGTT (%)	14 (44%)	151 (55%)	0.40

* P values represent comparisons between women who developed diabetes and those who did not using Student's t-test or a chi-squared test

BMI body mass index, *GA* gestational age, *OGTT* oral glucose tolerance test, *JSOG* Japan Society of Obstetrics and Gynecology, *PG* plasma glucose

Table 4 The association between the predictive variables and the postpartum development of diabetes in a univariate logistic regression analysis

Predictive Variables	Chi-square	P value
Maternal age (years)	2.15	0.14
Nulliparous (%)	1.47	0.22
Family history of diabetes (%)	0.0	0.99
Pre-pregnancy BMI (kg/m^2)	8.13	0.0044
Pre-pregnancy BMI $\geq$25 kg/m^2	8.77	0.0031
GA at OGTT (weeks)	0.13	0.71
JSOG criteria period[a]	0.19	0.66
OGTT results during pregnancy		
Fasting PG (mg/dl)	2.82	0.093
1-h PG (mg/dl)	3.66	0.056
2-h PG (mg/dl)	5.76	0.016
HbA1c (%) ($n = 269$)	16.3	<0.0001
Insulin therapy in pregnancy (%)	8.75	0.0031
Weight gain during pregnancy (kg)	0.13	0.72
Follow-up period (weeks)	0.74	0.39

BMI body mass index, *GA* gestational age, *OGTT* oral glucose tolerance test, *JSOG*, Japan Society of Obstetrics and Gynecology, *PG* plasma glucose
[a]adjusted for the follow-up period

criteria did not affect the percentage of women with postpartum glucose disorder (29.5% vs. 32.3%, respectively [10]. Because the number of women who were diagnosed in the IADPSG group was higher than that in the CC group, the IADPSG criteria could be superior for identifying women with postpartum glucose disorder who would have been missed by the CC criteria [10], even though the IADPSG criteria are based on only the perinatal outcomes and not on the risk of developing postpartum diabetes.

There is already evidence to show that women with a history of GDM are at significant risk for the development of type 2 diabetes; however, the follow-up tests after delivery have been suboptimal [11, 12], in spite of the current recommendations including early postpartum diabetic screening at 6–12 weeks postpartum and further follow-up tests [13–15]. In addition to the markedly low follow-up rates of only 16–48% that were reported in previous studies [16–19], the increase in the number of women with GDM after the adoption of the IADPSG criteria makes their postpartum follow-up screening more difficult. Under these conditions, it is very important to identify women with a high risk of developing postpartum diabetes.

A recent meta-analysis using a univariate model identified a large number of risk factors for the future progression of diabetes. These included BMI, a family history of diabetes, non-white ethnicity, advanced

Table 5 Results of the multiple logistic regression analysis to investigate the factors associated with the postpartum development of diabetes: The continuous variable model (n = 269)[a]

Variables included in the multivariate models	Model 1			Model 2[b]		
	RR	95% CI	P value	RR	95% CI	P value
Pre-pregnancy BMI (kg/m²)	1.04	0.96–1.13	0.29	1.08	0.98–1.20	0.13
2-h PG (mg/dl)	1.02	1.00–1.03	0.042	1.02	1.00–1.04	0.030
HbA1c (%)	5.38	1.64–19.06	0.0069	5.04	1.27–22.0	0.021
Insulin therapy during pregnancy (%)	1.92	0.71–5.78	0.22	1.92	0.66–6.46	0.24

[a] We used data from 269 women who had HbA1c test results available at the time of the diagnostic OGTT during pregnancy
[b] Adjusted for the maternal age, parity, family history of diabetes, GA at OGTT, fasting and 1-h PG, weight gain during pregnancy, and follow-up period
RR relative risk, *BMI* body mass index, *PG* plasma glucose, *OGTT* oral glucose tolerance test, *GA* gestational age

maternal age, an early diagnosis of GDM, the fasting and post-glucose load PG, the HbA1c level, the use of insulin, multiparity, hypertensive disorder, and preterm delivery [7]. Although we did not investigate obstetric complications, such as hypertension and preterm delivery, or the breastfeeding conditions in our study, the risk factors identified in the univariate analysis were similar to those reported in Rayanagoudar's study [7]. There were some differences between the studies regarding maternal age, family history, multiparity and GA at the time of their diagnosis. These differences are probably due to the small sample size of our study.

After controlling for confounders in the multivariate models, we identified two independent risk factors for the development of diabetes during a relatively long-term postpartum follow-up period of five years that were present during the index pregnancy: elevated 2-h PG and HbA1c values. Several authors have reported that the HbA1c level at the diagnosis of GDM during pregnancy is an independent predictor of the development of postpartum diabetes [20–22]. In a Swedish study [20] of 144 women with GDM who had high risk factors, including a first-degree family history of diabetes or previous GDM, the HbA1c and fasting PG values during pregnancy were found to be independent predictors in 43 cases (30.6%) in which women developed diabetes within 5 years postpartum. They found that an HbA1c level of ≥5.7% and a fasting PG level of ≥94 mg/dl (5.2 mmol/L) were associated with a 4.8- and 6.8-fold increase in the risk of developing postpartum diabetes,

respectively, in comparison to women whose HbA1c and fasting PG levels were below these cutoff values. In our study, the cutoff HbA1c value derived from the ROC was 5.6%, which is in line with that in the Swedish study. We did not find a significant association between fasting PG and diabetes; instead, 2-h PG was an independent predictor. This is probably due to several factors, including the difference in the study populations, especially the fact that the Swedish study only included high-risk women, the difference in the lengths of the follow-up periods and ethnicity [23]. Despite these differences, the HbA1c level of ≥5.7% and fasting PG level of ≥94 mg/d in the Swedish study [20], and the HbA1c level of ≥5.6% and the 2-h PG level of ≥183 mg/dl in our study were not comparable to the marked hyperglycemia that is seen in patients with pregestational diabetes. It is therefore important to consider that those modestly elevated HbA1c and glucose levels (either the fasting or the post-glucose load) during pregnancy are associated with the development of diabetes within 5 years postpartum. Several studies addressed HbA1c as a parameter for predicting postpartum diabetes in women with GDM among different races and ethnicities with different diagnostic criteria for GDM and follow-up duration [24–27]. Those studies found significant independent predictive cut-off values for the development of diabetes between 5.4% and 5.7%. Again, a modestly elevated level HbA1c seems to be a significant predictor regardless of race and ethnicity.

Table 6 Multiple logistic regression models to investigate the association between the risk factors and the postpartum development of DM: The categorical variable model (n = 269)[a]

Variables included in the multivariate models	Model 1			Model 2[b]		
	RR	95% CI	P value	RR	95% CI	P value
Pre-pregnancy BMI ≥25 (kg/m²)	1.62	0.67–3.91	0.28	2.31	0.84–6.56	0.11
2-h PG ≥183 (mg/dl)	5.29	2.15–13.27	0.0004	7.02	2.51–20.72	0.0002
HbA1c ≥5.6 (%)	6.18	2.22–20.47	0.0003	4.67	1.53–16.73	0.0061
Insulin therapy during pregnancy (%)	2.02	0.75–6.10	0.17	2.30	0.75–8.17	0.15

[a] We used data from 269 women who had HbA1c test results available at the time of the diagnostic OGTT during pregnancy
[b] Adjusted for the maternal age, parity, family history of diabetes, GA at OGTT, fasting and 1-h PG, weight gain during pregnancy, and follow-up period
RR relative risk, *BMI* body mass index, *PG* plasma glucose, *OGTT* oral glucose tolerance test, *GA* gestational age

In our previous study, we reported that both a lower insulingenic index, which exhibits decreased early-phase insulin secretion and insulin therapy during pregnancy are independent predictors for abnormal glucose tolerance, including both prediabetes and diabetes, in the early postpartum period [5].

Because we only measured insulin in half of the subjects in the current study, we were not able to address insulin dynamics during pregnancy. Kwak et al. [28] reported the difference in the characteristics between diabetic women with a history of GDM who were diagnosed in the early and late postpartum period. Interestingly, they suggested that women with the early development of diabetes had more pronounced defects in their beta-cell function, which might be explained by differences in their genetic predisposition [28].

The major strength of this study was the relatively high follow-up rate of up to 86%, which was very similar regardless of the diagnostic criteria used. As already mentioned, the previously reported postpartum follow-up rates were less than 50%. In our study, 75% of the subjects underwent at least two follow-up OGTTs and more than 50% of them were followed up beyond 12 months after their pregnancy (Table 2).

The present study is associated with several limitations. We did not address any postpartum factors, including postpartum weight change and breastfeeding. An increase in weight during the postpartum period is known to be a significant risk factor for the development of diabetes [2, 29, 30]. Although we controlled for the baseline obesity and weight gain in pregnancy in the multivariate analysis, we did not investigate the effect of the postpartum weight changes on the development of diabetes during the follow-up period. Breastfeeding is also expected to be a predictor of the postpartum development of diabetes in the general population [31] and in women with a history of GDM [32–34]. However, we did not investigate this factor because we could not obtain sufficient data on the subjects' breastfeeding practices due to the retrospective approach of our study. Because of the small sample size in this study, we were unable to conclude that other variables, including prepregnancy obesity and insulin therapy during pregnancy as well as fasting PG during the diagnostic OGTT for GDM, were not significant predictors for the development of postpartum diabetes. Because of the small sample size, we were unable to perform analyses limited to women were diagnosed under the IADPSG criteria. Although our results suggest that the IADPSG criteria are efficient at identifying women with GDM at risk of developing postpartum diabetes, further prospective cohort studies with a larger sample size are necessary to draw any definitive conclusions on this issue.

Conclusions

In conclusion, despite the diagnostic criteria, in women with a history of GDM, the elevation of the HbA1c and 2-h PG levels during pregnancy, at the time of the diagnostic OGTT, was independently associated with the development of diabetes within 5 years postpartum. Thus, to make an early diagnosis of postpartum diabetes, it is important to carefully pay attention to pregnant women with HbA1c and 2-h PG levels that are higher than the above-mentioned cutoff points of 5.6% and 183 mg/dl, respectively, despite the use of insulin.

Abbreviations

AUC: area under the curve; BMI: body mass index; CC: Carpenters-Coustan; CI: confidence interval; GA: gestational age; GDM: gestational diabetes; HbA1c: hemoglobin A1c; IADPSG: International Society of Diabetes and Pregnancy Study Group; JSOG: Japan Society of Obstetrics and Gynecology; OGTT: oral glucose tolerance test; PG: plasma glucose; ROC: receiver operating curve; RR: relative risk; SMBG: self-monitored blood glucose; WHO: World Health Organization

Acknowledgements

Not applicable.

Funding

There was no funding source for this study.

Availability of data and materials

The datasets used and/or analysed during the current study are available from the corresponding author on reasonable request.

Authors' contributions

Y.K., I.Y., and H.Y. wrote the initial research proposal and manuscript; Y.K., H.Y., S.Sugimi, Y.U.and S.Suga acquired data, Y.K. and H.Y., and I.Y analyzed data; M.F. and N.K. contributed to the discussion; Y.K. drafted the manuscript; I.Y. revised the manuscript and gave final approval of the version. All authors read and approved the final manuscript.

Competing interests

The authors declare that they have no competing interests.

References

1. Bellamy L, Casas P, Hingorani AD, Williams D. Type 2 diabetes mellitus after gestational diabetes: a systematic review and meta-analysis. Lancet. 2009; 373:1773–9.
2. O'Sullivan JB. Gestational diabetes: factors influencing rate of subsequent diabetes. Sutherland HW, Stowers JM (eds) In: Carbohydrate metabolism in pregnancy and the newborn. Springer-Verlag, New York, p. 429, 1978.
3. Matthews DR, Matthews PC. Type 2 diabetes as an 'infectious' disease: is this the black death of the 21st century? Diabet Med. 2011;28:2–9.

4. International Association of Diabetes and Pregnancy Study Groups. Recommendations on the diagnosis and classification of hyperglycemia in pregnancy. Diabetes Care. 2010;33:676–82.

5. Kugishima Y, Yasuhi I, Yamashita H, Fukuda M, Yamauchi Y, Kuzume A, Hashimoto T, Sugimi S, Umezaki Y, Suga S, Kusuda N. Risk factors associated with abnormal glucose tolerance in the early postpartum period among Japanese women with gestational diabetes. Int J Gynecol Obstet. 2015;129:42–5.

6. Morikawa M, Yamada T, Yamada T, Akaishi R, Nishida R, Cho K, Minakami H. Change in the number of patients after the adoption of IADPSG criteria for hyperglycemia during pregnancy in Japanese women. Diabetes Res Clin Pract. 2010;90:339–42.

7. Rayanagoudar G, Hashi AA, Zamora J, Khan KS, Hitman GA, Thangaratinam S. Quantification of the type 2 diabetes risk in women with gestational diabetes: a systematic review and meta-analysis of 95,750 women. Diabetologia. 2016;59:1403–11.

8. The Committee on Nutrition and Metabolism of the Japan Society of Obstetrics and Gynaecology. The committee report. Acta Obstet Gynaecol Jpn. 1984;36:2055–8.

9. World Health Organization (2006). Definition and diagnosis of diabetes mellitus and intermediate hyperglycemia: report of a WHOIDF consultation. World Health Org. http://www.who.int/iris/handle/10665/43588.

10. Assaf-Balut C, Bordiú E, del Valle L, Lara M, Duran A, Rubio MA, et al. The impact of switching to the one-step method for GDM diagnosis on the rates of postpartum screening attendance and glucose disorder in women with prior GDM. The San Carlos gestational study. J Diabetes Complicat. 2016; https://doi.org/10.1016/j.jdiacomp.2016.04.026.

11. McGovern A, Butler L, Jones S, van Vlymen J, Sadek K, Munro N, Carr H, de Lusignan S. Diabetes screening after gestational diabetes in England: a quantitative retrospective cohort study. Br J General Practice. 2014:e17–23.

12. Lawrence JM, Black ME, Hsu JW, Chen W, Sacks DA. Prevalence and timing of postpartum glucose testing and sustained glucose dysregulation after gestational diabetes mellitus. Diabetes Care. 2010;33:569–76.

13. National Institute for Health and Clinical Excellence. Diabetes in pregnancy: management of diabetes and its complications from pre-conception to the postnatal period: NICE; 2008. https://www.nice.org.uk/guidance/ng3/chapter/1-Recommendations.

14. ACOG Committee opinion #435. Postpartum screening for abnormal glucose tolerance in women who had gestational diabetes mellitus. American College of Obstetricians and Gynwcologists. Obstet Gynecol. 2009;113:1419–21.

15. Clinical Question 005-1: Diagnosis of glucose intolerance in pregnant women (in Japanese). Guidelines for Obstetrical Practice in Japan 2014 edition. Japan Society of Obstetrics and Gynecology (JSOG) and Japan Association of Obstetricians and Gynecologists (JAOG). 2014. pp. 19–23.

16. Smirnakis KV, Chasan-Taber L, Wolf M, Markenson G, Ecker JL, Thadhani R. Postpartum diabetes screening in women with a history of gestational diabetes. Obstet Gynecol. 2005;106:1297–303.

17. Russell MA, Phipps MG, Olson CL, Welch HG, Carpenter MW. Rates of postpartum glucose testing after gestational diabetes mellitus. Obstet Gynecol. 2006;108:1456–62.

18. Baker AM, Brody SC, Salisbury K, Schectman R, Hartmann KE. Postpartum glucose tolerance screening in women with gestational diabetes in the state of North Carolina. N C Med J. 2009;70:14–9.

19. Kwong A, Mitchell RS, Senoir PA, Chik CL. Postpartum diabetes screening: adherence rate and the performance of fasting plasma glucose versus oral glucose tolerance test. Diabetes Care. 2009;32:2242–4.

20. Ekelund M, Shaat N, Almgren P, Groop L, Berntorp K. Prediction of postpartum diabetes in women with gestational diabetes mellitus. Diabetologia. 2010;53:452–7.

21. Eades CE, Styles M, Leese GP, Cheyne H, Evans JMM. Progression from gestational diabetes to type 2 diabetes in one region of Scotland: an observational follow-up study. BMC Pregnancy Childbirth. 2015;15:11. https://doi.org/10.1186/s12884-015-0457-8.

22. Oldfield MD, Donley P, Walwyn L, Scudamore I, Gregory R. Long term prognosis of women with gestational diabetes in a multiethnic population. Postgrad Med J. 2007;83:426–30.

23. Hsu WC, Boyko EJ, Fujimoto WY, Kanaya A, Karmally W, Karter A, King GL, Look M, Maskarinec G, Misra R, Tavake-Pasi F, Arakaki R. Pathophysiologic differences among Asians, native Hawaiians, and other Pacific islanders and treatment implications. Diabetes Care. 2012;3:1189–98.

24. Claesson R, Ignell C, Shaata N, Berntorp K. HbA1c as a predictor of diabetes after gestational diabetes mellitus. Primary Care Diabetes. 2017;11:46–51.

25. Liu H, Zhang S, Wang L, Leng J, Li W, Li N, Li M, Qiao Y, Tian H, Tuomilehto J, Yang X, Yu Z, Hu G. Fasting and 2-hour plasma glucose, and HbA1c in pregnancy and the postpartum risk of diabetes among Chinese women with gestational diabetes. Diabetes Rec Clin Pract. 2016;112:30–6.

26. Kwon SS, Kwon JY, Park YW, Kim YH, Lim JB. HbA1c for diagnosis and prognosis of gestational diabetes mellitus. Diabetes Res Clin Pract. 2015;110:38–43.

27. Bartakova V, Malúšková D, Mužík J, Bělobrádková J, Kaňková K. Possibility to predict early postpartum glucose abnormality following gestational diabetes mellitus based on the results of routine mid-gestational screening. Biochem Med. 2015;25:460–8.

28. Kwak SH, Choi SH, Jung HS, Cho YM, Lim S, Cho NH, Kim SY, Park KS, Jang HC. Clinical and genetic risk factors for type 2 diabetes at early or late post partum after gestational diabetes mellitus. J Clin Endocrinol Metab. 2013;98: E744–52.

29. Liu H, Zhang C, Zhang S, et al. Prepregnancy body mass index and weight change on postpartum diabetes risk among gestational diabetes women. Obesity. 2014;22:1560–7.

30. Bao W, Yeung E, Tobias DK, et al. Long-term risk of type 2 diabetes mellitus in relation to BMI and weight change among women with a history of gestational diabetes mellitus: a prospective cohort study. Diabetologia. 2015;58:1212–9.

31. Stuebe AM, Rich-Edwards AW, Willett WC, Manson JE, Michels KB. Duration of lactation and incidence of type 2 diabetes. JAMA. 2005;294:2601–10.

32. Gunderson EP, et al. Lactation intensity and postpartum maternal glucose tolerance and insulin resistance in women with recent GDM: the SWIFT cohort. Diabetes Care. 2012;35:50–6.

33. Ziegler AG, Wallner M, Kaiser I, Rossbauer M, Harsunen MH, et al. Long-term protective effect of lactation on the development of type 2 diabetes in women with recent gestational diabetes mellitus. Diabetes. 2012;61:3167–71.

34. Gunderson EP, Hurston SR, Ning X, Lo JC, Crites Y, Walton D, Dewey KG, Azevedo RA, Young S, Fox G, Elmasian CC, Salvador N, Lum M, Sternfeld B, Quesenberry CP Jr, for the Study of Women, Infant Feeding and Type 2 Diabetes After GDM Pregnancy Investigators. Lactation and progression to type 2 diabetes mellitus after gestational diabetes mellitus: a prospective cohort study. Ann Int Med. 2015;163:889–92.

First and second trimester urinary metabolic profiles and fetal growth restriction: an exploratory nested case-control study within the infant development and environment study

Gauri Luthra[3*], Ivan Vuckovic[1], A. Bangdiwala[2], H. Gray[3], J. B. Redmon[4], E. S. Barrett[5], S. Sathyanarayana[6], R. H. N. Nguyen[7], S. H. Swan[8], S. Zhang[1], P. Dzeja[1], S. I. Macura[1] and K. S. Nair[9]

Abstract

Background: Routine prenatal care fails to identify a large proportion of women at risk of fetal growth restriction (FGR). Metabolomics, the comprehensive analysis of low molecular weight molecules (metabolites) in biological samples, can provide new and earlier biomarkers of prenatal health. Recent research has suggested possible predictive first trimester urine metabolites correlating to fetal growth restriction in the third trimester. Our objective in this current study was to examine urinary metabolic profiles in the first and second trimester of pregnancy in relation to third trimester FGR in a US population from a large, multi-center cohort study of healthy pregnant women.

Methods: We conducted a nested case-control study within The Infant Development and the Environment Study (TIDES), a population-based multi-center pregnancy cohort study. We identified 53 cases of FGR based on the AUDIPOG [Neonatal growth - AUDIPOG [Internet]. [cited 29 Nov 2016]. Available from: http://www.audipog.net/courbes_morpho.php?langue=en] formula for birthweight percentile considering maternal height, age, and prenatal weight, as well as infant sex, gestational age, and birth rank. Cases were matched to 106 controls based on study site, maternal age (± 2 years), parity, and infant sex. NMR spectroscopy was used to assess concentrations of four urinary metabolites that have been previously associated with FGR (tyrosine, acetate, formate, and trimethylamine) in first and second trimester urine samples. We fit multivariate conditional logistic regression models to estimate the odds of FGR in relation to urinary concentrations of these individual metabolites in the first and second trimesters. Exploratory analyses of custom binned spectroscopy results were run to consider other potentially related metabolites.

Results: We found no significant association between the relative concentrations of each of the four metabolites and odds of FGR. Exploratory analyses did not reveal any significant differences in urinary metabolic profiles. Compared with controls, cases delivered earlier (38.6 vs 39.8, $p < 0.001$), and had lower birthweights (2527 g vs 3471 g, $p < 0.001$). Maternal BMI was similar between cases and controls.

Conclusions: First and second trimester concentrations of urinary metabolites (acetate, formate, trimethylamine and tyrosine) did not predict FGR. This inconsistency with previous studies highlights the need for more rigorous investigation and data collection in this area before metabolomics can be clinically applied to obstetrics.

Keywords: Obstetrics, NMR spectroscopy, Fetal growth restriction

* Correspondence: gauri.luthra@gmail.com
[3]Department of Maternal Fetal Medicine, University of Minnesota, 606 24th Ave S #400, Minneapolis, MN 55454, USA
Full list of author information is available at the end of the article

Background

Fetal growth restriction (FGR) is a complication of pregnancy that has been associated with a variety of adverse perinatal outcomes including intrauterine fetal demise, neonatal morbidity, and neonatal death. Studies have revealed that growth-restricted fetuses are predisposed to the development of cognitive delay in childhood and diseases in adulthood such as obesity, type 2 diabetes mellitus, coronary artery disease, and stroke. [1] The FGR incidence is reported to be approximately 4% to 8% in developed countries, including the United States, and 6% to 30% in developing countries. [2] Routine prenatal care fails to identify a large proportion of women at risk; therefore, there is an imperative need to identify the risk of FGR early in pregnancy so that it might be prevented.

FGR is commonly defined as an estimated fetal weight that is less than the 10th percentile for gestational age. [3] In the research literature, FGR is often mistakenly interchanged with 'small for gestational age' (SGA, birthweight below the 10th percentile for the gestational age) [4] or 'low birthweight' (defined as birth weight less than 2500 g) [5], to describe the same phenomenon; however, these terms are not necessarily synonymous. It has been estimated that approximately one third of all SGA infants are growth restricted (hence two thirds are constitutionally small) [2]; additionally, not all growth restricted babies are SGA. For our study, we defined FGR as failure to achieve the individual baby's growth potential as defined by the specific growth potential formula from AUDIPOG. [6] Mamelle et al. [7] illustrates the benefits of using this formula along with a discussion clarifying the concepts of SGA and FGR and their relationships with one another.

In a 2014 article by Maitre et al. [8], the authors found a significant correlation between lower levels of four urinary metabolites (acetate, formate, tyrosine and trimethylamine) and a higher incidence of FGR by performing NMR spectroscopy on first trimester urinary samples of pregnant patients in a cohort from Greece. They applied the AUDIPOG growth potential formula to better identify growth restricted fetuses. The exact role that these four metabolites play in relation to possible pathology causing FGR is yet to be discovered though they have been associated with nutrition and colonic health and tyrosine associated with phenylketonuria. [9–11]

Metabolomics, the comprehensive analysis of low molecular weight molecules (metabolites) in biological samples, can provide new and earlier biomarkers of prenatal health. [12–15] Studies also have shown a possible link between metabolites and the intrauterine environment and the effect it can have on fetal development and physiological systems during gestation as well as later in life. [16, 17] As we learn more about the intrauterine environment and how it is influenced by metabolites, we hope to find an early, non-invasive way to identify pregnancies at risk of FGR.

Our objective in this current study was to examine urinary metabolic profiles in the first and second trimester of pregnancy in relation to third trimester FGR in a US population from a large, multi-center cohort study of healthy pregnant women.

Methods

We used data from The Infant Development and the Environment Study (TIDES) [18, 19] in which, from 2010 to 2012, pregnant women were recruited from obstetrical clinics affiliated with academic medical centers in four U.S. cities: Minneapolis, MN; Rochester, NY; San Francisco, CA; and Seattle, WA. The primary aim of the TIDES study was to examine prenatal phthalate exposure in relation to infant genital morphology. Participants gave a urine sample in each trimester, which was collected at a study visit and frozen. Participants also completed a questionnaire in each trimester regarding demographics and possible environmental exposures.

For our case-control study, we reviewed these questionnaires and de-identified previously collected data that included sociodemographic variables such as maternal age, maternal education, and woman's parity, along with known contributing factors to FGR, including smoking status of the mother during pregnancy, chronic hypertension, and pre-gestational diabetes. Though pre-gestational diabetes is most commonly associated with fetal overgrowth (macrosomia), there is a subset of patients where impaired growth is more common among women with diabetic vasculopathy due to impaired placental function as well as fetal demise. [20] Per The American College of Obstetricians and Gynecologists (ACOG), for patients with pre-gestational diabetes in the setting of hypertension and nephropathy, the risk of fetal intrauterine growth restriction is more than doubled. [21]

Identification of FGR cases and controls

FGR cases were determined using the AUDIPOG formula for the average predicted birthweight for an infant with specific characteristics of: maternal height, age, and prenatal weight, as well as infant sex, gestational age, and birth rank.

AUDIPOG formula [6]:

$$
\begin{aligned}
\text{avg\_pred\_bw} = {} & 10,228066774 - 0,646727171^{*}\text{GA} \\
& + 0,0259713417^{*}\text{GA}^{2} - 0,000291122 \\
& {}^{*}\text{GA}^{3} - 0,045467351^{*}\text{sex} + 0,0606013862 \\
& {}^{*}\text{rank} - 0,013592585^{*}\text{rank}^{2} + 0,0009109473 \\
& {}^{*}\text{rank}^{3} + 0,0003976103 * \text{MA} + 0,0019992269 \\
& {}^{*}\text{MH} + 0,0169049061^{*}\text{MW} - 0,000171266 \\
& {}^{*}\text{MW}^{2} + 5,8340462\text{E-}7^{*}\text{MW}^{3}
\end{aligned}
$$

The natural logarithm of this average predicted birthweight was used with the observed birthweight to determine a z-score and percentile for each infant.

If an infant fell into the 10th percentile for his or her given characteristics, then they were considered as having FGR. Otherwise they were considered in the pool of controls. Controls were matched to cases using a 2:1 ratio based on study site, maternal age (± 2 years), parity, and infant sex.

Metabolomic assays

Urine samples were shipped on dry ice and stored at − 80 °C at The Metabolomics Core Lab at Mayo Clinic in Rochester, MN, where their metabolic profiles were analyzed. The samples were prepared and NMR spectra were recorded according to Bruker IVDr (in vitro diagnostics) SOPs. [22] The samples were thawed on ice and mixed with Bruker VERBR urine buffer (phosphate buffer pH 7.4 containing 0.1% TSP-d_4) in 9:1 (v/v) ratio. Typically, a 550 μl urine aliquot was transferred to an Eppendorf tube, then 61.1 μl of buffer was added and the mixture was vortexed for 20 s. The sample was spun down at 5000 rpm and 600 μl of supernatant was transferred to 5 mm NMR tubes. Pool samples were prepared by combining 50 μL aliquots of all the samples. The NMR spectra were recorded on a Bruker 600 MHz Avance III HD spectrometer equipped with BBI room temperature probehead and SampleJet auto sampler (Bruker Biospin, Rheinstetten, Germany). The auto sampler temperature was regulated at 6 °C. Tuning, matching, shimming, and pulse calibration were performed in automation mode prior to acquisition. For each sample, two experiments were acquired: 1D noesy with presaturation (noesygppr1d) and homonuclear 2D J-resolved (jresgpprqf) at 300 K.^{1}H noesy spectral parameters were: p1 ~ 12 μs, ds 4, ns 32, td 64 k, sw 20 ppm (12,019 Hz), aq 2.73 s, d14s, d8 80 ms. The FIDs were multiplied by an exponential weighting function corresponding to a line broadening of 0.3 Hz prior to Fourier transformation. Spectra were automatically referenced and phase and baseline corrected using the Bruker IVDr protocol in the software program Topspin, version 3.5. The 2D J-resolved spectral parameters were: F1 domain td 40, sw 0.13 ppm (78 Hz), aq 0.26, F2 domain td 8 k, ds 12, ns 2, sw 16.7 ppm (10,026 Hz), aq 0.41 s, d1 2 s.

After acquisition, the spectra for the four metabolites of interest, were automatically uploaded and analyzed by the Bruker IVDr server. The reports, based on individual samples, and containing concentrations of 18 standard and 8 nonstandard metabolites, were created (Additional file 1). Three of these standard metabolites were the metabolites of interest (acetate, formate, trimethylamine). Tyrosine was not a standard metabolite and was quantified individually in the software program Chenomx NMR, suite 8.2, profiler mode, by fitting experimental spectra to resonant tyrosine peaks at δ 6.88 (d) and 7.18

(d). The concentrations were expressed as mmol/L of urine and mmol/mol of Creatinine (Additional file 2). The quantification of urine metabolites is based on an ERETIC signal generated at 12 ppm. (Additional file 3). The concentrations were normalized to creatinine in the urine due to fluctuations in hydration of the participants.

Exploratory metabolite identification

All NMR spectra were uploaded into the software program Chenomx NMR suite 8.2. The spectral region δ 0.5 to 9.4 ppm was divided in 216 custom bins, with region 4.69–4.86 containing residual water resonances excluded. The bin integrals were normalized to total peak area and subsequently used for statistical analysis (Additional file 4). As an alternative approach, we tried excluding the urea region δ 5.3–6.4 and PQN normalization, but it did not improve statistical analysis.

To explore if any other metabolites were associated with FGR, analyses were performed using SIMCA (Soft independent modeling of class analogy) software v14 (MKS Data Analytics Solutions, Umeå, Sweden) for multivariate data analysis. [23] Unsupervised principal component analysis (PCA) was run to detect any innate trends and potential outliers within the data. Supervised partial least squares discriminant analysis (PLS-DA) and orthogonal partial least squares discriminant analysis (OPLS-DA) were performed to obtain additional information on differences in the metabolite composition of groups. PLS-DA and OPLS-DA models were calculated with unit variance scaling, and the results were visualized in the form of score plots to show the group clusters. The VIP (variable importance in the projection) values and regression coefficients were calculated to identify the most important molecular variables for the clustering of specific groups.

Statistical analysis

Demographic variables (maternal age, maternal BMI, site, parity, gestational age, birthweight and infant gender) were summarized by mean (standard deviation) for continuous variables and N(%) for categorical variables. These characteristics were compared between cases and controls using T-tests and chi-square tests.

Four metabolites

The goal of the primary analysis was to determine if there exists an association between the four metabolite concentrations at either trimester with odds of FGR. This included multivariable conditional logistic regression for each of the four metabolites to determine. Demographic variables that were not used in calculating the outcome (maternal age, BMI, and parity) were considered for inclusion in the model along with metabolite concentration at each trimester. Interquartile odds ratios (IORs) with 95% confidence intervals (CIs) were calculated for FGR to produce estimates of ORs customized to a unit of change reflecting the difference between the 75th percentile and 25th percentile of each metabolite concentration.

Exploratory metabolites
The NMR spectra were custom binned into potential metabolite representatives so that each patient had one measure of "proportion of spectrum" in the first trimester and one in the second trimester for each potential metabolite. Median concentrations were estimated within each bin for each trimester and the difference in medians between cases and controls was calculated. For each trimester, the absolute differences were ranked in descending order and the 25 biggest were noted. For these 50 bins, within each bin and for each trimester, a nonparametric Wilcoxon rank sum test was performed to compare median "proportion of spectrum" between cases and controls. The Benjamini-Hochberg method was used to adjust for multiple testing. Results were then listed in order of ascending p-value and used to consider which metabolites may merit further exploration regarding an association with FGR.

P-values less than 0.05 were considered statistically significant and all analyses were conducted using SAS version 9.4 (Cary, NC).

The STROBE (Strengthening the Reporting of Observational Studies in Epidemiology) guidelines were used to ensure the reporting of this observational study. [24]

Results
The 53 cases were matched 2:1 to 106 controls for a total of 159 subjects resulting in a total of 318 urine samples. Of the original 159 patients, 158 had sufficient data to be included in the analysis (one subject had unreadable first trimester spectroscopy analysis results).

Demographic comparison results, as shown in Table 1, were as expected given the construction of the FGR formula and the matching on maternal age, site, parity, and infant gender. There was no difference in maternal or infant characteristics with the exception of infant gestational age and birthweight. Maternal BMI was similar between cases and controls. Cases had a statistically significantly lower gestational age at birth (38.6 vs 39.8, $p < 0.001$), and lower birthweight (2527 g vs 3471 g, $p < 0.001$).

Four metabolites
The median concentrations of the four metabolites are listed in Table 2. None of the demographic variables of interest differed significantly between cases and controls, and were not included in the model. The final model consisted of only the main effects of the metabolite

levels in each trimester. The resulting estimates of Interquartile ORs for each metabolite are displayed in Table 3; any association between each of the four metabolites and odds of FGR was found to be non-significant.

Exploratory metabolites
Metabolite identification (as described under Methods) was effective when comparing first trimester case samples to second trimester case samples and first trimester control samples to second trimester control samples, as in Fig. 1, a and b; however, when we compared case samples versus control samples within a trimester, good separation could not be visualized; see Fig. 1, c and d.

The custom binning of the NMR spectroscopy resulted in 215 bins expected to represent separate metabolites. The 25 largest differences in relative concentration between cases and controls in the first trimester ranged from 0.000256 to 0.006265. The 25 largest differences in relative concentration between cases and controls in the second trimester ranged from 0.000347 to 0.004184. After adjusting for multiple testing, none of the p-values were found to be significant. The bins that correlated with the largest differences in the first trimester were attributed to 1-Methylnicotinamide, Lysine, Proline betaine, 3-Hydroxybutyrate/3-Aminoisobutyrate, Creatinine and Guanidoacetate. The bins correlated with the largest differences in the second trimester were attributed to Xanthyrenate, Histidine, Acetate + N-Phenylacetyl glutamine, Urea and Carnitine. Again, none of these were of significance.

Discussion
We found no significant association between the relative concentration level of each of the four metabolites of interest and odds of FGR. In addition, results did not reveal any significant differences in the exploratory urinary metabolic profiles. As expected, compared with controls, cases delivered earlier (38.6 vs 39.8, $p < 0.001$), and had lower birthweights (2527 g vs 3471 g, $p < 0.001$).

Pregestational diabetes and chronic hypertension, other noted factors that can contribute to fetal growth restriction, were rare in this cohort (pre-gestational diabetes: 0/53 cases, 2/109 controls, chronic hypertension: 2/53 cases, 2/109 controls) and thus were not included in our analyses. Smoking among subjects was equally proportionate among cases and controls.

The strengths of our study include the large cohort of patients in the TIDES group (758 patients total enrolled), which allowed the relatively rare nature of fetal growth restriction to yield a large number of cases (53) with matched controls. The patients came from 4 different geographic areas of the country and this contributed to the diversity of the group. Additionally, our analysis involved conditional logistic regression which helps account for the bias inherent to a case-control study.

Table 1 Demographic data [mean(SD)]

Variable		Overall (n = 158)	FGR Case (n = 53)	Control (n = 105)	p-value*
Maternal Age	(yrs)	29.4 (6.2)	29.5 (6.4)	29.3 (6.1)	0.91
Maternal BMI	(kg/m²)	27.9 (7.0)	27.9 (7.6)	27.8 (6.7)	0.98
Site					1.0
	UCSF	29	10 (18%)	19 (19%)	
	UMN	21	7 (13%)	14 (13%)	
	URMC	93	31 (59%)	62 (58%)	
	UW	15	5 (10%)	10 (9%)	
Parity					0.86
	0	94	31 (58%)	63 (60%)	
	≥1	64	22 (42%)	42 (40%)	
Gestational Age at Birth	(wks)	39.4 (1.8)	38.6 (2.4)	39.8 (1.1)	< 0.0001
Birth weight	(g)	3154 .3 (621)	2526.5 (421)	3471.1 (448)	< 0.0001
Sex					0.96
	Male	75	25 (47%)	50 (48%)	
	Female	83	28 (53%)	55 (52%)	
Smoker at T1		14 (9%)	5 (10%)	9 (9%)	1.00
Cigarettes per wk. (n = 14)	Med (IQR)	21 (3–35)	28 (25–35)	7 (2–21)	0.14
Pregestational Diabetes		2	0	2 (2%)	0.55
Chronic Hypertension		4	2 (4%)	2 (2%)	0.60

*p-values for Maternal Age, BMI, Gestational Age, and Birthweight are from T-tests. P-values Site, Parity, Sex, and Smoker are from chi-square tests. P-value for Cigarettes per week is from Wilcoxon rank sum test. P-values for Pregestational Diabetes and Hypertension are from Fisher's exact test

Another strength was the emphasis on the accuracy of our data and our sample runs in the NMR spectroscopy lab at Mayo. Trial runs were performed on mock urine samples before initiating processing and NMR spectroscopy on our actual samples. This limited human error as well as machine error. Finally, given the sensitive nature of NMR spectroscopy, it is vital to assemble a team with members from the metabolomics lab as well as the clinical side to ensure data collection and results are valid and not the result of sample processing error, lab mishandling, software error or assumptions made on poor understanding of the spectra profiles. The collaborative

nature of this project with expert spectroscopists as well as clinicians allowed for accurate collection and analysis of data while at the same time maintaining a focus on the potential clinical significance of our findings.

NMR spectroscopy did confirm a significant metabolic shift between first and second trimesters through multivariate projection analysis such as principal component analysis (PCA) and orthogonal-partial least squares discriminatory analysis (OPLS-DA); however, the accessibility of inexpensive methods (eg. ultrasound) to determine

Table 2 Median [IQR] mmol/mol creatinine of each metabolite by trimester

Variable	Trimester	Overall	FGR Case	Control
Acetic Acid	1	11 [7–17]	10 [6–16]	11 [8–18]
	2	12 [7–17]	12 [7–19]	11 [7–17]
Trimethylamine	1	4 [3–6]	4 [3–5]	4 [3–6]
	2	4 [3–5]	3 [3–5]	4 [3–5]
Formic Acid	1	19 [13–29]	19 [12–31]	19 [14–28]
	2	25 [18–36]	25 [18–37]	25 [18–35]
Tyrosine[a]	1	17 [13–23]	16 [8–22]	18 [13–24]
	2	18 [13–25]	19 [12–24]	18 [13–25]

[a]Some subjects were missing tyrosine spectroscopy analysis results, thus n = 153 subjects were used in analysis of tyrosine

Table 3 Interquartile Odds Ratios of FGR for each metabolite

Variable	Trimester	Odds Ratio	95% CI Min	95% CI Max	p-value
Acetic Acid	1	0.93	0.77	1.11	0.42
	2	1.12	0.86	1.46	0.40
Trimethylamine	1	0.90	0.59	1.35	0.60
	2	1.20	0.80	1.79	0.38
Formic Acid	1	1.07	0.64	1.79	0.78
	2	1.06	0.74	1.53	0.73
Tyrosine[a]	1	0.74	0.49	1.10	0.14
	2	1.16	0.76	1.78	0.50

Interquartile ranges for acetic acid: 10, trimethylamine: 2.5, formic acid: 17, and tyrosine: 11
[a]Some subjects were missing tyrosine spectroscopy analysis results, thus n = 153 subjects were used in analysis of tyrosine

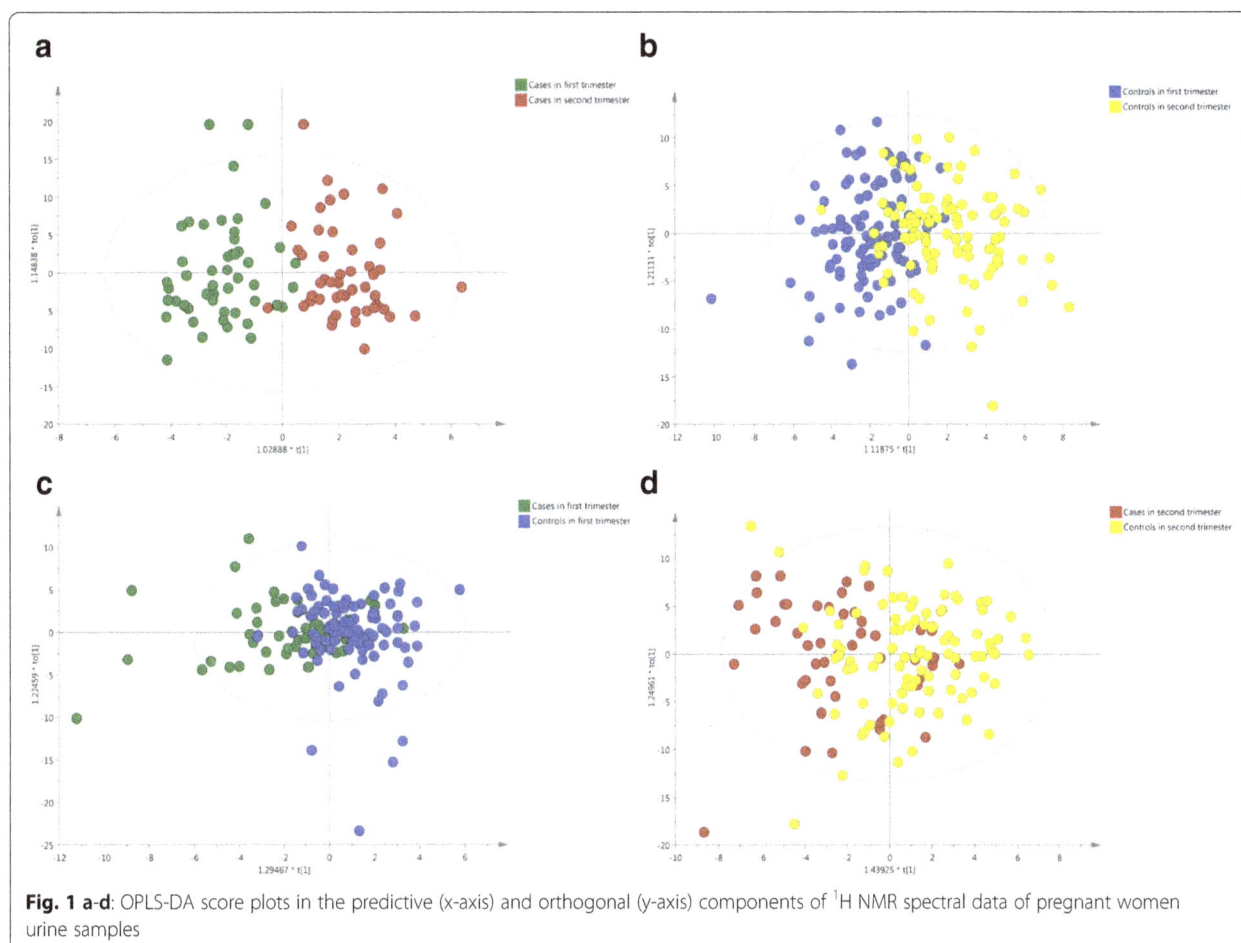

Fig. 1 a-d: OPLS-DA score plots in the predictive (x-axis) and orthogonal (y-axis) components of ¹H NMR spectral data of pregnant women urine samples

gestational age undermines the clinical usefulness of NMR spectroscopy to discern what trimester a pregnant patient is in. Still, this result does prove the technology reveals that the metabolites are undergoing a significant change. In another recent study, investigators found that a 50% increase in each of three separate third trimester urine metabolites is correlated with an increase in birth weight of 1%–2.4% (5-11 g). [25] Though these results may have statistical significance in that study, and might warrant further investigation, they too have little clinical value at this time, considering the small size of the increase.

The current results do not to show the metabolomics to offer potential biomarkers of FGR but do offer intriguing preliminary data to pursue further given the potential of metabolomics to yield clinically useful and individualized results from a low risk, non-interventional sample early in pregnancy. Further studies are warranted not only using NMR spectroscopy, but also applying highly sensitive tandem mass spectrometry based approaches utilizing timely collection of plasma samples. Though the gathering of non-interventional samples such as urine is very low cost, the running of urine samples by NMR spectroscopy is

very expensive; plasma based measurements applying sensitive and less expensive mass spectrometry based metabolomics approaches may be considered in the future to assist diagnosis of conditions in obstetrics.

The primary limitation to our study is the exploratory nature of this area. There is very little metabolomics literature available on pregnant patients. Conversely, this might also be considered the greatest strength; when a path is new, every step forward has a greater impact on the direction traveled. Also, the retrospective nature of our study was limiting to the extent that we could not control what data had already been collected. It would have been useful to have chosen a stricter definition of FGR (5th percentile or 3rd percentile). With a tighter definition, our specificity would increase, but at the expense of sensitivity. Given the exploratory nature of this work to assess if urinary metabolites are a plausible means by which to screen for FGR, we chose a higher cut off to achieve a data set that was interpretable. A sensitivity analysis was conducted with cases in the 5th percentile and we found similar results. Additionally, because it is not an ongoing study, we cannot add to our data to incorporate further subjects in future. It may have been useful to include Doppler information from ultrasounds with the focus on looking for signs of growth restriction had we been given the choice. This is the nature of studying rare outcomes with a lack of time and funding necessary for a prospective study. Our NMR spectroscopy data will be added to the Bruker company's database of labs using their machines.

Conclusions

In conclusion, we did not detect changed odds of FGR based on the concentration of urinary metabolites (acetate, formate, trimethylamine and tyrosine) in either trimester. Additionally, we did not detect differences in the first and second trimester urinary metabolic profiles of pregnant patients with FGR compared to controls. This contradicts prior work, and highlights the need for more rigorous investigation and data collection in this area before metabolomics can be clinically applied to obstetrics.

Additional files

Additional file 1: Bruker Analysis Report. Analysis report generated from Bruker software containing concentrations of 18 standard and 8 nonstandard metabolites for all samples. (PDF 99 kb)

Additional file 2: Tyrosine concentrations for all samples. Tyrosine was not a standard metabolite and was quantified individually in the software program Chenomx NMR, suite 8.2, profiler mode, by fitting experimental spectra to resonant tyrosine peaks at δ 6.88 (d) and 7.18 (d). The concentrations were expressed as mmol/L of urine and mmol/mol of Creatinine. (XLSX 135 kb)

Additional file 3: ^{1}H NMR Bruker IVDr spectrum of pooled urine sample. The quantification of urine metabolites is based on an ERETIC signal generated at 12 ppm. (PPTX 350 kb)

Additional file 4: Binned spectrum line using total area normalization. All NMR spectra were uploaded into the software program Chenomx NMR suite 8.2. The spectral region δ 0.5 to 9.4 ppm was divided in 216 custom bins, with region 4.69–4.86 containing residual water resonances excluded. The bin integrals were normalized to total peak area and subsequently used for statistical analysis. (XLSX 703 kb)

Abbreviations

ACOG: The American College of Obstetricians and Gynecologists; CI: Confidence interval; FGR: Fetal growth restriction; IOR: Interquartile odds ratio; IVD: In vitro diagnostics; OPLS-DA: Orthogonal partial least squares discriminant analysis; PCA: Principal component analysis; PLS-DA: Partial least squares discriminant analysis; SD: Standard deviation; SGA: Small for gestational age; SIMCA: Soft Independent Modeling of Class Analogy; STROBE: Strengthening the Reporting of Observational Studies in Epidemiology; TIDES: The Infant Development and the Environment Study; VIP: Variable importance in the projection

Acknowledgements

We express our gratitude to the Department of Maternal Fetal Medicine at the University of Minnesota for supporting this study. We also thank the NMR Spectroscopy lab at the Mayo Clinic in Rochester, MN for accommodating this project.

Funding

Funding provided by the U.S. Department of Health and Human Services, National Institutes of Health, National Institute of Diabetes and Digestive and Kidney Diseases, Grant number U24DK100469, as well as the University of Minnesota, School of Graduate Medical Education, Fellowship Research Fund. All researchers had independence from the funders.

Authors contributions

Author GL conceived the study, obtained TIDES samples for the study, worked in processing and analyzing samples in NMR lab, statistical analysis of the results as well as drafted the manuscript. Author IV participated in the design and coordination of the study, stored the samples for the study, conceived the protocol for processing/analyzing the samples, processed/ analyzed the samples, and was the primary source for all NMR spectroscopy aspects of the study. Author AB performed statistical analysis. Authors JBR, HG, RHN, SS, ES and SHS were involved in the original TIDES study and were involved in approving sample use for this study as well as approved the design of this study. Authors SZ, PD, SIM and KSN provided scientific advice on the process and interpretation of all samples. KSN acted as the primary liaison for Mayo Clinic collaboration, specifically the use of the NMR spectroscopy lab at the Mayo laboratories as well as the use of his laboratory for sample storage/processing. All authors read and approved the final manuscript.

Competing interests

The authors declare that they have no competing interests. All authors have completed the ICMJE uniform disclosure form at http:// www.icmje.org/coi_disclosure.pdf and declare: no support from any organisation for the submitted work other than what is listed under funding; no financial relationships with any organisations that might have an interest in the submitted work in the previous three years, no other relationships or activities that could appear to have influenced the submitted work.

Author details

[1]Nuclear Magnetic Resonance Facility, Mayo Clinic, Stabile SL-035, 200 First Street SW, Rochester, MN 55905, USA. [2]Clinical and Translational Science Institute, University of Minnesota, 717 Delaware Street SE, Second Floor, Minneapolis, MN 55414, USA. [3]Department of Maternal Fetal Medicine, University of Minnesota, 606 24th Ave S #400, Minneapolis, MN 55454, USA. [4]Division of Diabetes Endocrinology and Metabolism, 516 Delaware Street SE, MMC 101, Minneapolis, MN 55455, USA. [5]Environmental and Occupational Health Sciences Institute, Rutgers School of Public Health, 170 Frelinghuysen Rd, Piscataway, NJ 08854, USA. [6]Department of Pediatrics, University of Washington Seattle Children's Research Institute, CW8-6, PO Box 5371, Seattle, WA 98145-5005, USA. [7]Division of Epidemiology and Community Health, University of Minnesota, 1300 S. 2nd Street, Suite 300, Minneapolis, MN 55454, USA. [8]Department of Preventive Medicine, Icahn School of Medicine at Mount Sinai, 1 Gustave L. Levy Pl, New York, NY 10029, USA. [9]Metabolomics Core, Mayo Clinic Hospital, Saint Mary's Campus, Alfred Building, Fifth Floor, Room 417, 200 First St. SW, Rochester, MN 55905, USA.

References

1. DJP B. Adult consequences of fetal growth restriction. Clin Obstet Gynecol. 2006;49:270–83.
2. Kramer MS. Determinants of low birth weight: methodological assessment and meta-analysis. Bull World Health Organ. 1987;65:663–737.
3. American College of Obstetricians and Gynecologists. ACOG Practice bulletin no. 134: fetal growth restriction. Obstet. Gynecol. 2013;121:1122–33.
4. ICD-10 Version:2010 [Internet]. P051 Small Gestation. Age. [cited 19 Oct 2016]. Available from: http://apps.who.int/classifications/icd10/browse/2010/en#/P05.1.
5. ICD-10 Version:2010 [Internet]. P07 - Disord. Relat. Short Gestation Low Birth Weight ICD-10. [cited 19 Oct 2016]. Available from: http://apps.who.int/classifications/icd10/browse/2010/en.
6. Neonatal growth - AUDIPOG [Internet]. [cited 29 Nov 2016]. Available from: http://www.audipog.net/courbes_morpho.php?langue=en.
7. Mamelle N, Cochet V, Claris O. Definition of fetal growth restriction according to constitutional growth potential. Biol Neonate. 2001;80:277–85.

8. Maitre L, Fthenou E, Athersuch T, Coen M, Toledano MB, Holmes E, et al. Urinary metabolic profiles in early pregnancy are associated with preterm birth and fetal growth restriction in the Rhea mother-child cohort study. BMC Med. 2014;12:110.

9. Wong JMW, de Souza R, Kendall CWC, Emam A, Jenkins DJA. Colonic health: fermentation and short chain fatty acids. J Clin Gastroenterol. 2006; 40:235–43.

10. Smyth DH. The rate and site of acetate metabolism in the body. J Physiol. 1947;105:299–315.

11. Deon M, Sitta A, Faverzani JL, Guerreiro GB, Donida B, Marchetti DP, et al. Urinary biomarkers of oxidative stress and plasmatic inflammatory profile in phenylketonuric treated patients. Int. J. Dev. Neurosci. Off. J. Int. Soc. Dev Neurosci. 2015;47:259–65.

12. Lord RS, Bralley JA. Clinical applications of urinary organic acids. Part 2. Dysbiosis markers. Altern. Med. Rev. J. Clin Ther. 2008;13:292–306.

13. Horgan RP, Broadhurst DI, Walsh SK, Dunn WB, Brown M, Roberts CT, et al. Metabolic profiling uncovers a phenotypic signature of small for gestational age in early pregnancy. J Proteome Res. 2011;10:3660–73.

14. Diaz SO, Pinto J, Graça G, Duarte IF, Barros AS, Galhano E, et al. Metabolic biomarkers of prenatal disorders: an exploratory NMR metabonomics study of second trimester maternal urine and blood plasma. J Proteome Res. 2011;10:3732–42.

15. Pinto J, Barros AS, Domingues MRM, Goodfellow BJ, Galhano E, Pita C, et al. Following healthy pregnancy by NMR metabolomics of plasma and correlation to urine. J Proteome Res. 2015;14:1263–74.

16. Dai Z, Wu Z, Hang S, Zhu W, Wu G. Amino acid metabolism in intestinal bacteria and its potential implications for mammalian reproduction. Mol Hum Reprod. 2015;21:389–409.

17. Fowden AL, Giussani DA, Forhead AJ. Intrauterine programming of physiological systems: causes and consequences. Physiol Bethesda Md. 2006;21:29–37.

18. Sathyanarayana S, Grady R, Redmon JB, Ivicek K, Barrett E, Janssen S, et al. Anogenital distance and penile width measurements in the infant development and the environment study (TIDES): methods and predictors. J Pediatr Urol. 2015;11:76.e1–6.

19. Barrett ES, Sathyanarayana S, Janssen S, Redmon JB, Nguyen RHN, Kobrosly R, et al. Environmental health attitudes and behaviors: findings from a large pregnancy cohort study. Eur J Obstet Gynecol Reprod Biol. 2014;176:119–25.

20. Vambergue A, Fajardy I. Consequences of gestational and pregestational diabetes on placental function and birth weight. World J Diabetes. 2011;2:196–203.

21. Pregestational Diabetes Mellitus - ACOG [Internet]. [cited 3 Dec 2017]. Available from: https://www.acog.org/Resources-And-Publications/Practice-Bulletins/Committee-on-Practice-Bulletins-Obstetrics/Pregestational-Diabetes-Mellitus

22. Bruker: Overview - AVANCE IVDr - Clinical Screening and In Vitro Diagnostics (IVD) Discovery and Validation [Internet]. Bruker.com. [cited 21 Nov 2016]. Available from: https://www.bruker.com/products/mr/nmr/avance-ivdr/overview.html

23. Trygg J, Holmes E, Lundstedt T. Chemometrics in metabonomics. J Proteome Res. 2007;6:469–79.

24. von Elm E, Altman DG, Egger M, Pocock SJ, Gøtzsche PC, Vandenbroucke JP, et al. The strengthening the reporting of observational studies in epidemiology (STROBE) statement: guidelines for reporting observational studies. J Clin Epidemiol. 2008;61:344–9.

25. Maitre L, Villanueva CM, Lewis MR, Ibarluzea J, Santa-Marina L, Vrijheid M, et al. Maternal urinary metabolic signatures of fetal growth and associated clinical and environmental factors in the INMA study. BMC Med. 2016;14:177.

Development of a tailored strategy to improve postpartum hemorrhage guideline adherence

Suzan M. de Visser[1][*][†], Mallory D. Woiski[1][†], Richard P. Grol[2], Frank P. H. A. Vandenbussche[1], Marlies E. J. L. Hulscher[2], Hubertina C. J. Scheepers[3] and Rosella P. M. G. Hermens[2]

Abstract

Background: Despite the introduction of evidence based guidelines and practical courses, the incidence of postpartum hemorrhage shows an increasing trend in developed countries. Substandard care is often found, which implies an inadequate implementation in high resource countries. We aimed to reduce the gap between evidence-based guidelines and clinical application, by developing a strategy, tailored to current barriers for implementation.

Methods: The development of the implementation strategy consisted of three phases, supervised by a multidisciplinary expert panel. In the first phase a framework of the strategy was created, based on barriers to optimal adherence identified among professionals and patients together with evidence on effectiveness of strategies found in literature. In the second phase, the tools within the framework were developed, leading to a first draft. In the third phase the strategy was evaluated among professionals and patients. The professionals were asked to give written feedback on tool contents, clinical usability and inconsistencies with current evidence care. Patients evaluated the tools on content and usability. Based on the feedback of both professionals and patients the tools were adjusted.

Results: We developed a tailored strategy to improve guideline adherence, covering the trajectory of the third trimester of pregnancy till the end of the delivery. The strategy, directed at professionals, comprehending three stop moments includes a risk assessment checklist, care bundle and time-out procedure. As patient empowerment tools, a patient passport and a website with patient information was developed. The evaluation among the expert panel showed all professionals to be satisfied with the content and usability and no discrepancies or inconsistencies with current evidence was found. Patients' evaluation revealed that the information they received through the tools was incomplete. The tools were adjusted accordingly to the missing information.

Conclusion: A usable, tailored strategy to implement PPH guidelines and practical courses was developed. The next step is the evaluation of the strategy in a feasibility trial.

Trial registration: Clinical trial registration: The Fluxim study, registration number: NCT00928863.

Keywords: Implementation strategy, Postpartum hemorrhage, Substandard care, Tailor-made

* Correspondence: Suzan.deVisser@radboudumc.nl
†Equal contributors
[1]Department of Obstetrics and Gynecology, Radboud Institute for Health Science, Radboud University Medical Center, Geert Grootplein 10, P.O. Box 9101, 6500, HB, Nijmegen, the Netherlands
Full list of author information is available at the end of the article

Background

Worldwide postpartum hemorrhage (PPH) is the main cause of severe maternal morbidity (SMM). A recent study in the United States estimated PPH to be responsible for almost half of the cases of SMM (47,6%) [1]. Globally the incidence of PPH is estimated around 10,5% and in high resource countries an increasing trend in PPH incidence has been seen [2]. For example, in The Netherlands the incidence increased from 3% in 2003 to 8% in 2011 in second line care [3].

A review on PPH guideline adherence found that 38% of the women with ≥1500 ml blood loss received substandard care [4]. Substandard health care is often suggested as a possible cause for inadequate reduction of morbidity [5–7]. It seems that evidence-based guidelines are not optimally adhered to, leading to substandard care and a gap between evidence-based medicine and clinical application [8].

Guideline dissemination without a tailored implementation strategy to improve spread among professionals and adherence to guidelines is often ineffective [9]. A review evaluating implementation strategies within the field of obstetrics concludes that a prospective identification of efficient strategies and barriers to change is necessary to improve clinical practice guideline implementation [10]. The strategy choice needs to be tailored to the setting for best possible results, consisting of the right tools to increase guideline adherence. In this paper we describe the development of an implementation strategy for a high resource obstetric setting to improve guideline adherence regarding postpartum hemorrhage.

Methods

Setting

The current study is part of the FLUXIM trial [11]. In this trial we developed quality indicators on PPH care (a); studied the adherence of these indicators in actual care (b), and analyzed barriers and facilitators for optimal care among both professionals, women and their partners (c). In the last part of the Fluxim trial the outcomes of these data were aggregated and formed the basis of the development of a strategy to improve guideline adherence.

Development strategy

The development of the implementation strategy consisted of three phases (Fig. 1).

Phase one: The selection of the tools for the implementation strategy

In the first phase the selection of the tools to be included in the implementation strategy was performed by a multidisciplinary expert panel of eight obstetricians, two anesthesiologists and two opinion leaders on quality of care research through an iterative process.

The barriers and facilitators from the professional level chosen for the implementation strategy were those mentioned by at least three out of the four focus groups, and feasible to incorporate in our strategy. These barriers were discussed among the authors to determine which barriers were most likely to supply the greatest gain for improvement and were feasible to include. The same selection criteria were applied to the facilitators. On the patient level, through consensus among the authors, barriers and facilitators were identified as eligible for the strategy.

International literature was searched for evidence on effectiveness of strategies to serve as a base for the selection of the tools to address the barriers and to incorporate the identified facilitators (i.e. the potential tools). The search covered three areas: tools and strategies within the obstetric health care, effective tools outside the field of obstetrics and patient oriented tools. Articles were searched on Medline and experts in the field of implementation science were consulted for recent literature. The search was limited to only article in English, limited to research performed in high resource countries, and there was no date restriction. The search results were presented to the expert panel combined with the barriers and facilitators that were considered most important and the low adherence scores of the actual care study as described above in the setting section [12, 13].

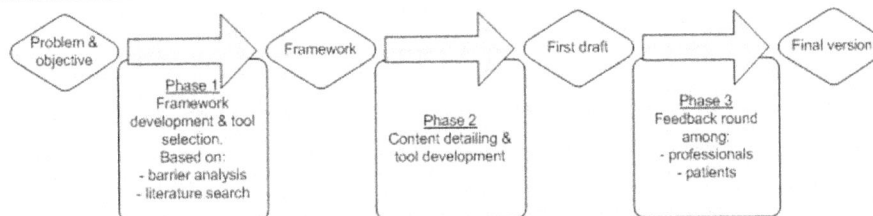

Fig. 1 The strategy development process. The three phases for the development of the implementation strategy to improve PPH guideline adherence. The first phase consisted of the analyses of barriers for guideline implementation and the search of international literature of strategy effectiveness, leading to the creating of the strategy framework. The second phase was the content detailing of the created framework and the development of the individual tools. After the first draft was made, a feedback round among professionals and patients was held to assess the content and usability of the tools

Phase two: The development of the tools and their content

In the second phase the selected potential tools were developed. The tool content was derived from international guidelines [14–20], ATLS-based courses (Advanced Trauma Life Support, e.g. the Managing Obstetric Emergencies and Trauma course) and international literature. They give recommendations based on the stage of delivery of the patient, and on the progression of the PPH. There are preventive measures, measures when the blood loss reaches 500 cm^3 and when there is ongoing blood loss above the liter or 2 l. These phases are also to be found in the division of the quality indicators. The tool set up and content follow this set up of PPH care, and places actions in relation to the stage of amount of blood loss of the patient.

According to both the Dutch and the international guidelines, identification of high-risk patients forms the basis of PPH care. However, most guidelines did not clearly define all risk factors for PPH and there was discrepancy between different guidelines. Therefore an additional search was performed using the Dutch PPH guideline, 6 international guidelines [15–20] and international literature. We searched for additional risk factors and odds ratios (OR's), and only OR's with confidence intervals available were considered. Medline was searched using the search terms 'PPH' and 'risk factors' and synonyms, followed by a snowballing search of the articles and reference lists of the guidelines if available. Furthermore, risk factors found in a multivariate analysis of the Netherlands Perinatal Registration (Dutch Perinatal Registration, DPR) by the LEMMoN study were considered as well (unpublished data, personal correspondence: J. Zwart, Severe Maternal Morbidity in the Netherlands. The LEMMoN study. 2009). Ultimately, all risk factors listed in the Dutch guideline were selected to be included in the tools, as well as all risk factors that were mentioned in at least two of the other six guidelines and found significant in either international literature or in the DPR analysis.

Phase 3: Feedback round expert panel and patients

In phase three, the developed tools, was presented in a feedback round among the expert panel. The nine members of the expert panel were asked to evaluate the tools on accuracy of the medical contents, clinical usability and control for inconsistencies with the current best evidence care as provided by the Dutch guideline, and to provide written feedback on these three items.

Patients were recruited to evaluate the patient materials developed for the strategy. Both high-risk patients and patients who experienced a PPH in the previous year were asked for the evaluation. High-risk patients were recruited from the obstetrics clinic in one of the participating hospitals. The patients having experienced a PPH were recruited by placing messages on childbirth forums. The women were asked to evaluate our website by means of a questionnaire. The questionnaire consisted of 37 questions, of which 29 were yes-no questions, evaluating six specific domains, and two general categories with eight open questions for points for improvement. The domains evaluated were the usability, speed of the website, website menu navigation, the completeness and clarity of the information provided, the layout and the risk-identification test available on the website.

Results

In the three steps described above we have created a strategy to improve the adherence to evidence based guidelines and the ATLS-based course for prevention and treatment of PPH. The strategy, shown in Fig. 2, consists of three stop moments, a checklist for PPH treatment for the professionals and two patient tools.

Setting

In short the results of the barriers and facilitators found for optimal PPH care and the current care analysis. The most important barriers experienced by professionals were lack of knowledge, team communication and leadership. They mentioned the use of checklists and flowcharts as factors to improve adherence to the guideline. Patients mentioned lack of information before, during and after the PPH as main barriers and an informative patient website and leaflet as main facilitator for optimal care [12]. Actual care was particularly not in accordance with guidelines with regard to the high risk identification and documentation of policy for PPH on the outpatient clinic and during labor, vital signs monitoring, and the different steps in the management of PPH. Furthermore, acts regarding management of PPH were only partly performed in time [13].

Phase one: The selection of the tools for the implementation strategy

The professionals' barriers and facilitators on which the expert panel reached consensus to include them in the tools, are listed in Table 1, those of the patients are shown in Table 2 [12].

When reviewing the literature on strategies for guideline implementation within the field of obstetrics, a systematic review [10] on evidence-based strategies for obstetric guideline implementation provided an overview of effective strategies. Of the tools they reviewed, educational tools showed mixed effects, audit & feedback was generally effective, strategies based on opinion leaders, quality improvement tools and academic detailing were ineffective or showed mixed effects. Reminders showed to be overall effective [10].

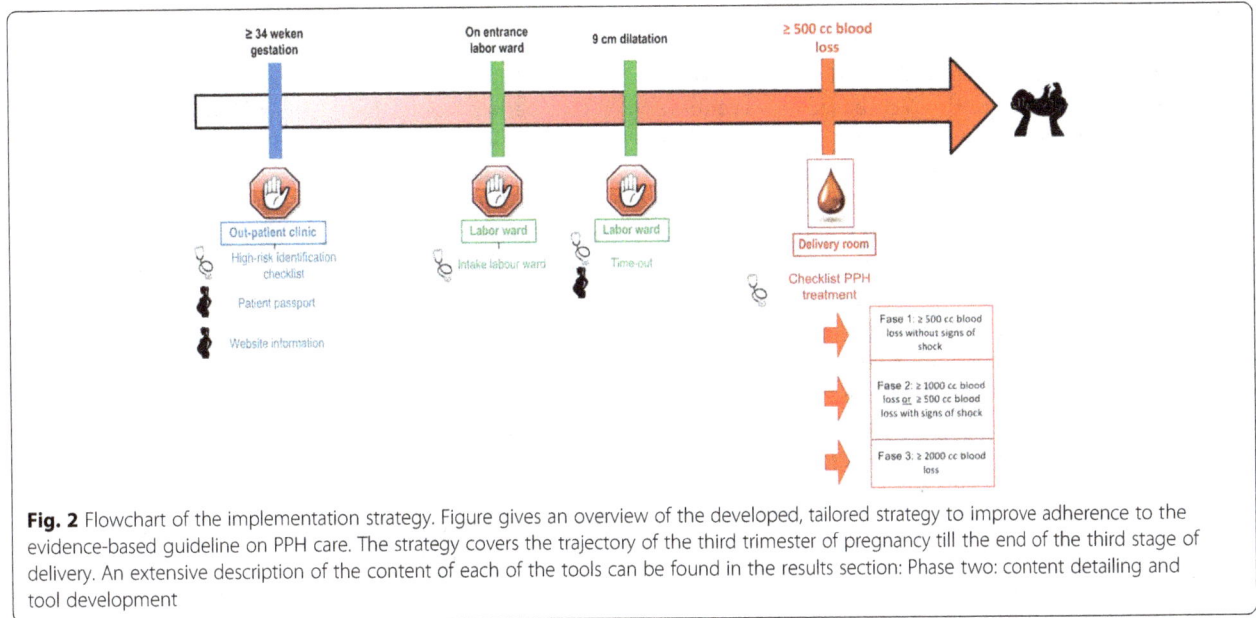

Fig. 2 Flowchart of the implementation strategy. Figure gives an overview of the developed, tailored strategy to improve adherence to the evidence-based guideline on PPH care. The strategy covers the trajectory of the third trimester of pregnancy till the end of the third stage of delivery. An extensive description of the content of each of the tools can be found in the results section: Phase two: content detailing and tool development

Table 1 Main barriers and facilitators addressed by professionals

	Barriers	N[a]
1	Lack of checklist/flowchart about PPH at the delivery rooms	4
2	The guideline is difficult to obtain the at the delivery ward	3
3	Recommendations and definitions in the guideline are unclear	3
4	Professionals overestimate their knowledge regarding identifying the patient-categories at risk for PPH and regarding the treatment of high-risk patients and patients with PPH	4
5	Professionals lack to detect high-risk patients at the outpatient clinic	4
6	Tools: need for practical tools for easier and practical use of the guideline	3
7	Lack of communication in the team responsible for the patient, about the risks, policy's, seriousness of the situations or actions that need to be taken	4
8	Unclearness in leadership trough lack of knowledge of each other's skills and ability, because of inexperienced professionals and the frequent change of team composition.	4
9	Disagreement between team members and with personnel of other disciplines about the seriousness of the situation (blood-bank personnel and anesthesiologists)	3
10	Lack of team collaboration, for orders are not followed and team members prefer following their own instincts in treatments that leads to inconsequent policy.	3
11	Presence of hierarchy leads to dread, for team members find it difficult to call in a gynecologist who is at home and speak freely against the supervisor when there is a disagreement about policy	3

	Facilitators	
1	The availability of a checklist/flowchart about PPH at the delivery rooms would improve care	4

[a] Amount of focus groups that mentioned the barrier or facilitator

Outside the field of obstetrics two types of effective tools were found that seemed applicable in an obstetric setting by the expert panel. The first were checklists, showing to be successful in reducing the complication rate in surgical settings [21–24], and revealing an increase in adherence to safety indicators and guidelines [21, 23]. Checklists can provide an overview in a complicated situation, and reduces room for human error and the number of omitted treatments. Furthermore, checklists can improve documentation of care, facilitate (team- and interdisciplinary) communication and leadership, and minimize information loss during transfer between professionals [23]. Secondly, care bundles, initiated of the Institute for Healthcare Improvement, have in multiple settings shown to increase compliance to quality indicators and reduced complications and mortality [25–27].

Patient empowerment is an important topic in health care and refers to the enhanced ability of patients to actively understand and influence their own health status

Table 2 Main barriers and facilitators addressed by patients

	Barriers
1	poor information supply to the patient about PPH
2	poor information supply to the partner and/or family about the medical condition, risks and procedures
3	lack of information material (e.g. folders or website)
4	patient's perception of delay in transfer to the operation room

	Facilitators
1	information about PPH before the delivery
2	a request for patient information material

and health care [28]. According to the WHO, interventions with empowerment characteristics have shown significant impact in improving health and quality of life in chronically ill patients [29]. Web-based interventions seem effective in empowering patients [30] and with a relative young target population a viable option for patient empowerment in PPH care.

Based on the barrier analysis and the literature, the expert panel decided on a multifaceted strategy with separate tools addressing different barriers at different levels, visualized in Fig. 2. The strategy encompassed the complete trajectory starting in the third trimester and ending after the third stage of delivery is finished and the patient is stable. For the professionals, it comprised three stop moments (with a risk assessment checklist, care bundle and time-out procedure), and a PPH treatment checklist. For the patients, a patient-passport was created to provide to high-risk patients and a website for both pregnant and postpartum women to provide preparation information before the delivery and information to process their recent experience.

Phase two: The development of the tools and their content

After selection, the individual tools were developed. Standard prototypes of the professional tools were developed based on the latest guidelines and literature.

These prototypes can be adjusted to local protocols (e.g. specific medication choice and dose, telephone numbers of emergency services) before disseminating and implementing them in the different Dutch hospitals. The content of the patient part was written by an obstetrician (MW) with expertise in PPH care. The text was checked by another obstetrician (HS) for accuracy and a layman (RH) for readability and understandability. As the strategy exists of four stop moments, four separate tools were created as can be seen in Fig. 2.

The first stop moment is at the outpatient clinic where the physician has to fill in a risk assessment checklist. The checklist could be filled in from 34 weeks of gestation or beyond. The checklist listed all identified risk factors for a PPH, thus enabling the user to identify high risk patients. It also listed the policy for high risk patients as a reminder for the user.

As described in the methods section a risk assessment checklist was developed by the Fluxim study as there is currently no such list available. To create the risk assessment checklist, in total 34 risk factors were selected for inclusion: 25 risk factors from the Dutch national guideline and an additional nine risk factors were found in at least two international guidelines with significant odds ratios. The risk factors could be divided into four categories: general health history, obstetric history, factors related to the current pregnancy and factors apparent during labor and delivery. The checklist is designed to

make the professionals aware of PPH risk factors, alert them on the increased risk and appropriate policy and remind them to inform the patient on the increased risk.

The patient tools that were created for the strategy could be used to inform the patient, facilitating the professional and ensuring consistent and comprehensive supply of PPH patient information. The tools consisted, as mentioned above, of a patient passport that allows patients to identify themselves as high-risk patient to professionals they meet later on in the pregnancy. It also provides written information about PPH and possible preventive measures professionals can take during the delivery. The second tool is a website available to all patients who attended the participating hospitals in the Fluxim trial for their antenatal care.

The second stop moment is upon entrance of the labor ward. At this stop moment professionals need to check if a risk assessment had been performed. In case it has not been done, the checklist has to be provided at that moment.

The third stop moment is near the end of the first stage of labor, closely before entering the second stage. During this stop moment the whole team has to be gathered in the room with the patient for a time-out procedure. It encompasses the checking of the patients' risk status and corresponding policy, and additional risk factors have to be listed (those that may arise during the first stage of delivery and those possibly arising during the second stage of delivery). As the time-out requires the team to come together in the room with the patient, it stimulates team communication and increases knowledge of all professionals working on the labor ward. The timing of the time-up is left upon the labor ward team, as this might differ per patient depending on the speed of dilatation. A care bundle consisting of preventive interventions (those identified as the active management of the third stage in the Dutch PPH guideline) was incorporated in the time-out, aiding in the standardizing of procedures.

As last of the professional tools, a checklist for PPH treatment was created. This checklist can be used by professionals at a blood loss of 500 ml and ongoing. It guides professionals through consecutive treatment options, gives advice on when to control for what factors (e.g. vital signs, coagulation status, etc), gives an indication of time elapsed and shows when to consult other professionals (i.e. an obstetrician or anesthesiologist). Furthermore, the checklist provides areas for the writing down of times of actions undertaken and vital signs; a procedure advised by ATLS-based courses for Obstetric emergencies.

Phase 3: Feedback round expert panel and patients

The expert panel was satisfied with the content and usability of the individual tools of the strategy and there were no points reported concerning inaccuracy of the medical contents, clinical unfeasibility or inconsistencies with the PPH guideline.

Sixteen patients evaluated the website. Of these, 6 were patients within their third trimester of the pregnancy and had an increased risk for PPH, 9 patients had experienced PPH in a recent delivery and of one returned questionnaire it was not clear if the correspondent was pregnant or post partum. Suggestions were made by the patients for improvement of the website, of which the most important improvement was the adding a section about recovery after PPH. All comments were taken into consideration for change and those that were feasible were changed. As some suggestions were not feasible they were not included in the adaptation process. An example of a non-feasible recommendation is the adding of percentages of increased risk per risk factor, which is not feasible as there is no consensus within the literature on the OR's of the risk factors. Information added to the website included information on the recovery after PPH, information for the partner and information about low-lying placentas. Other changes that were made were the adding of images and suggestion on clearer color schemes.

Discussion

We developed a tailored strategy to improve adherence to the evidence-based guideline on PPH care within secondary and tertiary care hospitals in the Netherlands. The strategy is based on current care, a barrier analysis and literature. A strategy with 3 stop moments was developed starting in the third trimester of the pregnancy and lasting till the end of the third stage of delivery. Tools used during the three stop moments are a checklist for risk assessment, patient empowerment tools and a time-out closely to the start of the second stage of delivery, with a PPH preventive care bundle incorporated in the time-out. Furthermore a checklist for PPH treatment was developed in case the blood loss exceeded 500 ml postpartum.

Safety checklists, such as the surgical safety checklists, have been derived from aviation and other high-risk industries where they have shown to be effective in reduction of adverse events. The Institute of Medicine published in 1999 the renowned report "To err is human" on medical errors, patient safety and the development of safety systems [31]. They made recommendations to reduce the reliance on human memory and to implement systems that standardize and simplify processes. A checklist is such a system that forces a time-out to summarize the situation and to prepare the professionals for what is coming. It facilitates leadership and open communication, and reduces reliance on memory and the number of omitted procedures. Various types of surgical safety checklists have proven that these systems can be translated to the

medical field and successfully reduce complications [21, 22, 24]. A delivery is an acute process where we heavily rely on the memory of the professionals, and where the room for error is large. A recent review on obstetric checklist development confirmed the need to standardize work in the maternity and labor ward, and listed PPH as 6th in their top ten areas that have high priority on checklist development [32].

Involving patients in the perinatal care process creates a shared responsibility and creates opportunity for women to take the lead in the creation of their own care plan. In 2010 an advisory committee ("pregnancy and birth") of the Dutch Ministry of Health has written a report with advice on how to approach pregnancy and childbirth healthcare from a current and reliable perspective [33]. The aim of the report is to improve (perinatal) health, not solely with the women are sick but in general thus preventing sickness, and to reduce health inequalities. The committee states seven cornerstones, two of which are related to patient empowerment (mother and child in the lead and well informed pregnant patients with shared responsibility). To reach this level of involvement of patients listening to patients and their needs is essential. Including patients in the barrier analysis gave us the opportunity to listen to patients carefully, leading to tools that are actually wanted by patients and filling the current information gap in perinatal care.

Currently, there is a discussion, outside the field of obstetrics, about the added effectiveness of multi-faceted strategies over single-faceted strategies. Although earlier reviews claimed that combinations of many different interventions are often effective [34, 35], Grimshaw found that a higher number of intervention components was not related to higher effectiveness [36].. It seems plausible that combined interventions are only more effective than single interventions, if these address different barriers at different levels. This is also the conclusion of Chaillet et al. [10] Their review shows that in the field of obstetrics multi-faceted strategies are more effective, with the prerequisite that each strategy facet is targeted at its own barrier. Furthermore they showed that a prospective identification of the barriers would enhance its effectiveness, a recurrent finding in reviews on strategy effectiveness [10, 34, 35]. We have created such a multi-faceted, tailor-made strategy with each separate tool developed to address specific barriers.

The framework of our strategy to improve the provision of optimal PPH care in high resource settings is based on barriers found among professionals and patients from the Netherlands, optimizing the strategy for the Dutch setting. However, we believe that the barriers are rather universal, and the framework would thus be applicable in similar obstetric setting in other countries.

We detailed the contents of the individual tools in accordance with the Dutch national PPH guideline, international guidelines and literature. As the focus of guideline committees per country can differ, and (conflicting) evidence in literature sometimes leaves room for interpretation, guidelines can vary between countries, organizations and in time. Developing a strategy that is flexible to content and thus adjustable to updates or different surroundings allows it to be constant up-to-date and adaptable for other high-resource countries. As the strategy is low in development cost and maintenance, it could be applicable in low-resource countries, though this still needs to be investigated.

The main strength of our strategy is the fact that it is tailor-made to the field of PPH. Professionals in the field suggested the barriers and facilitators, which most likely facilitates the acceptance of the strategy in a clinical setting.

Limitations of any strategy development lie within the scarce amount of knowledge available for strategy selection. It is known that tailor-made strategies perform better, yet there is no explicit model prescribing which strategy or tool is to be expected most effective in a certain setting. Furthermore limitations of our study are the fact that it is created developed based on barriers found in a high income country, thus limiting the generalization towards lower income countries. Also, our literature search on strategy development evidence was a systematic comprehensive search.

The aim of this article is to describe the process of development, however at this point we need more evidence as to rather the strategy will indeed improve adherence to the guidelines, and ultimately decrease the PPH incidence. Therefore the next steps are testing the feasibility and effectiveness of the strategy in the clinical practice. Before setting up a large randomized controlled trial to evaluate the effectiveness of the trial, a feasibility trial has to be conducted. In such a feasibility trial, the strategy has to be evaluated on usability, time consummation and possible points for improvement. Additionally, an indication towards possible effectiveness and costs can be received. This will allow for optimization of the strategy before testing its cost-/effectiveness in a robust study design.

Conclusion

In conclusion, to our knowledge, the developed tailored strategy is the first worldwide in the acute setting of obstetric care encompassing the whole process from prevention to treatment of PPH. Based on current barriers and facilitators nominated by professionals in the field combined with international literature we have aimed to create a usable, tailored strategy that can aid in the implementation of evidence-based guidelines into daily practice.

Abbreviations

ATLS: Advanced trauma life support; DPR: Dutch Perinatal Registration; OR: Odds ratio; PPH: Postpartum hemorrhage; SMM: Severe maternal morbidity; WHO: World Health Organisation

Acknowledgements

None.

Funding

The study was supported by a ZonMW grant. No. 80–82315–98-09003.

Authors' contributions

SV, MW, RG, HS and RH were involved with the conception and design of the strategy. All authors were involved with the analysis and interpretation of the literature for strategy and tool development. SV, MW, HS and RH were responsible for drafting the article, and RG, FV and MH all critically revised drafts and provided feedback. All authors approve of the version to be published.

Competing interests

The authors declare that they have no competing interests.

Author details

[1]Department of Obstetrics and Gynecology, Radboud Institute for Health Science, Radboud University Medical Center, Geert Grootplein 10, P.O. Box 9101, 6500, HB, Nijmegen, the Netherlands. [2]Department of IQ Healthcare, Radboud Institute for Health Science, Radboud University Medical Center, Nijmegen, Netherlands. [3]Department of Obstetrics and Gynecology, GROW School for Oncology and Developmental Biology, Maastricht University Medical Center, Maastricht, The Netherlands.

References

1. Grobman WA, Bailit JL, Rice MM, Wapner RJ, Reddy UM, Varner MW, et al. Frequency of and factors associated with severe maternal morbidity. Obstet Gynecol. 2014;123(4):804–10.
2. Knight M, Callaghan WM, Berg C, Alexander S, Bouvier-Colle MH, Ford JB, et al. Trends in postpartum hemorrhage in high resource countries: a review and recommendations from the international postpartum hemorrhage collaborative group. BMC Pregnancy Childbirth. 2009;9:55.
3. Registry tNP. Perinatale Zorg in Nederland. Utrecht: the Netherlands Perinatal Registry; 2003–2011.
4. Bouvier-Colle MH, Ould El Joud D, Varnoux N, Goffinet F, Alexander S, Bayoumeu F, et al. Evaluation of the quality of care for severe obstetrical haemorrhage in three French regions. BJOG. 2001;108(9):898–903.
5. McGlynn EA, Asch SM, Adams J, Keesey J, Hicks J, DeCristofaro A, et al. The quality of health care delivered to adults in the United States. N Engl J Med. 2003;348(26):2635–45.

6. Lawton B, MacDonald EJ, Brown SA, Wilson L, Stanley J, Tait JD, et al. Preventability of severe acute maternal morbidity. Am J Obstet Gynecol. 2014;210(6):557. e1–6.

7. van Dillen J, Mesman JA, Zwart JJ, Bloemenkamp KW, van Roosmalen J. Introducing maternal morbidity audit in the Netherlands. BJOG. 2010;117(4): 416–21.

8. Bodenheimer T. The American health care system–the movement for improved quality in health care. N Engl J Med. 1999;340(6):488–92.

9. Grol R, Wensing M. What drives change? Barriers to and incentives for achieving evidence-based practice. Med J Aust. 2004;180(6 Suppl):S57–60.

10. Chaillet N, Dube E, Dugas M, Audibert F, Tourigny C, Fraser WD, et al. Evidence-based strategies for implementing guidelines in obstetrics: a systematic review. Obstet Gynecol. 2006;108(5):1234–45.

11. Woiski MD, Hermens RP, Middeldorp JM, Kremer JA, Marcus MA, Wouters MG, et al. Haemorrhagia post partum; an implementation study on the evidence-based guideline of the Dutch Society of Obstetrics and Gynaecology (NVOG) and the MOET (managing obstetric emergencies and trauma-course) instructions; the Fluxim study. BMC Pregnancy Childbirth. 2010;10:5.

12. Woiski MD, Belfroid E, Liefers J, Grol RP, Scheepers HC, Hermens RP. Influencing factors for high quality care on postpartum haemorrhage in the Netherlands: patient and professional perspectives. BMC Pregnancy Childbirth. 2015;15:272.

13. Woiski MD. Quality of Postpartum Hemorrhage care. The need for standardization. [PhD thesis]. Nijmegen: Radboud University; 2016.

14. (NVOG) DSoOaG. Haemorrhagia Postpartum [Guideline]. 2006 [updated 22–03–2006. 2nd:[Available from: http://nvog-documenten.nl/index. php?pagina=/richtlijn/pagina.php&fSelectTG_62=75&fSelectedSub= 62&fSelectedParent=75.

15. (RCOG) RCoOaG. Prevention and Management of Postpartum Haemorrhage 2009 [updated april 2011. Available from: http://www.rcog.org.uk/files/rcog-corp/GT52PostpartumHaemorrhage0411.pdf.

16. ACOG Practice Bulletin: Clinical Management Guidelines for Obstetrician-Gynecologists Number 76, October 2006: postpartum hemorrhage 2006 [updated Oct. 2006/10/03:[1039-47]. Available from: http://www.ncbi.nlm. nih.gov/entrez/query.fcgi?cmd=Retrieve&db=PubMed&dopt=Citation&list_ uids=17012482.

17. Force CHT. OB Hemorrhage Care Guidelines: Checklist Format California Maternal Quality Care Collaborative; 2010 [Available from: http://www. cmqcc.org/ob_hemorrhage/ob_hemorrhage_care_guidelines.

18. Health NCCfWsaCs. NICE clinical guideline 55. Intrapartum care: care of healthy women and their babies during childbirth: National Institute for Health and Clinical Excellence; 2007 [updated september 2007. Available from: http://guidance.nice.org.uk/CG55.

19. Leduc D, Senikas V, Lalonde AB, Ballerman C, Biringer A, Delaney M, et al. Active management of the third stage of labour: prevention and treatment of postpartum hemorrhage. J Obstet Gynaecol Can. 2009;31(10):980–93.

20. Unit OaGCC. 9.1 Primary postpartum haemorrhage Perth, Australiaseptember 2010 [updated September 2010. Available from: http:// kemh.health.wa.gov.au/development/manuals/O&G_guidelines/sectionb/#9.

21. Haynes AB, Weiser TG, Berry WR, Lipsitz SR, Breizat AH, Dellinger EP, et al. A surgical safety checklist to reduce morbidity and mortality in a global population. N Engl J Med. 2009;360(5):491–9.

22. de Vries EN, Prins HA, Crolla RM, den Outer AJ, van Andel G, van Helden SH, et al. Effect of a comprehensive surgical safety system on patient outcomes. N Engl J Med. 2010;363(20):1928–37.

23. Thomassen O, Storesund A, Softeland E, Brattebo G. The effects of safety checklists in medicine: a systematic review. Acta Anaesthesiol Scand. 2014; 58(1):5–18.

24. Weiser TG, Haynes AB, Dziekan G, Berry WR, Lipsitz SR, Gawande AA. Effect of a 19-item surgical safety checklist during urgent operations in a global patient population. Ann Surg. 2010;251(5):976–80.

25. Nguyen HB, Corbett SW, Steele R, Banta J, Clark RT, Hayes SR, et al. Implementation of a bundle of quality indicators for the early management of severe sepsis and septic shock is associated with decreased mortality. Crit Care Med. 2007;35(4):1105–12.

26. Nguyen HB, Lynch EL, Mou JA, Lyon K, Wittlake WA, Corbett SW. The utility of a quality improvement bundle in bridging the gap between research and standard care in the management of severe sepsis and septic shock in the emergency department. Acad Emerg Med. 2007;14(11): 1079–86.

27. Resar R, Pronovost P, Haraden C, Simmonds T, Rainey T, Nolan T. Using a bundle approach to improve ventilator care processes and reduce ventilator-associated pneumonia. Jt Comm J Qual Patient Saf. 2005;31(5): 243–8.

28. Bruegel RB. Patient empowerment–a trend that matters. J AHIMA. 1998; 69(8):30–3. quiz 5-6

29. Wallerstein N. What is the evidence on effectiveness of empowerment to improve health? Copenhagen: World Health Organization, Regional Office for Europe, Health Evidence Network; 2006.

30. Samoocha D, Bruinvels DJ, Elbers NA, Anema JR, van der Beek AJ. Effectiveness of web-based interventions on patient empowerment: a systematic review and meta-analysis. J Med Internet Res. 2010;12(2):e23.

31. Kohn LT, Corrigan J, Donaldson MS. To err is human: building a safer health system. Washington, D.C: Committee on Quality of Health Care in America, Institute of Medicine, National Academy Press; 2000. p. xxi, 287.

32. Fausett MB, Propst A, Van Doren K, Clark BT. How to develop an effective obstetric checklist. Am J Obstet Gynecol. 2011;205(3):165–70.

33. Een goed begin. Veilige zorg rondom zwangerschap en geboorte.: Stuurgroep zwangerschap en geboorte; 2009.

34. Bero LA, Grilli R, Grimshaw JM, Harvey E, Oxman AD, Thomson MA. Closing the gap between research and practice: an overview of systematic reviews of interventions to promote the implementation of research findings. The Cochrane effective practice and Organization of Care Review Group. BMJ. 1998;317(7156):465–8.

35. Grimshaw JM, Shirran L, Thomas R, Mowatt G, Fraser C, Bero L, et al. Changing provider behavior: an overview of systematic reviews of interventions. Med Care. 2001;39(8 Suppl 2):II2–45.

36. Grimshaw JM, Thomas RE, MacLennan G, Fraser C, Ramsay CR, Vale L, et al. Effectiveness and efficiency of guideline dissemination and implementation strategies. Health Technol Assess. 2004;8(6):iii–v. 1-72

Avoiding late preterm deliveries to reduce neonatal complications: an 11-year cohort study

Noémie Bouchet[1], Angèle Gayet-Ageron[2], Marina Lumbreras Areta[1], Riccardo Erennio Pfister[3] and Begoña Martinez de Tejada[1*] (iD)

Abstract

Background: Late preterm (LPT) newborns, defined as those born between 34 0/7 and 36 6/7 gestational weeks, have higher short- and long-term morbidity and mortality than term infants (≥37 weeks). A categorization to justify a non-spontaneous LPT delivery has been proposed to distinguish evidence-based from non-evidence-based criteria. This study aims to describe rates and temporal trends of non-spontaneous LPT neonates delivered according to evidence-based or non-evidence-based criteria and to evaluate the number of avoidable LPT deliveries, including severe neonatal morbidity rates and associated risk factors.

Methods: Retrospective cohort study including all LPT neonates born at a Swiss university maternity unit between January 1, 2002 and December 31, 2012. Trends of LPT neonates and neonatal complications were assessed across time using Poisson regression and risk factors for neonatal complications by logistic regression.

Results: Among 40,609 singleton live births, 4223 (10.5%) were preterm and 2017 (4.9%) LPT. In the latter group, 26.2% were non-spontaneous (evidence-based: 12.0%; non-evidence-based: 14.2%). The most frequent indications for evidence-based non-spontaneous LPT delivery were severe preeclampsia (51.8%) and abnormal fetal tracing (24.7%). Indications for non-evidence-based non-spontaneous LPT deliveries were hemorrhage (36.2%) and mild preeclampsia (15.7%). LPT birth rates remained stable over time. The rate of neonatal complications after non-evidence-based LPT birth remained high over time (43.8% vs. 43.5% in 2002 and 2012, respectively; $P = 0.645$), whereas the annual proportion of neonatal complications overall showed a decreasing trend (from 38.0% in 2002 to 33.5% in 2012; $P = 0.051$).

Conclusions: LPT birth rates were stable over time, but neonatal complications remained high, particularly after non-evidence-indicated LPT birth. A total of 287 LPT births could have been potentially avoided if an evidence-based protocol for delivery indications had been used. Efforts should be made to avoid non-spontaneous LPT births in order to reduce neonatal complications.

Keywords: Late preterm birth, Delivery, Spontaneous, Non-spontaneous, Evidence-based, Trends, Neonatal complications

Background

Since the 1990s, the worldwide rate of preterm births (birth before 37 weeks' gestation) has been increasing and even represented up to 11% of all live births in 2010 in Europe and the USA [1, 2]. This trend is partly correlated with the rise of medically-indicated preterm delivery in order to reduce stillbirth [3, 4]. Preterm delivery may occur as a result of spontaneous preterm labor, including the preterm premature rupture of membranes (PPROM) or medical interventions, such as labor induction or elective cesarean, that are initiated to reduce poor outcomes associated with specific maternal or fetal conditions [5–7]. Late preterm (LPT) birth, defined as delivery between 34 0/7 and 36 6/7 weeks' gestation, represents two-thirds of all preterm births and impacts heavily on the rise of medically- indicated deliveries [8–11]. LPT neonates have long been wrongly considered as "near

* Correspondence: begona.martinezdetejada@hcuge.ch
[1]Obstetrics Unit, Department of Obstetrics and Gynecology, Geneva University Hospitals and Faculty of Medicine, 30 Boulevard de la Cluse, 1205 Geneva, Switzerland
Full list of author information is available at the end of the article

term". Beliefs about supposed "almost maturity" and the fear of stillbirth motivated weak indications for induced deliveries, such as isolated oligohydramnios or gestational hypertension [12–14].

It is now well established that LPT infants have an increased risk of morbidity and mortality compared to those born at term [15]. In the short term, they have a higher risk than term infants to suffer from respiratory distress syndrome, apnea, hypothermia, hypoglycemia, jaundice, hyperbilirubinemia, necrotizing enterocolitis and intraventricular hemorrhage [14, 16, 17]. This leads to frequent admissions to the neonatal intensive care unit (NICU) and a longer duration of hospitalization with high economic costs [18–20]. In the long term, LPT newborns appear to have an increased risk of cerebral palsy and mental retardation, as well as more behavioral abnormalities than their term peers [21, 22]. Learning disabilities and a lower socioeconomic level than their parents have also been described [23, 24]. Moreover, LPT birth and its consequences have a negative emotional and psychosocial impact on parents and families, which can last well beyond the initial period of hospitalization [25, 26].

Therefore, it is of crucial importance to determine the optimal time of delivery in order to reduce perinatal morbidity and mortality, while balancing neonatal and infant risks [27, 28]. Based on a review of the guidelines of the American College of Obstetricians and Gynecologists' [29], the obstetrics literature and published expert opinion [27], Gyamfi-Banneman et al. proposed a set of evidence-based (EB) indications to justify a LPT delivery [30, 31]. In the absence of sufficient scientific evidence, indications were considered weak to justify iatrogenic LPT delivery and were thus categorized as non-EB and included elective (non-medical) indications [13].

The aims of this study were to describe the trend of LPT births and their indications over an 11-year period according to the Gyamfi-Banneman categorization [31]. We also sought to assess neonatal complications related to LPT birth and the accompanying risk factors.

Methods

This retrospective cohort study was conducted at the maternity unit of Geneva University Hospitals, Geneva, Switzerland, and included all LPT births between January 1, 2002 and December 31, 2012. The local institutional ethics committee approved the research protocol.

Study population

The maternity unit is the largest in Switzerland with approximately 4000 deliveries per year, of which approximately 10% are preterm. We included all births of singletons between 34 + 0 and 36 + 6 weeks' gestation. Stillbirths and multiple gestations were excluded. We obtained the list of all newborns during the study period from the labor and delivery suite database and gathered maternal and neonatal data from the medical charts using a standardized report form. Relevant data were extracted from the following sources: the maternal and neonatal databases of the obstetrics service and the neonatal database of the pediatric department. All data were coded using a unique study number.

Outcomes

The primary outcome was the number of LPT births among spontaneous LPT, EB non-spontaneous LPT and non-EB non-spontaneous LPT deliveries. The secondary outcome was an adverse neonatal event defined by the presence of at least one of the following complications: neonatal death; NICU admission; need for ventilatory support; neonatal sepsis with bacteremia; and respiratory disease requiring oxygen or ventilatory support (composite outcome).

Variables

Data were described on an annual basis. We extracted the following maternal and obstetrical variables: maternal age; gestational age at delivery (based on the first trimester ultrasound); gravidity; parity; history and type of cesarean section; prior myomectomy; chronic hypertension; gestational hypertension; preeclampsia; cholestasis; PPROM; intrauterine growth retardation; abnormal fetal Doppler (umbilical and/or cerebral); abnormal fetal tracing; oligohydramnios; pulmonary maturation; pre-labor uterine rupture; delivery onset: spontaneous or non-spontaneous (labor induction or elective cesarean); indication for delivery; mode of delivery (vaginal delivery with or without instruments, elective or in-labor cesarean section); fetal presentation; and type of anesthesia.

Neonatal variables included gender; birth weight in grams; Apgar score at 5 min; umbilical arterial pH; growth retardation (<10th percentile growth for gestational age); use of ventilatory support by either non-invasive ventilation (continuous positive airway pressure) or invasive ventilation (intubation and mechanical ventilation); duration of hospitalization in days; hospitalization site (maternity, NICU); presence of respiratory pathologies (wet lung, respiratory distress syndrome); neonatal sepsis with positive bacteremia; neonatal malformation; chromosomal abnormalities; and neonatal death at less than 1 month.

We classified LPT birth as either spontaneous or non-spontaneous LPT. Spontaneous LPT birth was defined as the spontaneous onset of uterine contractions and cervical dilation. Women with PPROM and no other indication were included in this group. The non-spontaneous LPT birth group included women with induction of labor or elective cesarean section without contractions. This group was further subcategorized according to Gyamfi-Banneman et al. as either EB or non-EB management. Indications labeled EB were supported by strong scientific evidence based on the guidelines of the American College of Obstetricians and Gynecologists' [29], the obstetrics literature and published expert opinion [27]. EB indications for non-spontaneous LPT birth were severe preeclampsia or eclampsia, intrauterine growth retardation with abnormal testing (abnormal fetal Doppler or fetal heart tracing, oligohydramnios) or poor interval growth, acute abruption, non-reassuring fetal heart rate tracing, cholestasis, and uterine rupture prior to spontaneous initiation of labor. Indications labeled non-EB were not supported by sufficient scientific evidence and thus weaker to justify a non-spontaneous LPT delivery. Non-EB indications for LPT birth included chronic or gestational hypertension, mild preeclampsia, intrauterine growth retardation with normal testing and adequate interval growth, prior myomectomy or classic cesarean section, isolated oligohydramnios. Any other indication reviewed in medical records and not listed previously was classified as an elective delivery and categorized as non-EB LPT. These indications were in general debated within the clinical team and not supported by scientific evidence, but mainly explained by the wishes of the patient or care provider. In Gyamfi-Banneman et al., only cholestasis with bile acids >40 micromol/L was considered as EB. Cholestasis with bile acids <40 micromol/L were considered as non-EB. In our study, all women with cholestasis were included in the EB group as we did not have measurements of bile acid levels.

Statistical analysis

All continuous variables were described by their mean ± standard deviation, overall median and LPT group. Categorical variables were described by their frequencies, relative proportion overall and LPT group. A comparison of continuous variables between the three groups of LPT deliveries (i.e. between spontaneous LPT and non-spontaneous LPT or between EB and non-EB non-spontaneous LPT) was done using the Kruskal-Wallis test because of skewed distributions. Categorical variables were compared between the groups using either the Chi-square or Fisher's exact test. The overall number of complications were then stratified on the three groups of LPT and assessed across time using Poisson regression models.

Finally, we assessed the risk factors associated with the occurrence of at least one complication using a logistic regression model where the LPT group was the main predictor. We pre-specified the following variables as important risk factors for neonatal complications: mode of delivery (spontaneous, elective cesarean or cesarean during labor); pulmonary maturation (yes/no); gestational age strata (34 to 34/6 weeks, 35 to 35/6 weeks, and 36 to 36/6 weeks); maternal age strata (<20, 20–29, 30–34, 35–39 and > = 40 years); birth weight strata

(<10th, 10th to 50th, 50 to 90th, and >90th percentile); and gender. Logistic regression provided maximum likelihood estimates of the odds ratios (OR) and their 95% confidence intervals (CI). The goodness-of-fit of the model was verified using the Hosmer-Lemeshow test. The amount of variation in the likelihood of neonatal complications explained by the model was indicated by the Cox and Snell R^2. The discriminant capacity of the model was evaluated by the area under the curve assorted with its 95% CI. Statistical significance was defined as a two-sided P value of <0.05. Statistical analyses were performed using Stata IC 14 (STATA Corp., College Station, TX).

Results

A total of 40,609 live singleton deliveries were recorded during the 11-year study period. Among these, 4223 (10.5%) were preterm and 2017 (4.9%) LPT. Among the LPT deliveries, 1487 were classified as spontaneous LPT (73.7%) and 530 (26.2%) as non-spontaneous LPT. In the latter group, 243 (12.0%) were EB and 287 (14.2%) non-EB (Fig. 1). Maternal and obstetric characteristics are shown in Table 1. There were more women with a history of cesarean section ($P < 0.001$) and with chronic or gestational hypertension ($P < 0.001$ in both) in the non-spontaneous LPT than in the spontaneous LPT group. The cesarean section rate was higher in the non-EB non-spontaneous LPT (82.9%) than in the EB group (67.1%; $P < 0.001$). Globally, cesarean section during labor was more frequent in the non-spontaneous LPT group compared to spontaneous LPT cases (OR: 1.8; 95% CI: 1.36–2.39; $P < 0.001$). The proportion of each LPT subgroup remained stable over time ($P = 0.665$ for spontaneous LPT; $P = 0.532$ for EB non-spontaneous LPT; $P = 0.609$ for non-EB non-spontaneous LPT; Fig. 2).

The most frequent indications for EB non-spontaneous LPT were severe preeclampsia (51.8%), abnormal fetal tracing (24.7%) and intrauterine growth retardation with abnormal testing. For non-EB non-spontaneous LPT cases, the most common indications were hemorrhage without placenta abruption (36.2%) and non-severe preeclampsia (15.7%). Elective indications accounted for 34.5% of non-EB non-spontaneous LPT and included various diagnoses, such as iso-immunization, maternal life-threatening conditions (i.e. breast cancer, acute renal failure, maternal sepsis), severe fetal malformation (laparoschisis, major renal defect) and maternal psychological distress related to pregnancy. Few cases were "strictly elective" without any clearly reported medical indication.

The proportion of infants hospitalized in the NICU was significantly higher in the non-spontaneous LPT compared to the spontaneous LPT group (Table 1). The number of neonatal complications in the three LPT

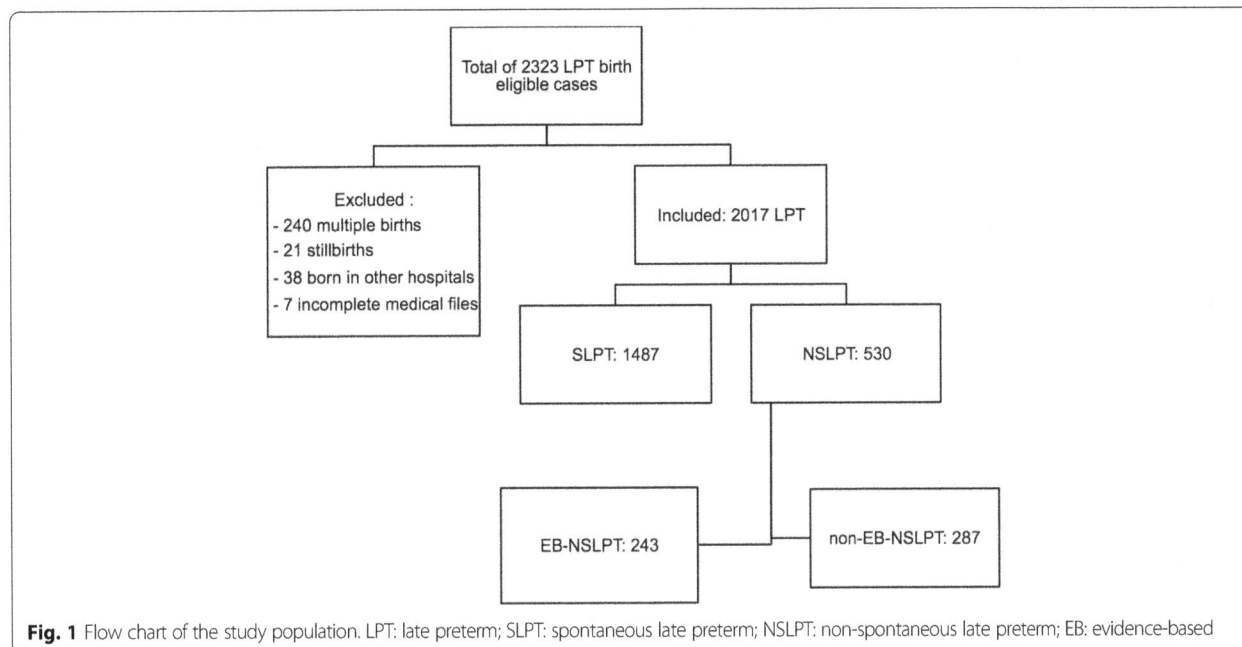

Fig. 1 Flow chart of the study population. LPT: late preterm; SLPT: spontaneous late preterm; NSLPT: non-spontaneous late preterm; EB: evidence-based

groups decreased over time, but the decrease was only statistically significant in the spontaneous LPT group ($P = 0.031$). The likelihood of neonatal complications was 3.66-fold (95% CI: 2.75–4.87) higher in EB non-spontaneous LPT compared to spontaneous LPT, 2.04-fold higher (95% CI: 1.58–2.63) in non-EB non-spontaneous LPT compared to spontaneous LPT, and 1.79-fold higher (95% CI: 1.26–2.55) in EB non-spontaneous LPT compared to non-EB non-spontaneous LPT (Fig. 3). After adjustment for the main confounders (Table 2), the likelihood of complications remained significantly higher among non-EB non-spontaneous LPT compared to spontaneous LPT cases ($P < 0.001$), but there was no significant difference between non-spontaneous non-EB LPT and EB LPT ($P = 0.225$). There was a trend for higher odds of complications in the non-spontaneous EB LPT group compared to spontaneous LPT. The odds of neonatal complications were also significantly and independently increased in the in-labor cesarean section group compared to vaginal deliveries, in boys compared to girls, and in neonates with a birth weight between the 10th to 50th percentile and below the 10th percentile compared to infants with a birth weight above the 90th percentile. The multivariable model was also adjusted for maternal age and lung maturation and demonstrated a good discriminant capacity with an area under the curve of 0.83 (95% CI: 0.81–0.85).

Discussion

Overall, approximately one-quarter of LPT deliveries at our center were iatrogenic. When stratified according to the classification proposed by Gyamfi-Banneman et al…, one-half were for non-EB indications [13]. In contrast to the current trend of increasing LPT delivery rates often attributed to non-spontaneous LPT birth, our rates remained stable over time and were slightly lower than those reported by other authors using the same criteria (17% by Gyamfi-Banneman et al. [13, 31] and 18% by Holland et al) [32]. Morais et al. reported a higher rate of 25.5% non-EB LPT, but included PPROM in this group [33]. By excluding PPROM, the rate decreased to 10.7%, the lowest reported so far.

In our study, the overall rate of neonatal complications in LPT tended to decrease, although the rate after non-EB LPT birth did not change over time. As guidelines for lung maturation during the late preterm period in women at risk of delivery have changed recently, we can expect a decreasing rate of respiratory morbidity in LPT neonates in the future [34, 35]. Nevertheless, newborns born after non-EB LPT management received lung maturation more often than the other two groups and the rate of complications was higher, thus emphasizing the importance of avoiding the occurrence of these cases.

Non-spontaneous LPT newborns require more neonatal care than spontaneous LPT as they are more frequently admitted to the NICU, have a longer hospital stay and require more ventilatory support [14]. The risk persisted after adjustment for independent risk factors of neonatal complications (mode of delivery, pulmonary maturation, gestational age, maternal, birth weight and gender). By strictly avoiding non-EB LPT (14.2% of LPT) deliveries, it might be possible to reduce the burden of neonatal morbidity up to a factor of two. We assume that potential supplementary factors may have influenced the obstetrical decision.

Table 1 Overall maternal and obstetric characteristics and type of late preterm delivery

	Overall	Spontaneous LPT (N = 1487)	EB-LPT (N = 243)	Non EB-LPT (N = 287)	P-value[a]	P-value[b]	P-value[c]
Obstetrical description							
Maternal age: mean (±SD, P50)	31.7 (±5.6; 32)	31.4 (±5.5; 32)	32.1 (±5.8; 32)	32.9 (±5.8; 33)	<0.001	0.06	<0.001
Mean gestational age in weeks (±SD, P50)	35.3 (±0.8; 36)	35.4 (±0.8; 36)	35.2 (±0.8; 35)	35.4 (±0.8; 36)	0.002	0.005	0.159
Gravidity, n (%)					<0.001	<0.001	0.625
Primigravida	714 (35.4)	531 (35.7)	110 (45.3)	73 (25.4)			
Multigravida	1303 (64.6)	956 (64.3)	133 (54.7)	214 (74.6)			
Parity, n (%)					<0.001	<0.001	0.399
Primiparous	1063 (52.7)	792 (53.3)	160 (65.8)	111 (38.7)			
Multiparous	954 (47.3)	695 (46.7)	83 (34.2)	176 (61.3)			
Prior caesarean section, n (%)					<0.001	<0.001	<0.001
No	1786 (88.5)	1360 (91.5)	217 (89.3)	209 (72.8)			
Segmental caesarean	213 (10.6)	117 (7.9)	23 (9.5)	73 (25.4)			
Non-segmental caesarean	18 (0.9)	10 (0.7)	3 (1.2)	5 (1.7)			
Prior myomectomy, n (%)	5 (0.3)	2 (0.1)	0 (0)	3 (1.0)	0.013	0.254	0.086
Chronic hypertension, n (%)	28 (1.4)	7 (0.5)	15 (6.2)	6 (2.1)	<0.001	0.016	<0.001
Gestational hypertension, n (%)	63 (3.1)	21 (1.4)	24 (9.9)	18 (6.3)	<0.001	0.126	<0.001
Preeclampsia, n (%)	212 (10.5)	39 (2.6)	128 (52.7)	45 (15.7)	<0.001	<0.001	<0.001
Severe preeclampsia, n (%)	127 (60.5)	0 (0)	127 (100.0)	0 (0)	<0.001	<0.001	<0.001
Cholestasis, n (%)	3 (0.2)	0 (0)	3 (1.2)	0 (0)	<0.001	0.096	0.004
Haemorrhage, n (%)					<0.001	<0.001	<0.001
No	1896 (94.0)	1480 (99.5)	233 (95.9)	183 (63.8)			
Placenta praevia	37 (1.8)	0 (0)	0 (0)	37 (12.9)			
Acute abruption	0 (0)	0 (0)	10 (4.1)	0 (0)			
Other, missing data	74 (3.7)	7 (0.5)	0 (0)	67 (23.3)			
Rupture of membranes, n (%)	1090 (54.0)	1079 (72.6)	43 (17.7)	0 (0)	<0.001	<0.001	<0.001
IUGR, n (%)	143 (7.1)	43 (2.9)	71 (29.2)	29 (10.1)	<0.001	<0.001	<0.001
Abnormal doppler, n (%)	42 (2.1)	0 (0)	36 (14.8)	6 (2.1)	<0.001	<0.001	<0.001
Oligohydramnios, n (%)	79 (3.9)	34 (2.3)	13 (5.4)	32 (11.2)	<0.001	0.019	<0.001
Abnormal fetal tracing, n (%)	73 (3.6)	0 (0)	73 (30.0)	0 (0)	<0.001	<0.001	<0.001
Lung maturation, n (%) (n = 1977)	373 (18.5)	220 (14.8)	48 (19.8)	105 (36.6)	<0.001	<0.001	<0.001
Uterine rupture, n (%)	0 (0)	0 (0)	0 (0)	0 (0)	–	–	–
Start of delivery, n (%)					<0.001	<0.001	<0.001
Spontaneous	883 (43.8)	880 (59.2)	3 (1.2)	0 (0)			
Induced	934 (46.3)	564 (37.9)	206 (84.8)	164 (57.1)			
Elective caesarean	200 (9.9)	43 (2.9)	34 (14.0)	123 (42.9)			
Mode of delivery, n (%)					<0.001	<0.001	<0.001
Vaginal	1278 (63.4)	1150 (77.3)	79 (32.5)	49 (17.1)			
Elective caesarean	200 (9.9)	43 (2.9)	34 (14.0)	123 (42.9)			
Cesarean in labour	539 (26.7)	294 (19.8)	130 (53.5)	115 (40.1)			
Presentation, n (%)					<0.001	<0.001	0.008
Cephalic	1325 (89.2)	983 (90.7)	175 (93.1)	167 (78.0)			
Breech	146 (9.8)	92 (8.5)	13 (6.9)	41 (19.2)			

Table 1 Overall maternal and obstetric characteristics and type of late preterm delivery *(Continued)*

	Overall	Spontaneous LPT (N = 1487)	EB-LPT (N = 243)	Non EB-LPT (N = 287)	P-value[a]	P-value[b]	P-value[c]
Other	15 (1.0)	9 (0.8)	0 (0)	6 (2.8)			
Type of anaesthesia, n (%)					<0.001	0.111	<0.001
Non	347 (17.2)	332 (22.3)	9 (3.7)	6 (2.1)			
Epidural	1629 (80.8)	1139 (76.6)	227 (93.4)	263 (91.6)			
General	41 (2.0)	16 (1.1)	7 (2.9)	18 (6.3)			
Neonatal description							
Female gender, n (%)	928 (46.0)	643 (43.2)	127 (52.3)	158 (55.1)	<0.001	0.521	<0.001
Birth weight (kg): mean (±SD, P50)	2.57 (±0.46, 2.56)	2.63 (±0.43, 2.61)	2.19 (±0.47, 2.14)	2.55 (±0.45, 2.56)	<0.001	<0.001	<0.001
Apgar <5, n (%)	14 (0.7)	10 (0.7)	2 (0.8)	2 (0.7)	0.966	0.999	0.769
Arterial pH < 7.10, n (%)	67 (3.5)	43 (3.1)	15 (6.4)	9 (3.3)	0.038	0.140	0.094
Growth retardation <p10, n (%)	173 (9.0)	72 (5.0)	77 (35.0)	24 (9.2)	<0.001	<0.001	<0.001
NICU stay, n (%)	828 (41.0)	518 (34.8)	161 (66.3)	149 (51.9)	<0.001	0.001	<0.001
Malformation, n (%)	46 (5.5)	24 (4.6)	7 (4.4)	15 (10.0)	0.033	0.054	0.138
Ventilatory support, n (%)					<0.001	0.428	<0.001
No	1733 (85.9)	1322 (88.9)	194 (79.8)	217 (75.6)			
Non-invasive	246 (12.2)	146 (9.8)	40 (16.5)	60 (20.9)			
Invasive	38 (1.9)	19 (1.3)	9 (3.7)	10 (3.5)			
Mean stay at NICU in days (±SD, P50) (n = 828)	12.1 (±14.2, 10)	11.4 (±13.7, 9)	13.3 (±13.4, 11)	13.0 (±16.5, 9)	0.226	0.067	0.006
Neonatal sepsis with bacteremia, n (%)	5 (0.6)	2 (0.4)	2 (1.2)	1 (0.7)	0.458	0.999	0.367
Respiratory diseases, n (%)	419 (21.1)	256 (17.5)	72 (30.6)	91 (32.2)	<0.001	0.711	<0.001
Neonatal death, n (%)	4 (0.2)	1 (0.07)	2 (0.8)	1 (0.35)	0.036	0.596	0.058
Presence of ≥1 complication*, n (%) (n = 2014)	829 (41.2)	518 (34.9)	161 (66.3)	150 (52.3)	<0.001	0.001	<0.001

LPT late preterm, *EB* evidence-based, *SD* standard deviation, *IUGR* intrauterine growth retardation, *NICU* neonatal intensive care unit, *SD* standard deviation
[a]Comparisons between the three groups of LPT birth; [b]comparisons between spontaneous LPT birth and EB plus non-EB-LPT birth; [c]comparisons between EB and non-EB-LPT birth
Complication *: neonatal death; NICU admission; need for ventilatory support; neonatal sepsis with bacteremia; and respiratory disease requiring oxygen or ventilatory support

Elective indications accounted for 34.5% of non-EB non-spontaneous LPT deliveries and included various diagnoses, such as maternal life-threatening conditions (i.e. breast cancer, acute renal failure, maternal sepsis), fetal malformation, etc. Although these indications are not considered as EB, their severity could explain the indication for delivery and the poor neonatal outcome [36].

Antepartum hemorrhage was a frequent indication for non-EB non-spontaneous LPT birth and included placenta praevia, vasa praevia, suspicion of uterine rupture and severe genital bleeding of unknown origin. Acute abruption and uterine rupture were considered EB non-spontaneous LPT indications. Placenta praevia indicated delivery between 35 5/7 weeks and 36 6/7 weeks in 37 cases, which is in agreement with recent recommendations from the American College of Obstetricians and Gynecologists Committee on Obstetric Practice [29]. Therefore, we suggest that the categorization of Gyamfi-

Banneman et al. should include placenta praevia as an EB indication for delivery during the late preterm period, possibly after 36 0/7 weeks if uncomplicated (no fetal growth restriction, no hemorrhage or repetitive bleeding, or no other additional EB indication). Fifteen cases were delivered due to suspected uterine rupture, although none was confirmed. By excluding the 52 cases (placenta praevia and suspicion of uterine rupture) where we disagree with the indications of Gyamfi-Banneman et al., we estimate that we could have potentially avoided 235 LPT deliveries.

The strengths of the present study are related to the use of the same categorization for LPT delivery as Gyamfi-Banneman et al., thus ensuring reproducible results and allowing to compare practices within institutions nationally and internationally. The study duration allowed to collect a large number of LPT cases (2017) with complete neonatal follow-up in a single center.

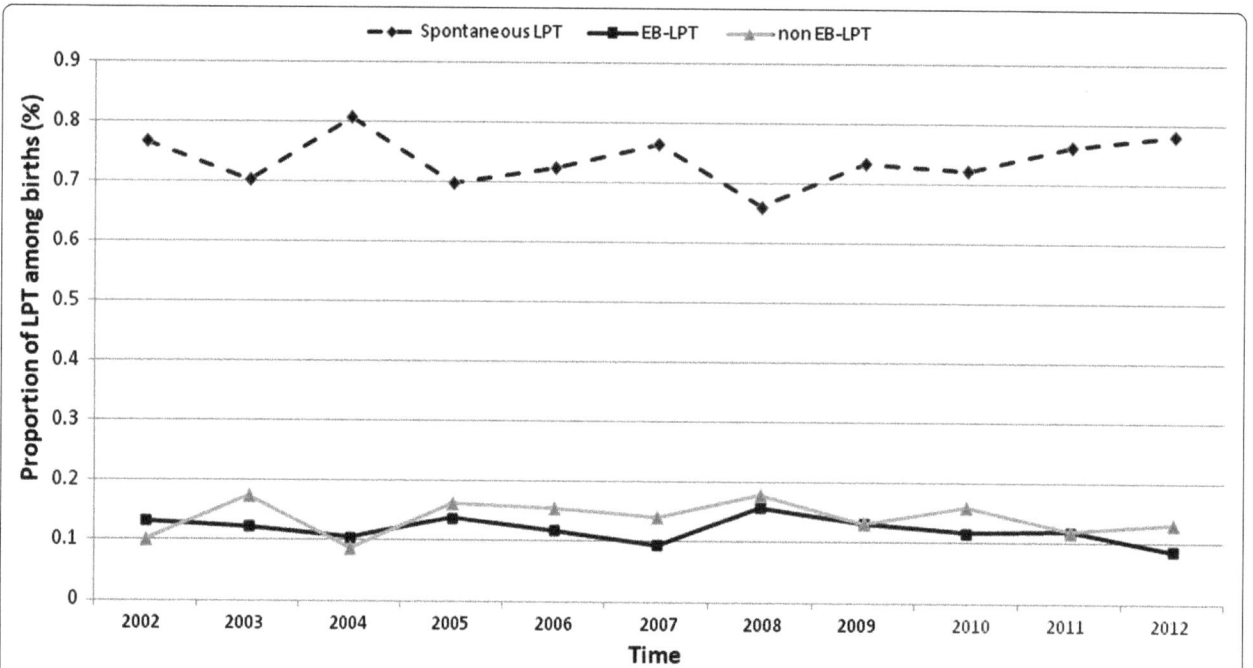

Fig. 2 Temporal trends of each type of late preterm birth: Geneva University Hospitals, 2002–2012. LPT: late preterm; EB: evidence-based

Our study has some limitations. First, its observational design means that the effect of unknown confounders could have impacted on the association between the LPT groups and neonatal complications. To account for this potential bias, we adjusted for the main known confounders. Second, we were unable to classify severe cholestasis as we did not measure bile acid and our three cases of cholestasis were classified as EB. Third, cases of PPROM were systematically induced from 34 weeks' gestation and classified as spontaneous LPT birth. However, based on recent evidence that an expectant management of PPROM provides more benefits without increasing the rate of neonatal sepsis [37], practices related to PPROM during the late preterm period have recently changed in our maternity unit. This subgroup represented quite a large number of cases (1076) and it would now be considered

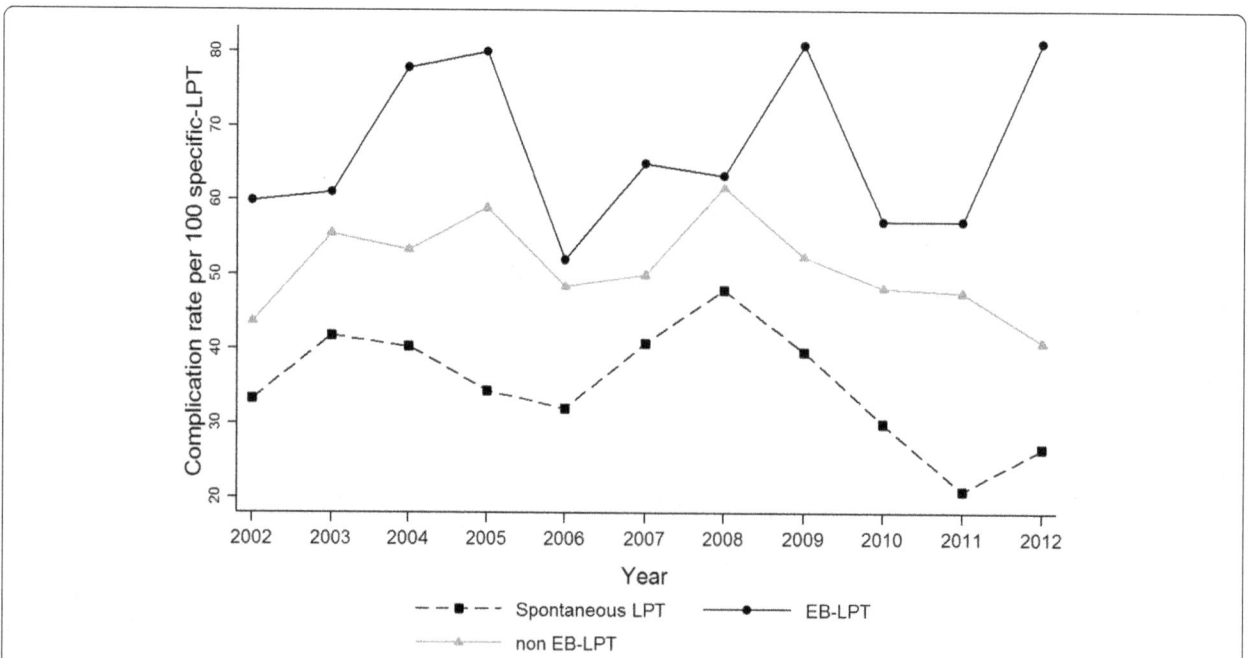

Fig. 3 Incidence rates of complications in the three late preterm birth groups. LPT: late preterm; EB: evidence-based

Table 2 Associated factors with the likelihood of neonatal complication (multivariate analysis)[a]

Variables	Odds ratio	95% confidence interval	P-value
Time periods (reference 2002–2004)			<0.001
2005–2006	0.83	0.59–1.15	0.258
2007–2008	0.96	0.68–1.36	0.830
2009–2012	0.47	0.34–0.64	<0.001
Group of LPT (reference spontaneous)			0.001
EB-LPT	1.49	0.99–2.22	0.051
Non EB-LPT	2.03	1.37–3.00	<0.001[a]
Mode of delivery (reference spontaneous)			0.0002
Elective caesarean	1.53	0.96–2.45	0.074
Caesarean during labour	1.80	1.36–2.39	<0.001
Lung maturation (reference no lung maturation)	1.01	0.75–1.37	0.941
Gestational age in weeks (reference [36])			<0.001
34	27.3	19.22–38.79	<0.001
35	3.15	2.41–4.10	<0.001
Mother's age in years (reference <20 years)			0.426
20–30	1.59	0.60–4.21	0.350
30–35	1.47	0.56–3.90	0.435
35–40	1.22	0.46–3.25	0.690
>=40	1.61	0.57–4.56	0.366
Weight percentile categories (reference >90th percentile)			<0.001
50-90th	1.08	0.76–1.53	0.665
10-50th	1.62	1.13–2.31	0.009
10th	16.18	9.46–27.67	<0.001
Boy (reference girl)	1.66	1.31–2.11	<0.001

LPT late preterm, EB evidence-based
[a]Amount of variation in the likelihood of neonatal complication explained by the model was 29%

PPROM without signs of complications as a non-EB indication for delivery, similar to Morais et al. [33].

Our aim was not to establish a new, strict and exhaustive classification of EB and non-EB criteria, but rather to support only EB indications. We also aimed to identify ways to reduce the number of non-spontaneous LPT deliveries in our setting and more generally. At present, this categorization is evolving and future research in the field of LPT management may help to improve the definition of EB and non-EB indications. In our setting, our study allowed to highlight that one-half of non-spontaneous LPT births could have been avoided if current recommendations had been applied. When possible, obstetrical settings should be encouraged to use this classification, which aims to improve the management of LPT births. A recent study reported that strengthening management policies of non-EB non-spontaneous LPT indications led to a decline in preterm birth [38]. Another study found that the presence of condition-specific obstetric protocols did not lead to detectable improvements in pregnancy outcomes [39]. Although Clark et al. reported that an association of protocols with a "hard stop" policy was the best way to improve EB medicine practices [40], the necessity for strict protocols in obstetric management remains a subject of debate among specialists.

Conclusions

The proportion of LPT births remained stable over the entire study period. One-quarter of LPT births were non-spontaneous and more than half of these were non-EB with a high risk of neonatal complications. Between 287 and 235 could have been avoided if strict criteria had been applied. Efforts should continue to reduce unnecessary LPT births in order to reduce neonatal morbidity.

Abbreviations
CI: Confidence interval; EB: Evidence-based; IUGR: Intrauterine growth retardation; LPT: Late preterm; NICU: Neonatal intensive care unit; OR: Odds ratio; PPROM: Preterm premature rupture of membranes; SLPT: Spontaneous late preterm delivery

Acknowledgements
We thank all research midwives and administrative staff at the obstetrics service of Geneva University Hospitals for their help with database development. We sincerely thank Rosemary Sudan for editorial assistance.

Funding
The project received institutional support from the Department of Gynaecology and Obstetrics and the Department of Pediatrics, Geneva University Hospitals. There was not funding for the study.

Authors' contributions
NB designed the study, contributed to data collection, and drafted the initial manuscript. AGA performed the statistical analyses and interpreted the results, critically reviewed and revised the manuscript. ML contributed to data collection, reviewed and revised the manuscript. REP coordinated data collection and critically reviewed the manuscript. BMdT conceived and designed the study and the data collection, coordinated and supervised data collection, and critically reviewed the manuscript. All authors read and approved the final manuscript as submitted.

Competing interests
The authors have no competing interest relevant to this article to disclose.

Author details

[1]Obstetrics Unit, Department of Obstetrics and Gynecology, Geneva University Hospitals and Faculty of Medicine, 30 Boulevard de la Cluse, 1205 Geneva, Switzerland. [2]Clinical Research Centre and Division of Clinical Epidemiology, Department of Community Health and Medicine, Geneva University Hospitals and Faculty of Medicine, 6 rue Gabrielle-Perret-Gentil, 1205 Geneva, Switzerland. [3]Neonatology Unit, Department of Pediatrics, Geneva University Hospitals and Faculty of Medicine, 30 Boulevard de la Cluse, 1205 Geneva, Switzerland.

References

1. Zeitlin J, Szamotulska K, Drewniak N, Mohangoo AD, Chalmers J, Sakkeus L, et al. Preterm birth time trends in Europe: a study of 19 countries. BJOG. 2013;120(11):1356–65.

2. Blencowe H, Cousens S, Oestergaard MZ, Chou D, Moller AB, Narwal R, et al. National, regional, and worldwide estimates of preterm birth rates in the year 2010 with time trends since 1990 for selected countries: a systematic analysis and implications. Lancet. 2012;379(9832):2162–72.

3. MacDorman MF, Mathews TJ, Martin JA, Malloy MH. Trends and characteristics of induced labour in the United States, 1989–98. Paediatr Perinat Epidemiol. 2002;16(3):263–73.

4. Ananth CV, Joseph KS, Oyelese Y, Demissie K, Vintzileos AM. Trends in preterm birth and perinatal mortality among singletons: United States, 1989 through 2000. Obstet Gynecol. 2005;105(5 Pt 1):1084–91.

5. Bassil KL, Yasseen AS 3rd, Walker M, Sgro MD, Shah PS, Smith GN, et al. The association between obstetrical interventions and late preterm birth. Am J Obstet Gynecol. 2014;210(6):538 e531–9.

6. Iams JD, Donovan EF. Spontaneous late preterm births: what can be done to improve outcomes? Semin Perinatol. 2011;35(5):309–13.

7. McParland PC. Obstetric management of moderate and late preterm labour. Semin Fetal Neonatal Med. 2012;17(3):138–42.

8. Raju TNK. Epidemiology of late preterm (near-term) births. Clin Perinatol. 2006;33(4):751–63.

9. Hui ASY, Lao TT, Leung TY, Schaaf JM, Sahota DS. Trends in preterm birth in singleton deliveries in a Hong Kong population. Int J Gynaecol Obstet. 2014; 127(3):248–53.

10. Davidoff MJ, Dias T, Damus K, Russell R, Bettegowda VR, Dolan S, et al. Changes in the gestational age distribution among U.S. singleton births: impact on rates of late preterm birth, 1992 to 2002. Semin Perinatol. 2006;30(1):8–15.

11. Lisonkova S, Hutcheon JA, Joseph KS. Temporal trends in neonatal outcomes following iatrogenic preterm delivery. BMC Pregnancy Childbirth. 2011;11:39.

12. Hankins GDV, Longo M. The role of stillbirth prevention and late preterm (near-term) births. Semin Perinatol. 2006;30(1):20–3.

13. Gyamfi-Bannerman C. Late preterm birth: management dilemmas. Obstet Gynecol Clin N Am. 2012;39(1):35–45.

14. Pike KC, Lucas JSA. Respiratory consequences of late preterm birth. Paediatr Respir Rev. 2015;16(3):182–8.

15. Boyle JD, Boyle EM. Born just a few weeks early: does it matter? Arch Dis Child Fetal Neonatal Ed. 2013;98(1):F85–8.

16. Engle WA, Tomashek KM. Wallman C: "late-preterm" infants: a population at risk. Pediatrics. 2007;120(6):1390–401.

17. Melamed N, Klinger G, Tenenbaum-Gavish K, Herscovici T, Linder N, Hod M, et al. Short-term neonatal outcome in low-risk, spontaneous, singleton, late preterm deliveries. Obstet Gynecol. 2009;114(2 Pt 1):253–60.

18. Bird TM, Bronstein JM, Hall RW, Lowery CL, Nugent R, Mays GP. Late preterm infants: birth outcomes and health care utilization in the first year. Pediatrics. 2010;126(2):e311–9.

19. Brown HK, Speechley KN, Macnab J, Natale R, Campbell MK. Neonatal morbidity associated with late preterm and early term birth: the roles of gestational age and biological determinants of preterm birth. Int J Epidemiol. 2014;43(3):802–14.

20. Khan K, Petrou S, Dritsaki M, Johnson S, Manktelow B, Draper E, et al. Economic costs associated with moderate and late preterm birth: a prospective population-based study. BJOG. 2015;122(11):1495–505.

21. Teune MJ, Bakhuizen S, Gyamfi Bannerman C, Opmeer BC, van Kaam AH, van Wassenaer AG, et al. A systematic review of severe morbidity in infants born late preterm. Am J Obstet Gynecol. 2011;205(4):e371–4.

22. Saigal S, Doyle LW. An overview of mortality and sequelae of preterm birth from infancy to adulthood. Lancet. 2008;371(9608):261–9.

23. Lipkind HS, Slopen ME, Pfeiffer MR, McVeigh KH. School-age outcomes of late preterm infants in new York City. Am J Obstet Gynecol. 2012; 206(3):e221–6.

24. Heinonen K, Eriksson JG, Kajantie E, Pesonen A-K, Barker DJ, Osmond C, et al. Late-preterm birth and lifetime socioeconomic attainments: the Helsinki birth cohort study. Pediatrics. 2013;132(4):647–55.

25. McGowan JE, Alderdice FA, Boylan J, Holmes VA, Jenkins J, Craig S, et al. Neonatal intensive care and late preterm infants: health and family functioning at three years. Early Hum Dev. 2014;90(4):201–5.

26. Rogers CE, Lenze SN, Luby JL. Late preterm birth, maternal depression, and risk of preschool psychiatric disorders. J Am Acad Child Adolesc Psychiatry. 2013;52(3):309–18.

27. Spong CY, Mercer BM, D'Alton M, Kilpatrick S, Blackwell S, Saade G. Timing of indicated late-preterm and early-term birth. Obstet Gynecol. 2011;118(2 Pt 1):323–33.

28. Mandujano A, Waters TP, Myers SA. The risk of fetal death: current concepts of best gestational age for delivery. Am J Obstet Gynecol. 2013;208(3):e201–8.

29. American College of Obstetricians & Gynecologists. ACOG committee opinion no. 560: medically indicated late-preterm and early-term deliveries. Obstet Gynecol. 2013;121(4):908–10.

30. Gyamfi-Bannerman C. Obstetric decision-making and the late and moderately preterm infant. Semin Fetal Neonatal Med. 2012;17(3):132–7.

31. Gyamfi-Bannerman C, Fuchs KM, Young OM, Hoffman MK. Nonspontaneous late preterm birth: etiology and outcomes. Am J Obstet Gynecol. 2011; 205(5):e451–6.

32. Holland MG, Refuerzo JS, Ramin SM, Saade GR, Blackwell SC. Late preterm birth: how often is it avoidable? Am J Obstet Gynecol. 2009;201(4):e401–4.

33. Morais M, Mehta C, Murphy K, Shah PS, Giglia L, Smith PA, et al. How often are late preterm births the result of non-evidence based practices: analysis from a retrospective cohort study at two tertiary referral centres in a nationalised healthcare system. BJOG. 2013;120(12):1508–14.

34. Gyamfi-Bannerman C, Thom EA, Blackwell SC, Tita AT, Reddy UM, Saade GR, et al. Antenatal betamethasone for women at risk for late preterm delivery. N Engl J Med. 2016;374(14):1311–20.

35. Society for Maternal-Fetal Medicine Publications Committee. Implementation of the use of antenatal corticosteroids in the late preterm birth period in women at risk for preterm delivery. Am J Obstet Gynecol. 2016;215(2):B13–5.

36. Kim SA, Lee SM, Kim BJ, Park CW, Park JS, Jun JK, Yoon BH. The risk of neonatal respiratory morbidity according to the etiology of late preterm delivery. J Perinat Med. 2017;45(1):129–134.1.

37. Morris JM, Roberts CL, Bowen JR, Patterson JA, Bond DM, Algert CS, et al. Immediate delivery compared with expectant management after preterm pre-labour rupture of the membranes close to term (PPROMT trial): a randomised controlled trial. Lancet. 2016;387(10017):444–52.

38. Gyamfi-Bannerman C, Ananth CV. Trends in spontaneous and indicated preterm delivery among singleton gestations in the United States, 2005-2012. Obstet Gynecol. 2014;124(6):1069–74.

39. Bailit JL, Grobman WA, McGee P, Reddy UM, Wapner RJ, Varner MW, et al. Does the presence of a condition-specific obstetric protocol lead to detectable improvements in pregnancy outcomes? Am J Obstet Gynecol. 2015;213(1):e81–6.

40. Clark SL, Frye DR, Meyers JA, Belfort MA, Dildy GA, Kofford S, et al. Reduction in elective delivery at <39 weeks of gestation: comparative effectiveness of 3 approaches to change and the impact on neonatal intensive care admission and stillbirth. Am J Obstet Gynecol. 2010;203(5):e441–6.

Permissions

List of Contributors

Paola Algeri, Francesca Pelizzoni, Francesca Russo, Maddalena Incerti, Sabrina Cozzolino, Salvatore Andrea Mastrolia and Patrizia Vergani
Department of Obstetrics and Gynecology, University of Milano-Bicocca, S. Gerardo Hospital, MBBM Foundation, Via Pergolesi 33, Monza, 20900 Monza, Monza e Brianza, Italy

Davide Paolo Bernasconi
Department of Health Sciences, Center of Biostatistic for Clinical Epidemiology, University of Milan-Bicocca, Via Pergolesi 33, Monza, 20900 Monza, Monza e Brianza, Italy

Masayuki Sekine and Takayuki Enomoto
Department of Obstetrics and Gynecology, Niigata University Graduate School of Medical and Dental Science, 1-757 Asahimachi-dori, Niigata 951-8510, Japan

Yoshiyuki Kobayashi and Tsutomu Tabata
Departments of Obstetrics and Gynecology, Mie University Graduate School of Medicine, Mie, Japan

Tamotsu Sudo and Ryuichiro Nishimura
Department of Gynecology, Hyogo Cancer Center, Hyogo, Japan

Koji Matsuo and Brendan H. Grubbs
Department of Obstetrics and Gynecology, University of Southern California, Los Angeles, CA, USA

Linnea Bärebring, Lena Hulthén, Anna Winkvist and Hanna Augustin
The Department of Internal Medicine and Clinical Nutrition, Sahlgrenska Academy, University of Gothenburg, Gothenburg, Sweden

Maria Bullarbo
Södra Älvsborg Hospital, Borås, Sweden

Maria Bullarbo
The Department of Obstetrics and Gynecology, Sahlgrenska Academy, University of Gothenburg, Gothenburg, Sweden

Anna Glantz
Department of Antenatal Care, Närhälsan, Primary Care, Gothenburg, Sweden

Joy Ellis
Department of Antenatal Care, Närhälsan, Primary Care, Södra, Bohuslän, Sweden

Inez Schoenmakers
MRC Human Nutrition Research, Nutrition and Bone Health Group, Cambridge, UK
The Department of Medicine,Faculty of Medicine and Health Sciences, University of East Anglia, Norwich, UK

Tom Witteveen, Athanasios Kallianidis, Jos van Roosmalen and Thomas van den Akker
Department of Obstetrics, Leiden University Medical Center, building 1, room K-6-P-35, 2300 RC Leiden, The Netherlands

Athanasios Kallianidis
Department of Obstetrics and Gynecology, Haga Teaching Hospital, Els Borst-Eilersplein 275, 2545 AA Den Haag, The Netherlands

Joost J. Zwart
Department of Obstetrics and Gynecology, Deventer Ziekenhuis, Nico Bolkesteinlaan 75, 7416 SE Deventer, The Netherlands

Kitty W. Bloemenkamp
Department of Obstetrics, Wilhelmina Children's Hospital Birth Centre, University Medical Centre Utrecht, Lundlaan 6, 3584 EA Utrecht, The Netherlands

Jos van Roosmalen
Athena Institute, Faculty of Science, VU University Amsterdam, De Boelelaan 1085, 1081 HV Amsterdam, The Netherlands

Yuan Jiang, Jie Chen, Huaijun Zhou and Ying Hong
Department of Obstetrics and Gynecology, Nanjing Drum Tower Hospital, Nanjing Medical University, Nanjing 210008, China

Yuan Jiang, Jie Chen, Huaijun Zhou, Mingming Zheng, Ke Han, Jingxian Ling, Xianghong Zhu, Xiaoqiu Tang, Rong Li and Ying Hong
Department of Obstetrics and Gynecology, Nanjing Drum Tower Hospital, Affiliated Hospital of Nanjing University Medical School, Nanjing 210008, China

Chayatat Ruangkit
Chakri Naruebodindra Medical Institute, Faculty of Medicine Ramathibodi Hospital, Mahidol University, Samut Prakan, Thailand

Matthew Leon, Kasim Hassen, Katherine Baker, Debra Poeltler and Anup Katheria
Neonatal Research Institute at Sharp Mary Birch Hospital for Women and Newborns, 8555 Aero Dr., Suite 104, San Diego, CA 92123, USA

Daniele Bolla, Saskia Vanessa Weissleder, Anda-Petronela Radan, Maria Luisa Gasparri, Luigi Raio, Martin Müller and Daniel Surbek
Department of Obstetrics and Gynaecology, Inselspital, Bern University Hospital, University of Bern, Effingerstrasse 102, CH-3010 Bern, Switzerland

Martin Müller
Departments of Obstetrics, Gynaecology and Reproductive Sciences, Yale University School of Medicine, New Haven, USA

Eva A. R. Goedegebure, Eva Stekkinger and Joost J. Zwart
Department of Obstetrics and Gynaecology, Deventer Hospital, Deventer, the Netherlands

Sarah H. Koning
Department of Endocrinology, University of Groningen, University Medical Center Groningen, 9700 RB Groningen, the Netherlands

Klaas Hoogenberg
Department of Internal Medicine, Martini Hospital, Groningen, the Netherlands

Fleurisca J. Korteweg
Department of Obstetrics and Gynaecology, Martini Hospital, Groningen, the Netherlands

Helen L. Lutgers
Department of Internal Medicine, Medical Center Leeuwarden, Leeuwarden, the Netherlands

Mattheus J. M. Diekman
Department of Internal Medicine, Deventer Hospital, Deventer, the Netherlands

Paul P. van den Berg
Department of Obstetrics and Gynaecology, University of Groningen, University Medical Center Groningen, Groningen, the Netherlands

George Daskalakis, Panagiotis Fotinopoulos, Mariana Theodora, Panagiotis Antsaklis, Michail Sindos and Dimitrios Loutradis
1st Department of Obstetrics and Gynecology, Athens Medical School, Alexandra General Hospital, 9 Aristeidou Street, 17563 P. Faliro, Athens, Greece

Vasilios Pergialiotis and Nikolaos Papantoniou
3rd Department of Obstetrics and Gynecology, Athens Medical School, Attikon General Hospital, Athens, Greece

Amy Jean Bannatyne, Peta Stapleton, Bruce Watt and Kristen MacKenzie-Shalders
School of Psychology, Bond University, 14 University Drive, Robina, QLD 4229, Australia

Amy Jean Bannatyne and MacKenzie-Shalders
Faculty of Health Sciences and Medicine, Bond University, 14 University Drive, Robina, QLD 4229, Australia

Roger Hughes
School of Medicine, University of Tasmania, 17 Liverpool Street, Hobart, TAS 7001, Australia

Wei Chen, Li Li, Yan Li and Yue Zhang
Clinical College of Ophthalmology, Tianjin Medical University, No.4, Gansu Road, Tianjin City, People's Republic of China

Hongyuan Zhang and Xu Chen
Tianjin Central Hospital of Gynecology and Obstetrics, Tianjin, China

Rosario Valdez Santiago, Luz Arenas Monreal, Anabel Rojas Carmona and Mario Sánchez Domínguez
Center for Health Systems Research, The National Institute of Public Health in Mexico, Av. Universidad 655, Col. Santa María Ahuacatitlán, 62100 Cuernavaca, Morelos, Mexico

S. W. E. Baijens
Gynaecology and Obstetrics Department, Meander Medical Hospital, Maatweg 3, 3813 TZ Amersfoort, the Netherlands

A. G. Huppelschoten
Gynaecology and Obstetrics Department, Jeroen Bosch Hospital, Henri Dunantstraat 1, 5223 GZ 's-Hertogenbosch, the Netherlands

J. Van Dillen and J. W. M. Aarts
Gynaecology and Obstetrics Department, Radboudumc, Geert Grooteplein Zuid, 10 6525 GA Nijmegen, the Netherlands

Bekir Kahveci
Department of Obstetrics and Gynecology, Diyarbakır Gazi Yaşargil Training and Research Hospital, 21010 Diyarbakır, Turkey

Rauf Melekoglu
Faculty of Medicine, Department of Obstetrics and Gynecology, The University of Inonu, 44280 Malatya, Turkey

Ismail Cuneyt Evruke and Cihan Cetin
Faculty of Medicine, Department of Obstetrics and Gynecology, The University of Cukurova, 01330 Adana, Turkey

Ahmad Sameer Sanad, Ahmad E. Mahran, Mahmoud Elmorsi Aboulfotouh, Hany Hassan Kamel, Hashem Fares Mohammed, Haitham A. Bahaa, Reham R. Elkateeb, Alaa Gamal Abdelazim, Mohamed Ahmed Zeen El-Din and Hossam El-Din Shawki
Obstetrics and Gynecology, Faculty of Medicine, Minia Maternity University Hospital, Minia University, Minia, Egypt

Alison Peel
London School of Hygiene and Tropical Medicine, London, UK

Abhishek Bhartia
Sitaram Bhartia Institute of Science and Research, New Delhi, India

Neil Spicer and Meenakshi Gautham
Department of Global Health and Development, Faculty of Public Health and Policy, London School of Hygiene and Tropical Medicine, London, UK

Hailemariam Berhe Kahsay
School of Nursing, Mekelle University, Mekelle, Ethiopia

Fikre Enquselassie Gashe and Wubegzier Mekonnen Ayele
School of Public Health, Addis Ababa University, Addis Ababa, Ethiopia

Somayya M. Sadek, Reda A. Ahmad, Hytham Atia and Adel G. Abdullah
Obstetrics and Gynecology Department, Faculty of Medicine, Zagazig University, Zagazig, Egypt

Serawit Lakew
Department of Nursing and Midwifery, Arbaminch University, Arba Minch, Ethiopia

Alaso Ankala
Department of Nursing and Midwifery, Arba Minch College of Health Sciences, Arba Minch, Ethiopia

Fozia Jemal
Department of Obstetrics and Gynecology, Tikur Anbesa Specialized Hospital, Addis Ababa University, Addis Ababa, Ethiopia

Stefania Cappello, Eleonora Piccolo, Luisa Casadei, Emilio Piccione
Department of Biomedicine and Prevention, Obstetrics and Gynecological Clinic, University of Rome "Tor Vergata", via Montpellier 1, 00133 Rome, Italy

Francesco Cucinelli and Maria Giovanna Salerno
Department of Woman's and Child's Health, Obstetrics and Gynecological Unit, San Camillo-Forlanini Hospital, Circonvallazione Gianicolense 87, 00152 Rome, Italy

Amanual Getnet Mersha
Department of Gynecology and Obstetrics, School of Medicine, College of Medicine and Health Sciences, University of Gondar, Gondar, Ethiopia

Yukari Kugishima, Ichiro Yasuhi, Hiroshi Yamashita, So Sugimi, Yasushi Umezaki, Sachie Suga, Masashi Fukuda and Nobuko Kusuda
Department of Obstetrics and Gynecology, NHO Nagasaki Medical Center, 1001-1 2-chome Kubara, Omura City, Nagasaki 856-8562, Japan

Ivan Vuckovic, S. Zhang, P. Dzeja and S. I. Macura
Nuclear Magnetic Resonance Facility, Mayo Clinic, Stabile SL-035, 200 First Street SW, Rochester, MN 55905, USA

A. Bangdiwala
Clinical and Translational Science Institute, University of Minnesota, 717 Delaware Street SE, Second Floor, Minneapolis, MN 55414, USA

Gauri Luthra and H. Gray
Department of Maternal Fetal Medicine, University of Minnesota, 606 24th Ave S #400, Minneapolis, MN 55454, USA

J. B. Redmon
Division of Diabetes Endocrinology and Metabolism, 516 Delaware Street SE, MMC 101, Minneapolis, MN 55455, USA

E. S. Barrett
Environmental and Occupational Health Sciences Institute, Rutgers School of Public Health, 170 Frelinghuysen Rd, Piscataway, NJ 08854, USA

S. Sathyanarayana
Department of Pediatrics, University of Washington Seattle Children's Research Institute, CW8-6, Seattle, WA 98145-5005, USA

R. H. N. Nguyen
Division of Epidemiology and Community Health, University of Minnesota, 1300 S. 2nd Street, Suite 300, Minneapolis, MN 55454, USA

S. H. Swan
Department of Preventive Medicine, Icahn School of Medicine at Mount Sinai, 1 Gustave L. Levy Pl, New York, NY 10029, USA

K. S. Nair
Metabolomics Core, Mayo Clinic Hospital, Saint Mary's Campus, Alfred Building, Fifth Floor, Room 417, 200 First St. SW, Rochester, MN 55905, USA

Suzan M. de Visser, Mallory D. Woiski and Frank P. H. A. Vandenbussche
Department of Obstetrics and Gynecology, Radboud Institute for Health Science, Radboud University Medical Center, Geert Grootplein 10, 6500, HB, Nijmegen, the Netherlands

Richard P. Grol, Marlies E. J. L. Hulscher and Rosella P. M. G. Hermens
Department of IQ Healthcare, Radboud Institute for Health Science, Radboud University Medical Center, Nijmegen, Netherlands

Hubertina C. J. Scheepers
Department of Obstetrics and Gynecology, GROW School for Oncology and Developmental Biology, Maastricht University Medical Center, Maastricht, The Netherlands

Noémie Bouchet, Marina Lumbreras Areta and Begoña Martinez de Tejada
Obstetrics Unit, Department of Obstetrics and Gynecology, Geneva University Hospitals and Faculty of Medicine, 30 Boulevard de la Cluse, 1205 Geneva, Switzerland

Angèle Gayet-Ageron
Clinical Research Centre and Division of Clinical Epidemiology, Department of Community Health and Medicine, Geneva University Hospitals and Faculty of Medicine, 6 rue Gabrielle-Perret-Gentil, 1205 Geneva, Switzerland

Riccardo Erennio Pfister
Neonatology Unit, Department of Pediatrics, Geneva University Hospitals and Faculty of Medicine, 30 Boulevard de la Cluse, 1205 Geneva, Switzerland

Index

A
Ablatio Placentae, 101
Anova, 3-4, 138-139
Antenatal Care (ANC), 160
Artificial Reproduction Techniques, 54, 57

B
Breast Cancer, 8-12, 194, 197

C
C- Reactive Protein, 55
Cardiotocography, 40, 116
Central Placenta Previa, 106-107, 110-111
Cervical Cancer, 8-12, 143, 148, 151
Chi Square Test, 3, 84, 109
Chorioamnionitis, 54-58
Colostomy, 22

D
Delayed Interval Intertwin Delivery, 54, 57
Delayed Umbilical Cord Clamping, 33, 38
Delphi Method, 59-60, 62, 74

E
Early Cord Clamping, 33, 38
Eclampsia, 3, 5, 7, 19, 21, 47, 76, 78, 102-105, 124-125, 127, 132, 194
Ectrodactyly, 155-156, 158
Edge To Os Distance (EOD), 133

F
Fetal Growth Restriction, 157, 176-177, 182-183
Fisher's Exact Test, 1, 3, 21, 41, 48, 180, 194

G
Gestational Diabetes, 2-3, 5-7, 36, 38, 45, 47, 49-50, 52-53, 65, 99, 101-104, 123-124, 127, 129-130, 168-169, 174-175, 177
Gestational Hypertension, 2-3, 99-103, 123, 125, 132, 194, 196
Glucose Intolerance, 3, 51, 102, 175

H
Hematoma, 21, 23, 35
Herlyn -werner-wunderlich Syndrome (HWWS), 155
Heterotopic Interstitial Pregnancy, 27-31

Hyperbilirubinaemia, 48, 50
Hypertensive Disorders, 2-3, 80, 102, 107, 123-132
Hysterectomy, 21-24, 28, 33-36, 106, 109-111, 155, 157

I
Implementation Strategy, 184-187
Induction of Labour, 39, 41, 43-44, 47, 50-51
Induction-to-vaginal Delivery Interval (IDI), 41
Intertwin, 54, 56-57
Intrauterine Fetal Death, 16, 19
Intraventricular Hemorrhage, 55, 102, 193

L
Laparoscopic Cornual Resection, 27, 29, 31
Laparotomy, 20-25, 27-29, 31
Late Preterm, 99, 101-104, 192, 195-200
Logistic Regression Analyses, 15, 149
Lower Uterine Segment, 106-108, 134-135, 138-140
Lymphoma, 8, 10

M
Macular Ct, 75, 77-79
Magnetic Resonance Imaging, 11-12, 156, 158
Mann-whitney Test, 41
Misoprostol Vaginal Insert, 39-41, 43-44
Misoprostol Vaginal Tablets, 39, 41-43

N
Neonatal Intensive Care Unit (NICU), 100
Nmr Spectroscopy, 176, 179-182
Nulliparity, 4, 23, 99-100, 124, 131

O
Obstetric Violence, 81-82, 88-89
Obstructed Hemivagina, 155, 157-159
Optical Coherence Tomography, 75, 79-80
Oral Glucose Tolerance Test (OGTT), 168-169

P
Placenta Previa, 100-103, 106-107, 109-111, 133-134, 139, 141
Placental Pathology, 34
Postpartum Hemorrhage, 22-24, 33, 36, 38, 106, 110, 134, 157, 184-185, 190-191
Pre-gestational Body Mass Index (PBMI), 1

Preeclampsia, 2-3, 5, 7, 14, 16-17, 40, 43-48, 50-52, 80, 99-102, 104-105, 107-108, 123-125, 127, 130, 132, 192-194, 196

Pregnancy-induced Hypertension, 36, 47, 50, 52

Preterm Delivery, 1-2, 4-6, 9, 13-18, 47-48, 50, 54-55, 99-104, 192, 196-197, 199-200

Preterm Premature Rupture of Membranes (PPROM), 192

R

Respiratory Distress Syndrome, 3, 5-6, 55-57, 102, 193

S

Selective Embryo Reduction, 27, 29, 31

Severe Acute Maternal Morbidity, 20-21, 24-25, 191

Shared Decision-making (SDM), 91

Singleton Pregnancy, 1, 33, 100, 129

Student's T-test, 34, 41, 109, 170-172

T

Tachysistole, 39, 41-42

Tachysytole, 39, 41, 43

Therapeutic Interventions, 21, 27, 29

Transvaginal Ultrasound, 27-29, 133-134

U

Uterine Artery Ligation, 106-107, 110-111

Uterine Atony, 34-36, 111

Uterine Surgery, 100, 109

Utero Didelphys, 155